UROGYNECOLOGIC SURGERY

Principles and Techniques in Gynecologic Surgery
Series Editor, Luis E. Sanz, MD

Associate Professor
Department of Obstetrics and Gynecology
Georgetown University School of Medicine
Washington, DC

Urogynecologic Surgery
W. Glenn Hurt, MD, Editor

Operative Laparoscopy: The Masters' Techniques
Richard M. Soderstrom, MD, Editor

Principles
and
Techniques
in
Gynecologic
Surgery

Luis E. Sanz, MD, Series Editor

UROGYNECOLOGIC SURGERY

Edited by

W. Glenn Hurt, MD

Professor of Obstetrics and Gynecology
Medical College of Virginia
Virginia Commonwealth University
Richmond, Virginia

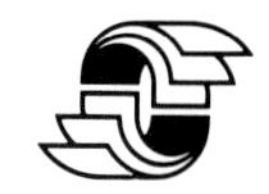

AN ASPEN PUBLICATION®
Aspen Publishers, Inc.
Gaithersburg, Maryland
1992

Library of Congress Cataloging-in-Publication Data

Urogynecologic surgery / W. Glenn Hurt.
p. cm.— (Principles and techniques in gynecologic surgery)
Includes bibliographical references and index.
ISBN: 0-8342-0339-1
1. Urogynecologic surgery. I. Hurt, W. Glenn, 1938— II. Series.
[DNLM: 1. Genital Diseases, Female—surgery. 2. Urinary Incontinence—surgery. WJ 190 U775]
RG484.U75 1992
617.4'6'0082—dc20
DNLM/DLC
for Library of Congress
92-7378
CIP

Editorial Services: Ruth Bloom
Library of Congress Catalog Card Number: 92-7378
ISBN: 0-8342-0339-1

Printed in the United States of America

1 2 3 4 5

To

H. Hudnall Ware, Jr, MD
(1898–1973)
Richmond, Virginia

and

C. Paul Hodgkinson, MD
(1907–)
Detroit, Michigan

Dr. Ware delivered me, trained me, and introduced me to Dr. Hodgkinson. Dr. Hodgkinson, who made many major contributions to urogynecology, taught me the importance of a urodynamic investigation and how it should be performed. He also taught me many of the principles and techniques of urogynecologic surgery.

Table of Contents

Contributors

Editor

W. Glenn Hurt, MD
Professor
Department of Obstetrics and Gynecology
Medical College of Virginia
Virginia Commonwealth University
Richmond, Virginia

Rodney A. Appell, MD
Professor and Vice-Chairman
Department of Urology
Louisiana State University School of Medicine
New Orleans, Louisiana

R. Peter Beck, MD
Director, Benign Gynecology
Professor
Department of Obstetrics and Gynecology
Medical College of Virginia
Richmond, Virginia

Alfred E. Bent, MD
Director, Division of Urogynecology
Department of Obstetrics and Gynecology
Greater Baltimore Medical Center
Towson, Maryland

Jerry G. Blaivas, MD
Professor and Vice-Chairman
Department of Urology
College of Physicians and Surgeons
Columbia University
New York, New York

Michael B. Chancellor, MD
Assistant Professor of Urology
Director of Neuro-Urology
Department of Urology
Jefferson Medical College
Thomas Jefferson University
Philadelphia, Pennsylvania

John O.L. DeLancey, MD
Assistant Professor
Division of Gynecology
Department of Obstetrics and Gynecology
University of Michigan School of Medicine
Ann Arbor, Michigan

Mickey M. Karram, MD
Director of Urogynecology
Good Samaritan Hospital
and
Assistant Professor
Department of Obstetrics and Gynecology
University of Cincinnati
School of Medicine
Cincinnati, Ohio

Raymond A. Lee, MD
Chair, Division of Gynecologic Surgery
Mayo Clinic and Mayo Foundation
and
Professor
Department of Obstetrics and Gynecology
Mayo Medical School
Rochester, Minnesota

Edward J. McGuire, MD
Professor and Chief
Section of Urology
Department of Surgery
University of Michigan School of Medicine
Ann Arbor, Michigan

Tim H. Parmley, MD
Professor
Department of Obstetrics and Gynecology
University of Arkansas for Medical Sciences
Little Rock, Arkansas

Manuel A. Penalver, MD
Associate Professor
Division of Gynecologic Oncology
Department of Obstetrics and Gynecology
University of Miami School of Medicine
Miami, Florida

A. Cullen Richardson, MD
Associate Clinical Professor
Department of Gynecology and Obstetrics
Emory University School of Medicine
Atlanta, Georgia

Jack R. Robertson, MD
Chief of Urogynecology and Clinical Professor
Department of Obstetrics and Gynecology
University of Nevada Medical School
Las Vegas, Nevada

Luis E. Sanz, MD
Associate Professor
Department of Obstetrics and Gynecology
Georgetown University School of Medicine
Washington, D.C.

Hugh M. Shingleton, MD
J. Marion Sims Professor and Chairman
Department of Obstetrics and Gynecology
University of Alabama-Birmingham
Birmingham, Alabama

Julian Wan, MD
Fellow, Section of Urology
Department of Surgery
University of Michigan School of Medicine
Ann Arbor, Michigan

Series Foreword

I have chosen the first book in the series *Principles and Techniques in Gynecologic Surgery* to focus on the ever-growing and important area of urogynecologic surgery. As just one indication of the increasing interest and patient population needing expertise in this area, the Residency Review Committee of the Accreditation Council for Graduate Medical Education now requires an increase in the training and exposure to urogynecology in all gynecologic residency programs. This text provides a thorough analysis of the problems in urogynecology and their surgical management. My hope is that it will serve as a reference source for residents and physicians not only in obstetrics/gynecology but urology as well.

Urogynecologic Surgery presents a comprehensive view of urogynecology. It begins with developmental anatomy and embryology and follows with the pertinent surgical anatomy. Preoperative evaluation of urinary incontinence is addressed with attention given to the appropriate diagnostic tests available and necessary. Different corrective surgical procedures for stress urinary incontinence and for total incontinence are then presented in detail with a discussion of urinary tract problems and complications that may arise from these urologic problems and surgical procedures.

Dr. Hurt, the editor of this first book in the series, has recruited excellent and accomplished urogynecologic surgeons to write chapters for the book. Each chapter is well illustrated and includes an extensive bibliography. Unique in its presentation in that the complete management of urogynecologic problems can be found in one text, this book provides an all-encompassing standard reference for both the gynecologist and the urologist.

Luis E. Sanz, MD
Associate Professor
Department of Obstetrics and Gynecology
Georgetown University School of Medicine
Washington, DC

Preface

In women, the embryogenesis, anatomy, and function of the lower urinary and genital systems are so interrelated that physicians must be knowledgeable about the possible effects that a pathologic condition or surgical procedure involving one system will have on the function of the other. In many ways, it is unfortunate that for certification purposes medical specialties have been divided along anatomic lines, resulting in the formation of The American Board of Obstetrics and Gynecology and The American Board of Urology. Currently, neither of these specialties is providing its postgraduates with adequate training in that area of practice best described as *urogynecology*. That is one of the problems that resulted in the preparation of this textbook.

The chapters in this textbook were written by surgeons, either gynecologists or urologists, who have extensive experience in their field and who have published articles or chapters in books dealing with the topic assigned to them. Their emphasis is placed on establishing a precise preoperative diagnosis, understanding the specific goals of each operative procedure, and performing the procedure that is most likely to effect a permanent cure.

Physicians who wrote about the treatment of stress urinary incontinence were asked to provide a historical basis and a sense of evolution of current procedures before giving a detailed description of their particular surgical techniques. The background material should be of educational benefit to surgeons who perform continence procedures, for "unless we know history, we are destined to repeat it."

This textbook gives a brief history of urogynecology in America. The chapter on the embryologic development of the female genital tract is written for its clinical relevance. The chapter on anatomy of genital support describes in detail those pelvic support systems that are responsible for the anatomic relations and physiologic function of the pelvic organs. Other chapters are devoted to the diagnosis and the surgical treatment of the various types of urinary incontinence (especially genuine stress and detrusor instability urinary incontinence), urethral diverticulum (and other urethral abnormalities), lower urinary tract injuries, and genitourinary fistulas. The final chapters concern postoperative bladder drainage and permanent forms of urinary diversion.

I would like to express my sincere appreciation to all who contributed to this textbook. I hope that their interpretation of surgical literature and their explanation of various surgical procedures will reduce the complications and improve the cure rates of persons who must undergo urogynecologic surgery.

W. Glenn Hurt, MD

1

Urogynecology: A Historical Perspective

Jack R. Robertson

Since the beginnings of medical writing, urologic and gynecologic problems have been associated. The Kahun papyrus, of approximately 2000 BC, was devoted to the diseases of women and included a discussion on diseases of the urinary bladder. Urinary fistula is an example of a problem that is the result of the intimate relation between the female urinary and genital systems. Henhenit was one of six women attached to the court of Menuhotep II, of the 11th dynasty, who reigned in Egypt about 2050 BC. Her mummy was found in 1935; radiography revealed she had an extensive genitourinary fistula.[1]

Modern gynecology and urogynecology were born at the same time. Although John Peter Mettauer, of Virginia, reported six successful closures of vesicovaginal fistulas in the years 1838 to 1847,[2] by using metallic sutures and draining the bladder with a catheter, his publication received little attention. J. Marion Sims published his monumental work on the treatment of vesicovaginal fistula in 1852[3]; it was he who established the interrelation of urology and gynecology. Sims' tenacity, sacrifice, and devotion to completing the job became an epic in surgical history. J. Marion Sims is known today as "The Father of Modern Gynecology."

Sims began his medical practice in Lancaster, South Carolina. His first two patients were infants who died of cholera. He became depressed and moved his practice to Mt. Meigs, Alabama, where he earned the reputation of being a great surgeon.

As a young leader in the community, Sims' practice thrived. He had a cabin at the back of his property, which he used for his Negro patients. One day a woman was thrown from her horse and was brought to Sims with a painful, impacted, retroverted uterus. The other local physicians had been unable to help her. Remembering the advice of his mentor, Professor Picoleau of the Charleston Medical College, Sims placed the patient in the knee-chest position and applied pressure within the vagina. The vagina ballooned with air, and the impacted uterus yielded.

Sims had seen several slave women with vesicovaginal fistulas, and he wondered about the possibility of examining these patients in this manner. He placed the next patient who had such a fistula in the knee-chest position and, subsequently, wrote in his autobiography

> Before I could get the bent spoon handle into her vagina, the air rushed in with a puffing noise, dilating the vagina to its fullest extent. Introducing the bent handle of the spoon, I saw everything as no man has ever seen before. The fistula was as plain as the nose on a man's face. The edges were measured as accurately as if it had been cut out of a piece of plain paper [Figure 1-1].[4]

This examination convinced Sims that vesicovaginal fistulas could be cured. It took 4 years of trial and error,

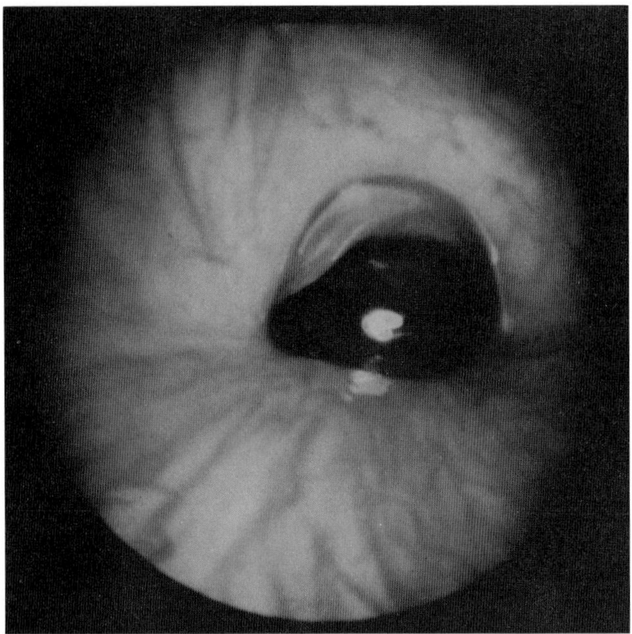

Figure 1-1 Fistula. Sims' use of knee-chest position gave him a good view. Today, with help of endoscopy, a better view is seen on intravesical side.

but he refused to give up. He enlarged the slave shack to two stories and began looking for patients. He wrote the following to his brother-in-law:

> If I live, I am bound to succeed; and I am as sure that I shall carry this thing through to success as I am that I now live, or as sure as I can be of anything. I have done too much already, and I am too near the accomplishment of the work to give it up now. My patients are all perfectly satisfied with what I am doing for them. I cannot depend on the doctors, and so I have trained the patients to assist me in the operations. I am going on with this series of experiments to the end. It matters not what it costs, if it costs me my life. For, if I shall fail, I believe somebody would be raised up to the work where I lay it down and carry it on to successful issue.[4]

In his attempts to close vesicovaginal fistulas, Sims had used silk sutures held with lead shot, but this maneuver had failed. One of the three slave girls he had operated on repeatedly was due for her 30th operation. This time Sims used silver wire sutures made by his jeweler. Her recovery was uncomplicated, and she was cured. In 1852, Sims published on the cure of 252 fistulas, the result of 320 attempts.[3]

Sims moved to New York and helped found Woman's Hospital, which was on the current site of the Waldorf Astoria Hotel. In a speech to the New York Academy of Medicine, Sims stated that the use of silver wire sutures was the greatest contribution made to surgery during that century. He toured Europe, where he operated with success on noted people in several countries. He returned to New York to find his colleagues had taken over his practice. He became bitter, and, in 1883, he died. Royster wrote that Sims was a genius because he took infinite pains in his work; developed the capacity for hard work and kept doggedly after it; and did one thing well, not merely to win success but to deserve it.[5]

Howard A. Kelly, the first Professor of Gynecology at the Johns Hopkins Medical School, believed that gynecology and female urology were too closely related to be separated. He believed that one could not be trained in either field and ignore the other. Time has proved that Kelly was right.

In 1893, Kelly devised a cystoscope. It was a hollow tube with a handle and a glass partition, which prevented water (used for distention) from running out of the bladder. Light was reflected from a head mirror. The patient was placed in the knee-chest position for examination[6] (Figure 1-2).

One day, Kelly's cystoscope was dropped accidentally and the glass shattered. Kelly knew that the vagina would balloon with air if the patient were placed in the knee-chest position. He wondered whether the bladder might also react in the same way. He inserted the broken cystoscope; when he removed the obturator, the bladder filled with air. He asked for a ureteral catheter. Howard Kelly, a gynecologist, inserted a ureteral catheter under direct vision. As Kelly also laid the groundwork for extraperitoneal nephrectomy, he could be credited as a

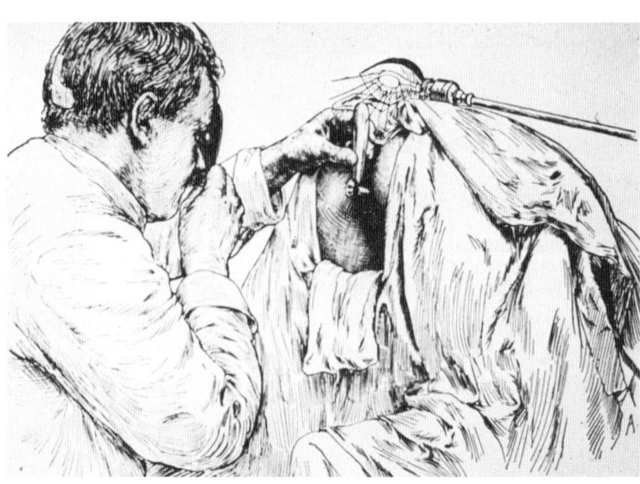

Figure 1-2 Howard Kelly was youngest member of Johns Hopkins "Big Four." He is shown examining patient in knee-chest position. *Source*: Reprinted from *Genitourinary Problems in Women* (p 11) by J Robertson with permission of Charles C Thomas, © 1978.

founder of the specialty of urology, although the American Urological Association was not formed until 20 years later. In 1914, Howard A. Kelly and Curtis F. Burnam, another gynecologist, coauthored a textbook, *Diseases of the Kidney, Ureters, and Bladder*, which was illustrated by Max Brodel.

Johns Hopkins' Department of Gynecology continued as the stronghold of female urology. Kelly's successor, Guy L. Hunner, described Hunner's ulcer, called today *interstitial cystitis*, while observing the bladder through a Kelly cystoscope.[7] Houston S. Everett succeeded Hunner and described many of the urinary tract complications that are associated with cervical cancer. His contributions enriched gynecologic oncology. He wrote *Gynecological and Obstetrical Urology* in 1943 and coauthored *Female Urology* with John H. Ridley in 1968.

Female urology continued as an integral part of gynecology at Johns Hopkins under the chair of Richard W. TeLinde. Water endoscopy was introduced, although the air cystoscope continued to be used. In 1978, TeLinde wrote, "It is difficult for me to conceive of doing first class gynecology without a knowledge of female urology."[8]

Unfortunately, many other gynecologic training programs offered little or no exposure to female urology. In 1987, the American Board of Obstetrics and Gynecology announced that resident education must include the diagnosis and management of lower urinary tract dysfunction in women. It is noteworthy that this pronouncement occurred 100 years after Howard Kelly established the first residency program in which he taught both gynecology and urology.

ENDOSCOPY IN UROGYNECOLOGY

Air cystoscopy, although a simple, inexpensive method of examining the female bladder, had three disadvantages: poor external illumination, no lens system, and need for the patient to be examined in the knee-chest position. John H. Ridley published a method of indirect air cystoscopy, with the use of techniques of both the air and the water methods.[9] The patient was placed in the knee-chest position, and the bladder was inflated with air. The conventional water cystoscope was used for inspection of the bladder.

I (Jack R. Robertson) reported a similar method of cystoscopy with the use of the culdoscope, which had an optical system for use through air.[10] My method was an office procedure for visualizing the bladder. It had two important disadvantages: (1) the vesical neck and the urethra could not be visualized because of the right-angled lens and (2) heat was emitted from the light bulb.

I modified the Kelly air cystoscope to overcome these obstacles. The female urethroscope I designed had optical glass fibers enclosed between the double wall of a stainless steel barrel. An electric source in the handle transmitted cold light around the circumference of the distal end. This allowed magnification at the proximal end. A vent allowed a closed system by placing a finger tip over the vent.[11]

The development of fiberoptic telescopes revolutionized endoscopy and made many changes in the practice of gynecology. I developed a new female urethroscope with a direct-view telescope, which locks into an open-barreled tube.[12] The first carbon dioxide endoscopy cystometer was developed for me, so that urethral and bladder pressure studies could be made during endoscopy.

Endoscopy has had a major impact on gynecology. Endoscopic procedures increased from 0.5% of all gynecologic surgical cases in 1968 to its explosive prevalence today. In 1976, laparoscopy accounted for most of these procedures.[13] Now hysteroscopy, pelviscopy, colposcopy, and urethroscopy share popularity with gynecologists.

URODYNAMICS AND PHARMACEUTICAL TREATMENT

Urodynamics began with Goren Enhörning's work in 1961.[14] Confirming his work, Tanagho and colleagues found that the highest urethral pressure of the female urethra was in the midurethral segment, with the intrinsic smooth muscle reinforced by the striated muscle. The normal pressure in the midurethra was approximately 100 centimeters of water (cm H_2O). By blocking each component of the urethral sphincter in succession, they showed that, with blocking of only the striated muscle component with curare, the urethral pressure was lowered by one third. When, in addition, the smooth muscle component was blocked, the urethral pressure dropped by two thirds. It was believed that the remaining one third of the urethral pressure was due to resistance of the physical elements within the urethral wall.[15]

Urodynamics has experienced a rocky road of conflicting conclusions and dubious equipment. A recent article, entitled "Consumers' Guide to Urodynamic Equipment," warns of 10% to 14% inaccuracies in equipment results. They recommend ambulatory monitoring (discussed in Chapter 4), concluding that detrusor instability (DI) and even genuine stress incontinence (GSI) are diagnosed more frequently with this method.[16]

Drugs are being developed for the treatment of lower urinary tract dysfunction. At best, drug therapy for the unstable bladder is helpful in only 50% of cases. The smooth muscle relaxants, oxybutynin chloride (Ditropan) and flavoxate hydrochloride (Urispas), and a tricyclic antidepressant, imipramine hydrochloride (Tofranil), have often effected dramatic cures. For the clinician in the office setting, if genitourinary fistula, urethral diverticulum, and GSI can be ruled out, these drugs have made conservative treatment of DI possible and have often prevented unnecessary and ineffective surgery.

BEHAVIORAL THERAPY

Although Arnold H. Kegel was not the first to discover the benefits of perineal exercises, he became such a champion in the education of the laity and the medical profession that his treatment became known as Kegel's exercises.[17]

Bladder re-education, also referred to as *bladder training* and *bladder drills*, is a scheduling regimen that progressively increases the voiding interval. T.N.A. Jeffcoate and W.J.A. Francis used bladder drills to break the urgency–frequency syndrome and increase bladder capacity.[18] J. Andrew Fantl and co-workers had patients keep a urinary diary and increase their voiding intervals to 2, 3, or 4 hours. They found that these regimens significantly reduced the number of incontinent episodes, regardless of whether the diagnosis was DI or GSI.[19]

SURGERY TO CORRECT FEMALE INCONTINENCE

The first serious surgical procedure recommended for the cure of stress incontinence was that of Howard Kelly, who, with W.A. Dumm, reported success in treating 16 of 20 cases by vaginal plication of the vesical neck.[20] This was the first vaginal plication operation. Innumerable modifications have been described.

In 1913, Kelly wrote:

> There is a peculiar form of incontinence of urine in women which either follows childbirth or comes on about middle age and is not associated with any visible lesion of the urinary tract. Sometimes the most suggestive picture that can be seen by a cystoscope is a gaping internal sphincter orifice which closes sluggishly. A little urine runs out when she coughs, laughs, sneezes, lifts anything, or steps high. For a long time surgeons have tried to relieve this condition by a variety of operations, some of them more or less bizarre, designed to act upon the external urethral orifice by contracting it, or to resect the vagina at the internal orifice, or to kink the urethra or in one way or another to tighten it. These operations rarely succeed. I have seen many patients subjected to them, but none relieved. The key to successful treatment lies at the internal orifice of the urethra and in the sphincter muscle which controls the canal at this point.[21]

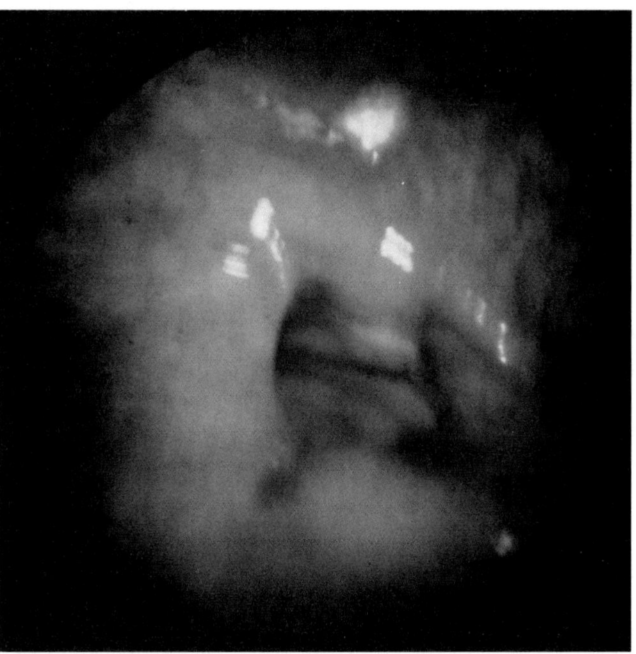

Figure 1-3 A "drain-pipe" urethra after multiple incontinence operations.

More than 150 operations have been described for the cure of stress incontinence. Many are urethropexies or colposuspensions, that is, Marshall-Marchetti-Krantz procedures, Burch procedures, or Richardson's paravaginal repair. Suburethral slings and F. Brantly Scott's artificial sphincter[22] have been used in patients who have a functionless "drain-pipe" urethra related to multiple operations (Figure 1-3).

In 1949, Victor F. Marshall, a urologist, and Andrew A. Marchetti and Kermit E. Krantz, two gynecologists, reported a new operation for stress incontinence. They had performed their operation on 50 patients,[23] 25 of whom had undergone previous unsuccessful operations, and they obtained excellent results in 82%. This operation, or one of its many modifications, has been used extensively, giving cure rates higher than those obtained with vaginal plastic procedures.

The Marshall-Marchetti-Krantz (MMK) operation was quickly adopted by urologists; most gynecologists preferred the anterior vaginal repair. A problem exists, however, in that patients often have genital as well as urinary problems, and genital problems may benefit by surgical correction at the time of surgery for urinary problems. In addition, whenever a urethropexy or urethral colposuspension is performed, the anterior displacement of the vagina directs the intra-abdominal pressure into the posterior cul-de-sac and predisposes the patient to the development of an enterocele. These problems may result in patients needing another operation, which should have been accomplished at the time of the initial procedure. Many modifications of the MMK procedure have developed as complications from the first operation became apparent. Those of Jack L. Lapides, T. Sundin with S. Petersson, and R.B. Quattlebaum failed primarily because of poor urethral suspension.[24–26] Kermit Krantz, himself, has discontinued suturing the bladder to the anterior wall of the abdomen.[27]

Richard A. Lee and Richard E. Symmonds[28] and Krantz[27] have recommended opening the bladder during MMK procedures to prevent sutures being placed in the urethra or the bladder and to visualize the proper elevation of the vesical neck. This method is especially helpful during repeat retropubic procedures. More recently, suprapubic endoscopy has been used for the same purpose. It requires a very small incision in the anterior wall of the bladder, affords an excellent view of the inside of the bladder, and may prevent a later fistula. M. Leon Tancer, in reviewing the repair of 96 vesicovaginal fistulas, found that 22% of patients who had undergone repair of their fistula had had a previous bladder injury for which the bladder had been opened and repaired.[29]

When it was recognized that MMK procedure failures might be due to the use of absorbable suture, permanent suture material was substituted. In several modifications of the MMK procedure permanent fixation has been used by placing sutures in holes drilled through the symphysis pubis. Some surgeons have recommended electrocautery, the use of talc powder, or scraping of the posterior aspect of the symphysis pubis to promote scar formation in the retropubic space.[30,31]

James A. O'Leary reported that in approximately 3% of patients osteitis pubis develops after the MMK procedure. Occasionally, this leads to prolonged disability or degenerative arthritis.[32]

John C. Burch described a modification of the MMK procedure to prevent some of these complications.[33] His operation was a colposuspension that attached the vagina to Cooper's ligament, thus elevating the urethrovesical junction to its proper retropubic position. This has become a popular procedure. Its primary complication is postoperative urinary retention, which is the result of excessive elevation of the vesical neck. For this reason, routine postoperative suprapubic bladder catheter drainage is recommended.

C. Paul Hodgkinson modified the Burch procedure by placing only one pair of permanent sutures on either side of the urethrovesical junction,[34] and Emil A. Tanagho discouraged dissection anterior to the urethra and encouraged placement of the suspending sutures 1 to 2 cm lateral to the urethrovesical junction to prevent needless trauma to the delicate urethral musculature.[35]

In 1959, Armand J. Pereyra recommended the first needle procedure for the cure of stress incontinence.[36] The modified Pereyra procedure, as currently performed, is a vaginal retropubic urethropexy.[37] It is generally used when other vaginal procedures are indicated for the repair of cystocele, rectocele, enterocele, or vaginal vault prolapse (or a combination of these conditions). A urethropexy procedure is contraindicated in the patient who has good urethral support. Occasionally, this is the case. The retropubic pubourethral ligament is the tissue Pereyra used for repositioning the urethra into the abdominal zone of pressure. Endoscopic visualization is recommended to ensure that there is no bladder injury (Figure 1-4). Thomas A. Stamey, Shlomo Raz,

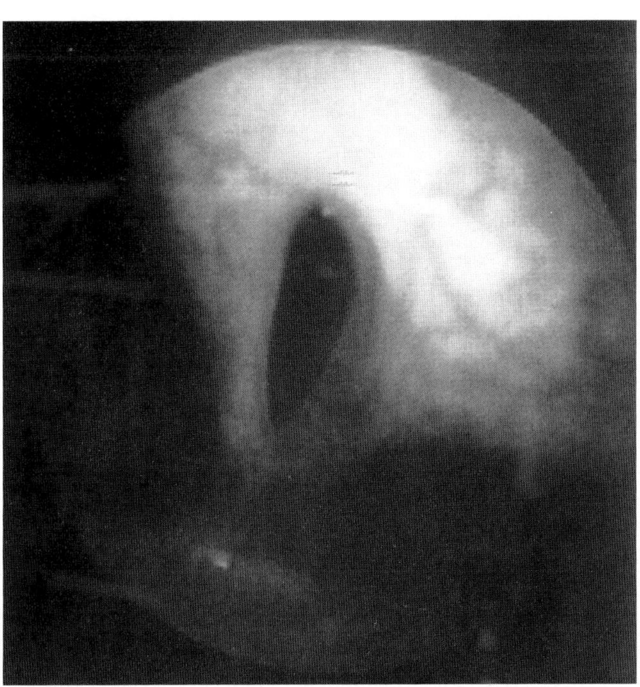

Figure 1-4 This patient was able to void only in standing position after Burch procedure. Intravesical sutures have been epithelialized. Sutures were cut endoscopically, and she was relieved.

Dominic Muzsnai, and Rubin F. Gittes have suggested modifications of the Pereyra procedure.[38–41]

Lee, Symmonds, and Goldstein placed permanent sutures through the fibrocartilage of the symphysis pubis instead of through the thin periosteum. They prefer this modification to the Stamey procedure of hanging tissues by permanent sutures to the rectus fascia.[42]

Most sling procedures are used only for patients who have had failed previous abdominal retropubic procedures. Recently Nicholette S. Horbach and colleagues have recommended a sling procedure for patients with a urethral closure pressure of less than 20 cm H_2O, because these patients respond less well to the usual operation for GSI.[43]

Reports on paravaginal repairs emphasize the importance of case selection. A. Cullen Richardson and coworkers recommend attaching the paravaginal fascia to the white line on the pelvic side wall.[44] Their operation is based on anatomic study findings, and the reported results are excellent.

A problem exists in the evaluation of many of these procedures. There is a lack of preoperative and postoperative studies for the documentation of diagnosis and cure. Only one proper randomized prospective study, that of Arieh Bergman and associates, has been reported.[45] They compared vaginal repair, the Pereyra procedure, and the Burch colposuspension. The best long-term results were achieved with the Burch procedure.

Axel Ingleman-Sundberg, working at the Karolinska Institute, Stockholm, Sweden, has been a pioneer in the field of urogynecology. He added much information about the functional anatomy and pathophysiology of stress urinary incontinence. His greatest contributions have been in surgical techniques, such as partial denervation of the bladder for the patient with an unstable bladder who does not respond to medical therapy.[46]

A major step in the cure of posthysterectomy vesicovaginal fistulas was taken by William Latzko in 1914.[47] His contribution is especially important today, because, in the United States, most vesicovaginal fistulas occur after hysterectomy. His simple method of cure consists of a partial colpocleisis. Because of better obstetric care, and especially because of the high incidence of cesarean section, in the United States obstetric fistulas are rare.

Working with Allan Lichtman, I investigated the incidence of urethral diverticula in women.[48] We reported successful cures with the use of the Spence procedure[49] to marsupialize the diverticulum when it is located distal to the point of the peak urethral closure pressure. Direct dissection is necessary if the location is proximal to this area and the ostium is small with periurethral tissue that is not inflamed. Tancer and colleagues devised a partial ablation technique for use when peridiverticular and urethral inflammation is present.[50]

CONCLUSION

The development of new instrumentation and endoscopic techniques has made the female urethra the most accessible portion of the urinary tract for examination. The urethra may be examined as easily as the cervix. It is time the female urethra is placed back in the pelvis, where it belongs.

Still, in 1992, the gynecologic cliches endure: "You always do a vaginal repair first. If that does not work, you can go from above," or, "While I am doing the hysterectomy, I will do an anterior or posterior repair, so that she does not have to return for further surgery later on." These cliches must be laid to rest. Why not do the proper operation the first time? The success rate progressively decreases after each unsuccessful operation, and a woman who does not need a repair should not have one. She may be unable to void or end up with a significant urinary residual.

Originally, female urology was recognized as a part of gynecology. The Kelly school of gynecology has disappeared; obstetrics and gynecology has become subspecialized; and general gynecology, especially surgical gynecology, has been de-emphasized. The focus has been placed on obstetrics.

A turf battle has developed between the disciplines of urology and obstetrics and gynecology. The American Board of Obstetrics and Gynecology has begun including urologic questions on its examinations. Urologists, however, claim gynecologic surgeons have limited knowledge of, and training in, urology. At the same time, urologists have started giving courses in female urology, including repair of cystocele and rectocele and vaginal hysterectomy. The patient has suffered from this turf battle.

Today, women with urinary symptoms are being treated by a gynecologist who has no knowledge of, or training in, urology. On the other hand, urologists, without any special knowledge of, or training in, gynecology, are doing surgical procedures that may adversely affect the female genital tract. Cooperation between urologists and gynecologists is needed. Treatment would be greatly improved if pelvic surgeons were trained in both of these closely related systems.

The American Association of Urologists began in 1917. The British Association of Urological Surgeons was formed in 1945. Both Richard Turner-Warwick, a

British urologist, and Stuart L. Stanton, a British urogynecologist, agree that urogynecology should be done by any urologist or gynecologist who has taken the time and made the effort to master this new subspecialty. An outstanding British urologist, T. Millen, is quoted as saying, "If the patient is to be made water tight, the urologist and gynecologist must not stay in water tight compartments."

In Great Britain, urogynecology is a subspecialty of obstetrics and gynecology. Despite recognition by the American Board of Obstetrics and Gynecology, this has not happened in the United States. Donald R. Ostergard started a urogynecologic fellowship in 1978, affiliated with the Department of Obstetrics and Gynecology, University of California, Irvine. In 1992, there are only seven urogynecologic fellowship programs in the United States.

The International Urogynecology Society was founded in Mexico in 1976 at the time of the world meeting of the International Federation of Gynecology and Obstetrics (FIGO). Axel Ingelman-Sundberg was the first president of the organization. The American Uro-Gynecologic Society (AUGS) held its first meeting in New Orleans in 1980, and I was its first president.

Nearly 2% of gynecologic pelvic surgery is the cause of some ureteral injury. No specialty includes more endoscopy than gynecology. Now that the 21st century is nearing, and the gynecologists are removing tumors and organs by pelviscopy, it is time that no patient whose surgery might jeopardize the lower urinary tract be allowed to leave the operating room until the gynecologist has looked through the endoscope to ensure that both ureters are intact and functioning.

New and highly technical equipment is appearing, such as flexible and extremely slim fiberoptic endoscopes and optic needles having built-in cameras with the images viewable on video monitors. These and other new devices, designed to be used in the physician's office or in the operating room, are aiding in the urogynecologic diagnosis of the patient as well as facilitating methods of surgery.

REFERENCES

1. Derry DE. Note on five pelves of women of the 11th dynasty in Egypt. *J Obstet Gynaecol Br Emp*. 1935;42:490–495.

2. Mettauer JP. On vesico-vaginal fistula. *Am J Med Sci*. 1847;14:117–121.

3. Sims JM. On the treatment of vesico-vaginal fistula. *Am J Med Sci*. 1852;23:59–82.

4. Sims JM. *The Story of My Life*. New York, NY: Appleton; 1894.

5. Royster HA. Biography of Marion Sims. *Surg Gynecol Obstet*. 1922;35:237–239.

6. Kelly HA. *Medical Gynecology*. New York, NY: Appleton; 1908.

7. Hunner GL. Elusive ulcer of the bladder. Further notes of a rare type of bladder ulcer, with a report of twenty-five cases. *Am J Obstet*. 1918;78:374–395.

8. TeLinde RW. Foreword in Robertson JR, *Genitourinary Problems in Women*. Springfield, Ill: Charles C Thomas Publisher; 1978.

9. Ridley JH. Indirect air cystoscopy. *South Med J*. 1951; 44:114–121.

10. Robertson JR. Office cystoscopy: substituting the culdoscope for the Kelly cystoscope. *Obstet Gynecol*. 1966;28:219–220.

11. Robertson JR. Air cystoscopy. *Obstet Gynecol*. 1968;32:328.

12. Robertson JR. Gynecologic urethroscopy. *Am J Obstet Gynecol*. 1973;115:986–990.

13. Wheeless CR. Laparoscopy. *Clin Obstet Gynecol*. 1976; 19:277.

14. Enhörning G. Simultaneous recording of intravesical and intraurethral pressure. *Acta Chir Scand (Suppl)*. 1961;276:5–12.

15. Tanagho EA, Meyers FH, Smith DR. Urethral resistance: its components and implications. I. Smooth muscle component. II. Striated muscle opponent. *Invest Urol*. 1969;7:136–149.

16. Barnes DG, Ralph D, Lewis CA, Shaw PJ, and Worth PH. Consumers' guide to commercially available urodynamic equipment. *Br J Urol*. 1991;68(2):138–143.

17. Kegel AH, Powell TH. The physiologic treatment of stress incontinence. *J Urol*. 1950;63:808.

18. Jeffcoate TNA, Francis WJA. Urgency incontinence in the female. *Am J Obstet Gynecol*. 1966;94:604–618.

19. Fantl JA, Wyman JF, McClish DK, et al. Efficacy of bladder training in older women with urinary incontinence. *JAMA*. 1991;265(S):609–613.

20. Kelly HA, Dumm WM. Urinary incontinence in women without manifest injury to the bladder. *Surg Gynecol Obstet*. 1914; 18:444–450.

21. Kelly HA. Incontinence of urine in women. *Urol Cutan Rev*. 1913;17:291–293.

22. Scott FB, Bradley WE, Timm GW. Treatment of urinary incontinence by an implantable prosthetic sphincter. *Urology*. 1973;1:252–259.

23. Marshall VF, Marchetti AA, Krantz KE. The correction of stress incontinence by simple vesicourethral suspension. *Surg Gynecol Obstet*. 1949;88:509–518.

24. Lapides JL. Simplified operation for stress incontinence. *J Urol*. 1971;105:262–264.

25. Sundin T, Petersson S. Anterior urethropexy according to Lapides in stress urinary incontinence. *Scand J Urol Nephrol*. 1975;9:28–31.

26. Quattlebaum RB. Successful management of female stress incontinence. *Urology*. 1976;7:501–503.

27. Krantz KE. The Marshall-Marchetti-Krantz procedure. In: Stanton SL, Tanagho EA, eds. *Surgery of Female Incontinence*. Berlin: Springer-Verlag; 1980.

28. Lee RA, Symmonds RE. Repeat Marshall-Marchetti procedure for recurrent stress urinary incontinence. *Am J Obstet Gynecol*. 1975;122:219–229.

29. Tancer ML. Post-hysterectomy vesicovaginal fistula repair, MVP Video. *J Obstet Gynecol*. 1988;1:7.

30. Hutch JA. Modification of the Marshall Marchetti Krantz operation. *J Urol*. 1968;99:607–612.

31. Gaker LB, Smith KM, Helfman H. Preliminary report on modified vesicourethropexy. *J Urol*. 1961;85:781–784.

32. O'Leary JA. Osteitis pubis following vesical suspension. *Obstet Gynecol*. 1963;24:73–77.

33. Burch JC. Urethrovaginal fixation to Cooper's ligament for the correction of stress incontinence, cystocele, rectocele, and prolapse. *Am J Obstet Gynecol*. 1961;82:281–290.

34. Hodgkinson CP. Stress urinary incontinence. *Am J Obstet Gynecol*. 1970;108:1141–1168.

35. Tanagho EA. Colpocystourethropexy: the way we do it. *J Urol*. 1976;116:751–753.

36. Pereyra AJ. A simplified surgical procedure for the correction of stress incontinence in women. *West J Surg*. 1959;67:223–226.

37. Pereyra AJ, Lebherz TB, Growdon WA, Powers JA. Pubourethral supports in perspective: modified Pereyra procedure for urinary incontinence. *Obstet Gynecol*. 1982;59:643–648.

38. Stamey TA. Endoscopic suspension of the vesical neck for urinary incontinence. *Surg Gynecol Obstet*. 1973;136:547–554.

39. Raz S. Modified bladder neck suspension for female stress incontinence. *J Urol*. 1981;17:82–84.

40. Muzsnai D, Carrillo E, Dubin C, Silverman I. Retropubic vaginoplasty for correction of urinary stress incontinence. *Obstet Gynecol*. 1982;59:113–117.

41. Gittes RF, Loughlin KR. No-incision pubovaginal suspension for stress incontinence. *J Urol*. 1987;183:568–570.

42. Lee RA, Symmonds RE, Goldstein RA. Surgical complications and results of modified Marshall-Marchetti-Krantz procedure for urinary incontinence. *Obstet Gynecol*. 1979;53:447–450.

43. Horbach NS, Blanco JS, Ostergard DR, et al. A suburethral sling procedure with polytetrafluoroethylene for the treatment of genuine stress incontinence in patients with low urethral closure pressure. *Obstet Gynecol*. 1988;71:648–652.

44. Richardson AC, Edmonds PB, Williams NL. Treatment of stress urinary incontinence due to paravaginal fascial defect. *Obstet Gynecol*. 1981;57:357–362.

45. Bergman A, Ballard CA, Koonings PP. Comparison of three different surgical procedures for genuine stress incontinence: prospective randomized study. *Am J Obstet Gynecol*. 1989;160: 1102–1106.

46. Ingelman-Sundberg A. Vaginal partial resection of the inferior hypogastric plexus. In: Youssef AF, ed. *Gynecological Urology*. Springfield, Ill: Charles C Thomas Publisher; 1960.

47. Latzko W. Postoperative vesicovaginal fistulas: genesis and therapy. *Am J Surg*. 1942;58:211–228.

48. Lichtman AS, Robertson JR. Suburethral diverticula treated by marsupialization. *Obstet Gynecol*. 1976;47:203–206.

49. Spence HM, Duckett JW. Diverticulum of the female urethra: clinical aspects and presentation of a single operative technique for cure. *J Urol*. 1970;104:432–437.

50. Tancer ML, Moopan MMU, Pierre-Louis C, et al. Suburethral diverticulum: treatment by partial ablation. *Obstet Gynecol*. 1983;62:511–513.

2

Embryologic Development of the Female Genital Tract

Tim H. Parmley

The purpose of this chapter is to make embryology, and specifically the embryologic development of the female genital and urinary tracts, relevant to clinicians. Embryology is legitimately difficult because it requires three- or four-dimensional thinking. It has been made unnecessarily difficult, however, by the use of one set of terms by embryologists and another set by anatomists. The following list is provided to clarify the confusion:

Coelomic membrane—peritoneum
Coelomic cavity—peritoneal cavity
Paired müllerian ducts—fallopian tubes
Fused müllerian duct—uterus, cervix, and upper portion of vagina
Vaginal plate—lower portion of vagina
Urogenital sinus—urachus, bladder, urethra, and vestibule
Wolffian duct—epithelial remnants or persistent ducts found

1. in the retroperitoneal space from the level of the kidney, along the course of the ureter, to the edge of the broad ligament;
2. along the tube in the mesosalpinx to the body of the uterus;
3. along the lateral wall of the uterus in the broad ligament;
4. within the body of the cervix along the base of the endocervical clefts; and
5. along the lateral wall of the vagina to the hymenal ring.

DEVELOPMENT OF THE EMBRYO

At implantation, the human blastocyst is a fluid-filled cyst.[1] The cyst wall is composed of a single cell layer, the *trophoectoderm*. Attached to the inner surface of the cyst, in a localized area, is a small collection of cells termed the *inner cell mass*. This is the embryo. The portion of the inner cell mass that is attached to the trophoectoderm becomes the dorsal surface of the embryo. Usually the inner cell mass is attached to that portion of the wall of the blastocyst that implants first.

During the second week of embryonic life, the inner cell mass becomes organized into a bilaminar disc[1] (Figure 2-1). The cells facing the lumen of the blastocyst are arranged in a single cell layer, the *endoderm*, which is thus the first germ layer to differentiate. This cell layer then extends beyond the inner cell mass to line a portion of the cavity of the blastocyst, the *yolk sac*. The rest of the cells of the inner cell mass become organized into a single cell layer, the *ectoderm*, forming the dorsal layer of the bilaminar disc. A cavity, the *amniotic cavity*, develops between the ectoderm and the trophoectoderm. The ectoderm is continuous at the edge of the embryo with the epithelium, the amnion that lines this cavity.

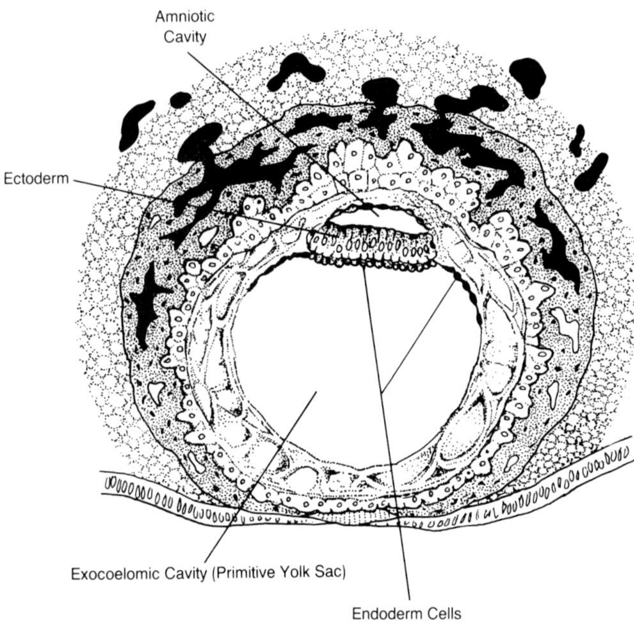

Figure 2-1 Twelve days from fertilization blastocyst is deeply embedded in endometrium. Embryo consists of two cell layers separating amniotic cavity and yolk sac. *Source:* Adapted from *Medical Embryology*, ed 3 (p 42) by J Langman with permission of Williams & Wilkins Company, © 1975.

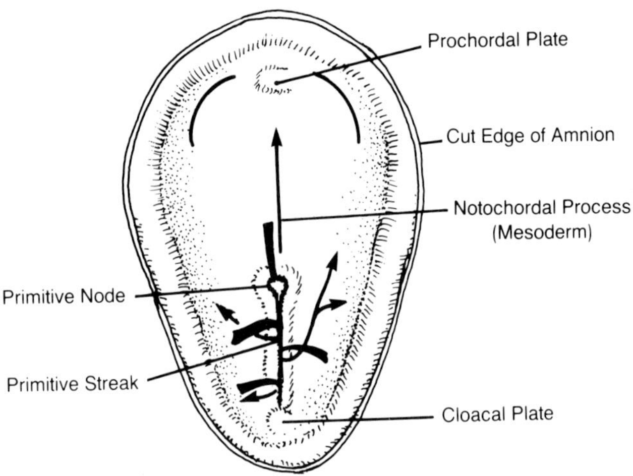

Figure 2-2 As arrows indicate, ectodermal cells sink into space between ectoderm and endoderm along linear groove, the *primitive streak*. This newly formed mesoderm then spreads between two layers, separating them except at prochordal and cloacal plates. *Source:* Adapted from *Medical Embryology*, ed 3 (p 52) by J Langman with permission of Williams & Wilkins Company, © 1975.

During the third week of embryonic life, the bilaminar disc becomes a trilaminar disc (Figure 2-2). The endoderm induces the formation of the third layer, the *mesoderm*, from the ectoderm.[2,3] The mesoderm forms a continuous layer between the ectoderm and the endoderm except at two sites. The ectoderm and the endoderm are tightly fused and are not separated by mesoderm anteriorly in the disc at a small oval site termed the *prochordal plate* and posteriorly at another small oval site termed the *cloacal plate*. These two plates will become, respectively, the oral orifice and the anogenital orifices.

The germ layers are important because tissues derived from a common germ layer tend to share biologic properties that they do not share with tissues derived from other germ layers. Certainly this is a generalization to which there are many exceptions, but it is nevertheless often clinically useful. For example, it may be assumed that any tissue derived from the mesoderm will be responsive to the sex steroids estrogen and progesterone, although the doses required to stimulate a response may vary greatly.

During the fourth week of embryonic life, the trilaminar disc balloons upward resulting in three-dimensional folding. This is due primarily to faster growth in the anterocentral portion of the disc than elsewhere.[2,4] The result is the formation of a tubular embryo. The folding process results in the internalization of the endoderm where it lines a continuous tube. This tube runs from the prochordal plate (ie, the oral orifice) to the cloacal plate where it then turns forward and runs to the umbilicus (Figure 2-3). The portion from the prochordal plate to the cloaca will become the gastrointestinal tract. The portion from the cloacal plate to the umbilicus is the *urogenital sinus* and will become the urachus, bladder, urethra, and vestibule.

The folding process also results in the externalization of the ectoderm. The mesoderm separates the ectoderm and the endoderm and will exhibit more subsequent growth than either. Therefore the ectoderm and the endoderm tend to become progressively separated except at the mouth and the cloacal orifices.

DEVELOPMENT OF THE UROGENITAL RIDGE

The mesoderm becomes organized in roughly three parallel columns on each side of the median axis of the embryo.[1] The two most medial columns, the *para-axial mesoderm*, give rise to much of the musculoskeletal system. The two next most medial columns, the *intermediate mesoderm*, become the urogenital ridge in the posterior wall of the coelomic or peritoneal cavity. The most lateral columns of mesoderm, the *lateral plate mesoderm*, develop a cavity within them that becomes the peritoneal or coelomic cavity. As this cavity

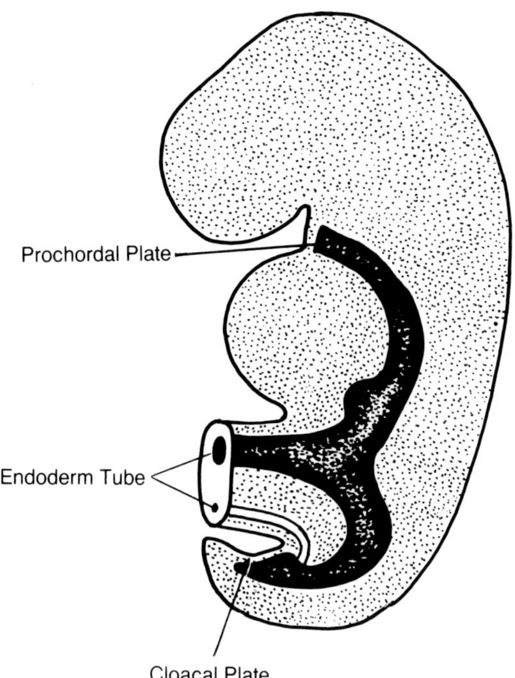

Figure 2-3 Three-dimensional folding of trilaminar disc has resulted in internalization of endoderm.

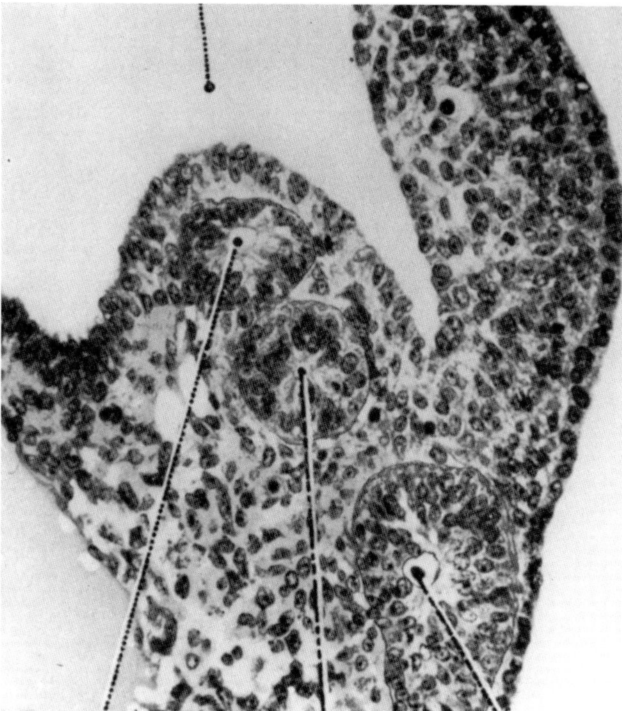

Figure 2-4 Mesonephric duct and tubule constitute most of intermediate mesoderm in this photomicrograph (× c. 250). They form a mass, which bulges into expanding peritoneal or coelomic cavity. Somite is posterior. *Source:* Reprinted from *Hamilton, Boyd, and Mossman's Human Embryology*, ed 4 (p 380) by WJ Hamilton and HW Mossman with permission of Williams & Wilkins Company, © 1972.

expands, the column of intermediate mesoderm becomes a bulge in its posterior wall (Figure 2-4).

The epithelium lining the coelomic or peritoneal cavity is derived by local differentiation from the same cells that make up the subepithelial stroma of the cavity.[1] Therefore both epithelium and stroma are derived from the mesoderm. This is in contrast to systems with which most clinicians are more familiar, such as the bowel or the skin, in which the epithelium is derived from one germ layer and the underlying stroma from another. Thus the epithelium of the coelomic cavity shares more biologic properties with its underlying stroma than is characteristic of the epithelium of skin or the bowel.

By the end of the fourth week, the intermediate mesoderm has enlarged to the extent that it forms a vertical ridge in the posterior wall of the coelomic cavity on each side of the midline.[1] This ridge, the *urogenital ridge*, projects into the coelomic cavity. It is composed mostly of mesonephric glomeruli. The glomeruli are connected in series by the mesonephric duct, which runs vertically, parallel to the long axis of the ridge. The mesonephric duct runs in the urogenital ridge all the way into the pelvis and then enters the urogenital sinus at that level where the future urethra will enter the vestibule. This is an important junction because the duct, *mesodermal epithelium*, enters a cavity, the *urogenital sinus*, lined by an endodermal epithelium (Figure 2-5).

During the fourth, fifth, and sixth weeks of embryonic life, the primordial germ cells migrate from the wall of the yolk sac, through the hindgut mesentery into a subepithelial site on the medial surface of the urogenital ridge.[5] Here they elicit a proliferation of the surface epithelial cells, which will give rise to the specialized gonadal epithelium. Male differentiation consists of the arrangement of the proliferating epithelial cells into radial cords that run from near the surface of the urogenital ridge into the medullary portion of the ridge, the future hilum of the gonad. The germ cells are incorporated within these cords, and this is an important feature of their development. Germ cells that are not incorporated die in most cases. The cords eventually become the testicular tubules, and the epithelial cells become the Sertoli cells. Germ cells depend on a close association with Sertoli cells throughout life. The Sertoli cells by an as yet unknown mechanism, maintain the long-term health of the germ cells.

The stroma between the testicular tubules develops a population of steroid hormone–producing cells, the

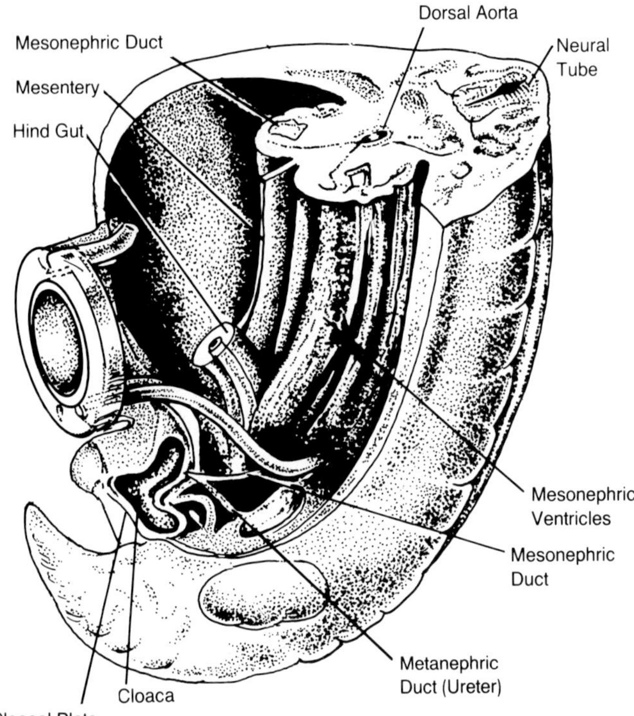

Figure 2-5 In this cut-away view, mesonephric duct runs down through urogenital ridge into pelvis and enters cloaca in its anterior or ventral portion. Shortly before doing so, it gives rise to ureter. *Source:* Adapted from *Hamilton, Boyd, and Mossman's Human Embryology*, ed 4 (p 384) by WJ Hamilton and HW Mossman with permission of Williams & Wilkins Company, © 1972.

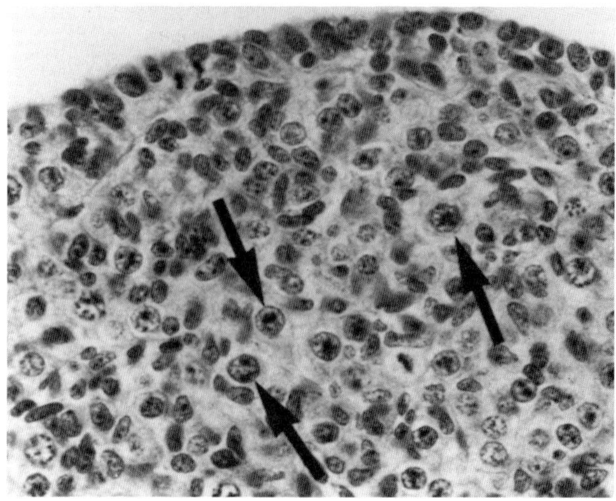

Figure 2-6 Small cells in this cellular mass become follicular epithelium and envelop large cells (*arrows*), which are germ cells. *Source:* Reprinted from *Blaustein's Pathology of the Female Genital Tract*, ed 3 (p 7) by RJ Kurnan (editor) with permission of Springer-Verlag, © 1987.

interstitial cells, which produce androgen and respond to the elevated gonadotropin levels that occur early in pregnancy.[6] The intrauterine male fetus therefore experiences a large surge of testosterone production near the end of the first trimester. This testosterone production results in male-type differentiation of the fetal central nervous system. Its absence will result in female-type differentiation. The early development of the testes is also associated with the production of müllerian duct inhibitory factor, a peptide that prevents development of the müllerian duct structures and actually causes regression of any preliminary development that has occurred.

In the case of female differentiation, the initial proliferation of epithelium and germ cells does not become organized into cords within the interior of the urogenital ridge but remains peripheral on its surface. Continuous proliferation results in an increasingly thick cortex on the surface of the urogenital ridge (Figure 2-6). Subsequently, the connective tissue in the hilum of the gonad invades this cortical mass of epithelial and germ cells.[7] It progressively divides them into smaller and smaller collections of cells. Eventually the collections are so small that they contain only a single germ cell, and a few epithelial cells, a *primordial follicle*. As this process begins in the hilum, it is more advanced in the interior of the ovary than on its surface at any given point in time. At birth, only a few nests of undivided germ cells and epithelial cells persist on the ovarian surface. Rarely, two germ cells are encapsulated into a single follicle.

FORMATION OF THE LOWER URINARY TRACT

In the middle of the urogenital ridge mesonephric glomeruli develop in a sequential manner, the cephalad ones first. They are close to the mesonephric duct that runs parallel to the long axis of the ridge and near its lateral surface. As it descends, it connects to each glomerulus. Eventually it extends into the caudad end of the embryo and enters the urogenital sinus at the level where the future urethra will enter the vestibule (Figure 2-7). (See also Figure 2-5.) Because the urethral orifice is immediately above the hymenal ring, the site of entry of the wolffian duct into the vestibule is also immediately superolateral to the hymenal ring. That this is the most caudad point the wolffian duct ever reaches is clinically important because it marks the caudad limit of anomalies that result from persistent wolffian ducts such as ectopic ureters and Gartner's duct cysts.

Just before the wolffian duct enters the urogenital sinus it gives off a diverticulum, the *ureteral diverticulum*. The diverticulum migrates back into the most caudad portion of the urogenital ridge and there induces the glomeruli and tubules, which will make up the

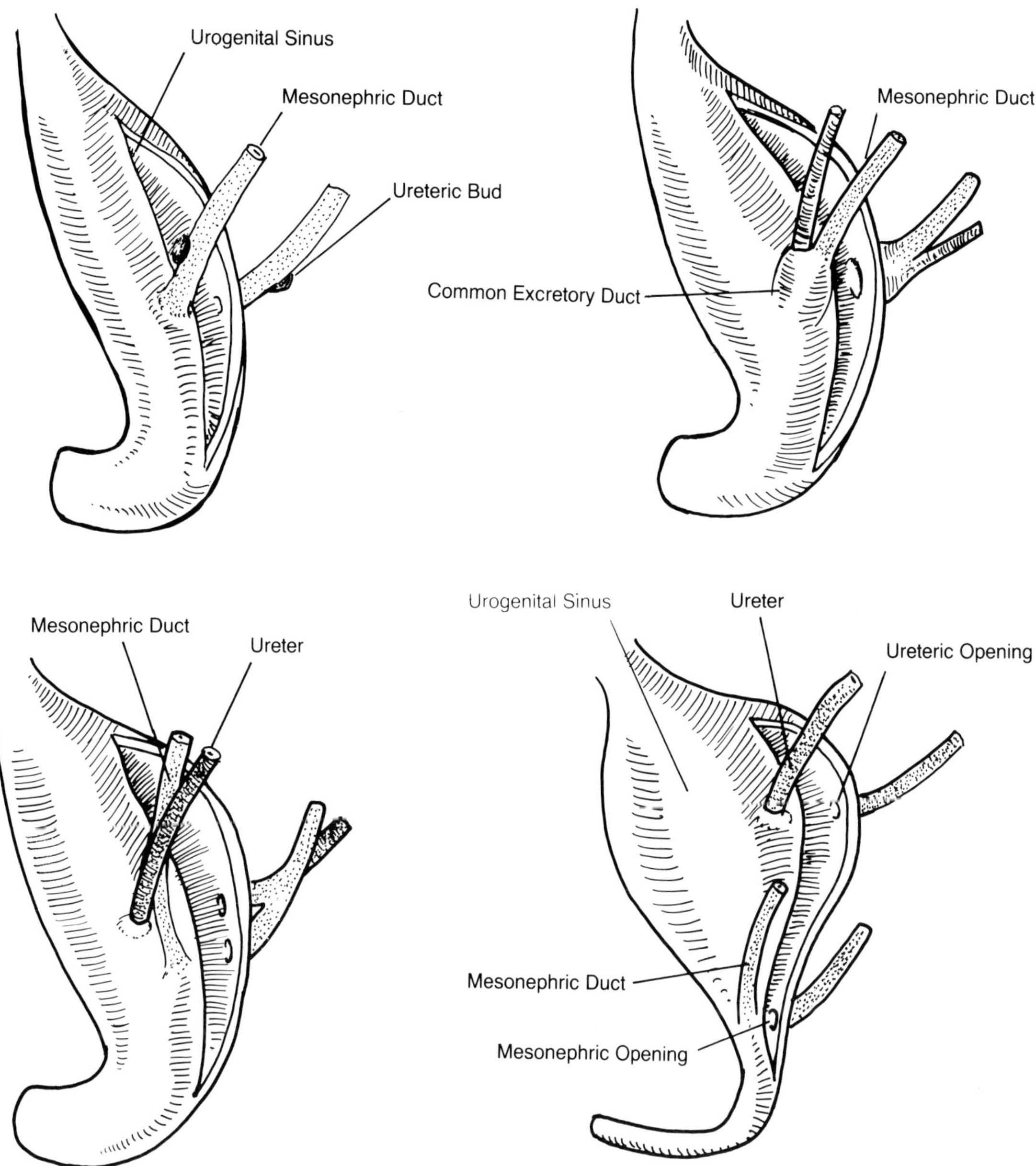

Figure 2-7 As mesonephric duct is everted into urogenital sinus, ureter and mesonephric duct develop separate orifices, and tissue between orifices becomes mesodermal. That portion of urogenital sinus below orifice of the mesonephric duct becomes the vestibule. *Source:* Adapted from *Hamilton, Boyd, and Mossman's Human Embryology*, ed 4 (p 396) by WJ Hamilton and HW Mossman with permission of Williams & Wilkins Company, © 1972.

mature kidney or metanephros.[1] (See Figures 2-5 and 2-7.)

The wolffian duct is mesodermal, and the urogenital sinus is endodermal. Therefore this junction is composed of tissue from two different germ layers. This is an important issue because, with subsequent growth, the wolffian duct is everted more and more into the urogenital sinus. In this manner, mesodermal, wolffian duct tissue is inserted like a patch into the posterior wall of the urogenital sinus[8] (Figure 2-8). (See also Figure 2-7.) When this eversion process reaches the level of the ureteral diverticulum, this structure develops a separate orifice in the urogenital sinus, and this orifice is displaced upward in the sinus. Eventually it is displaced to the level of the corners of the trigone of the bladder, but the original wolffian duct orifice remains low where the urethra enters the vestibule. From this process, then, the trigone of the bladder and the posterior wall of the urethra are mesodermal as they develop from the patch of mesoderm inserted into the posterior wall of the urogenital sinus by eversion of the wolffian duct into the urogenital sinus.

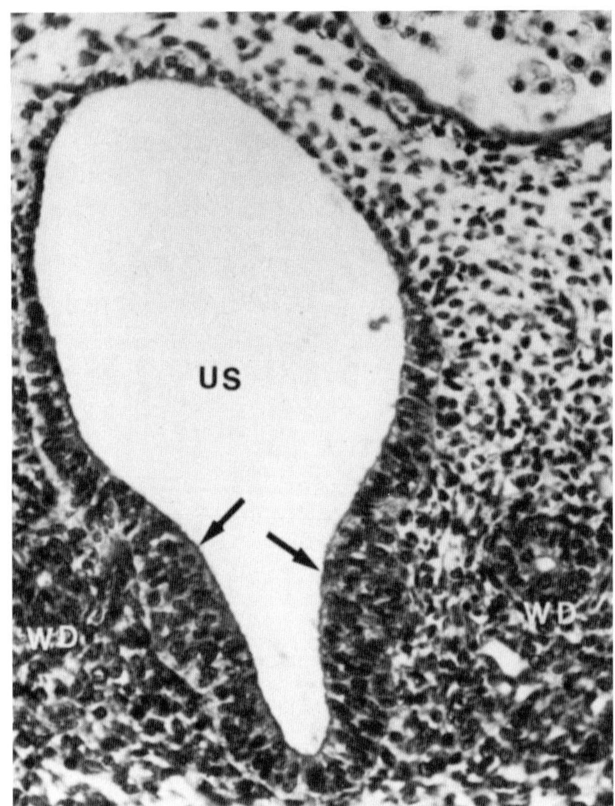

Figure 2-8 Anterior wall of urogenital sinus (US) is composed of low cuboidal epithelium. Posterior wall (*arrows*) is composed of more columnar epithelium similar to that in wolffian (mesonephric) ducts (WD). One of latter is entering sinus on left. *Source:* Reprinted from *Blaustein's Pathology of the Female Genital Tract*, ed 3 (p 4) by RJ Kurnan (editor) with permission of Springer-Verlag, © 1987.

If a portion of the mesonephric kidney continues to function and the wolffian duct persists, the duct forms an ectopic ureter that opens into the vestibule or higher in the vagina. This rarely occurs, however. More commonly, wolffian duct remnants persist in the retroperitoneal space as only microscopic curiosities. Anywhere along their course, however, they may result in the development of cysts, which in the vagina, to add to the confusion, are known as Gartner's duct cysts.

The fact that the trigone of the bladder and the posterior wall of the urethra are of mesodermal origin is clinically important as it determines that these tissues respond in common with the vagina to sex steroids. When estrogen deficiency occurs in a postmenopausal woman, these tissues also atrophy. The symptomatic result is urgency and dysuria, and posterior urethral caruncles may develop. Estrogen can be used successfully to treat both caruncles and symptoms. (Interestingly, estrogen can also be used to treat prolapsed urethras in small children.)

DEVELOPMENT OF THE VAGINAL PLATE

A further important result of the insertion of mesoderm into the posterior wall of the urogenital sinus is that it results in the portion of the urogenital sinus wall that lies between the orifices of the two wolffian ducts being mesoderm. As the lower aspect of the vagina, or the *vaginal plate*, develops from this site, the lower part of the vagina is mesoderm and responds to sex steroids. The vaginal plate develops as follows.

When the müllerian ducts develop during the fifth week of embryonic life, they begin as multiple evaginations on the lateral surface of the urogenital ridge.[1] Here they are lateral to the wolffian duct. It is the coalescence of these multiple evaginations that results in the fimbriated end of the tube. Failure of one or more evaginations to coalesce with the others results in a hydatid of Morgagni or an accessory lumen or diverticulum. Once coalescence has occurred, each müllerian duct forms a discrete tube whose tip is so closely applied to the wolffian duct epithelium that many believe it to be within the basement membrane of the wolffian duct.[9] Maintaining this close relation, the müllerian duct tip migrates along the wolffian duct tip into the pelvis. This is presumably an example of a mechanism increasingly demonstrated in embryology, one in which the direction of the movement of a cell or cells is dictated by the underlying matrix on which it moves.

When the müllerian duct reaches the pelvis, its tip moves anteriorly over the wolffian duct and then lies on the medial side of this structure (Figure 2-9). Because the embryo is tiny and all the spaces being discussed are quite small, when the two müllerian ducts are both medial to their respective wolffian ducts they are in close apposition to each other. The most caudad portion of the ducts fuse, side to side. By the end of the 10th embryonic week, the fused tip of the müllerian duct abuts on the posterior wall of the urogenital sinus immediately between the two orifices of the wolffian duct. This is where the wall of the urogenital sinus has been converted into mesoderm by the prior insertion of wolffian duct tissue.[8] When induced by the fused tip of the müllerian duct, the mesodermal tissue at this site begins to produce a column of squamous tissue, the *vaginal plate*. This tissue separates the tip of the müllerian duct from the posterior wall of the urogenital sinus, which is the future vestibule (Figure 2-10). Achieving patency, the vaginal plate becomes the lower aspect of the vagina early in the second trimester.[10,11]

When the tip of the müllerian duct breaks down and continuity is established among the vaginal plate, the

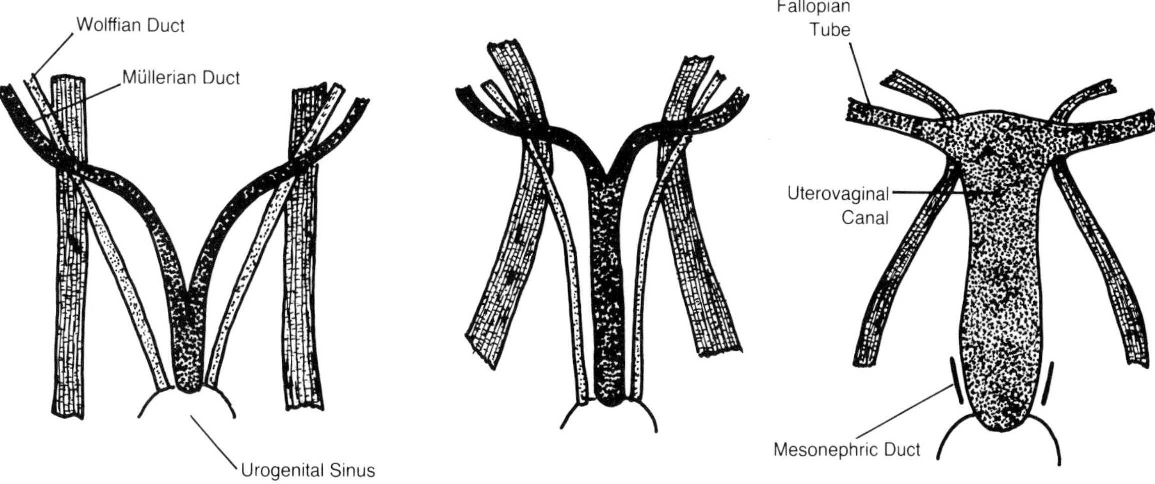

Figure 2-9 Müllerian duct begins lateral to wolffian (mesonephric) duct but crosses it anteriorly and fuses with opposite müllerian duct in midline. *Source:* Reprinted from *Illustrated Human Embryology*, Vol 2 (p 90) by H Tuchmann-Duplessis and P Haegel with permission of Springer-Verlag, © 1974.

lower vagina, and the lumen of the müllerian duct, the columnar epithelium of the upper vaginal müllerian duct is replaced from caudad to cephalad by a stratified squamous epithelium.[12] This process of squamous metaplasia terminates at the anatomic external os of the cervix, resulting in an epithelial squamocolumnar junction. It is not clear why this process begins or ends when it does, but it is presumed that something in the external environment (ie, the vagina) induces the process of squamous metaplasia, which effects this change.

The presumption is based on three reasons. First, results of studies with injections of dilute silicone in human embryos demonstrate that the endocervical canal is patent before 26 weeks, but not after that time.[11] There is no true obstruction, but differentiation in the cervical stroma has resulted in sufficient rigidity, so that the endocervical canal is functionally obstructed to a solution that would previously pass through it. It is at the same time (ie, between 20 and 25 weeks) and at the expected site (ie, the external os of the cervix) that squamous metaplasia ceases.

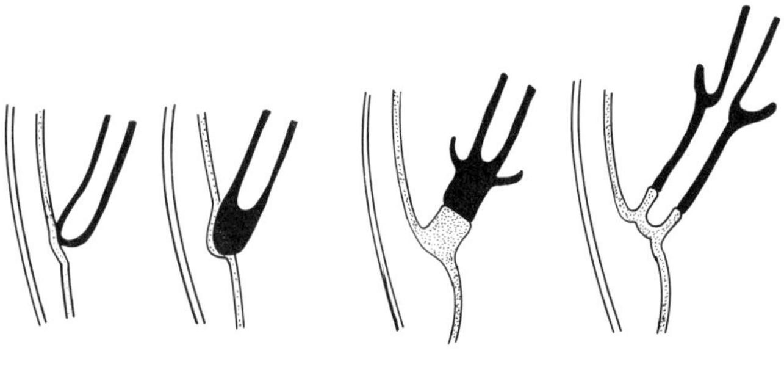

Figure 2-10 Tip of müllerian duct induces vaginal plate from posterior wall of urogenital sinus. Vaginal plate becomes lower aspect of vagina. *Source:* Adapted from *Illustrated Human Embryology*, Vol 2 (p 91) by H Tuchmann-Duplessis and P Haegel with permission of Springer-Verlag, © 1974.

Second, when complete transverse vaginal septa persist, the upper vaginal chamber is lined by a columnar, mucus-secreting epithelium.[13] Finally, when, at any future point, the endocervical mucosa is everted into the vagina, the process of squamous metaplasia begins again. This occurs prominently at birth, at puberty, and at the time of the first pregnancy.

EFFECTS OF DIETHYLSTILBESTROL

Diethylstilbestrol characteristically has three effects on the previously discussed embryologic events.[14] First, it inhibits the development of the vaginal plate, so that the müllerian duct contribution to the vagina ends up closer to the hymenal ring than would otherwise be the case. Second, it prevents conversion of the müllerian duct epithelium to a stratified squamous epithelium. The mechanism for this effect is unknown. Potentially, it stimulates enough secretion from the müllerian duct epithelium, so that this tissue is relatively protected from the vaginal environment.

Finally, diethylstilbestrol disorganizes the stromal differentiation, which produces the rigid body of the cervix. As it is the rigid body of the cervix that results in the functional obstruction of the endocervical canal that apparently defines the site of the squamocolumnar junction (as described earlier), the anomalies described in patients exposed to diethylstilbestrol in utero are not accurately viewed as specific structures but as the absence of structure. Although occurring after differentiation of the cervix, differentiation of the walls of the uterus and the fallopian tubes is a similar process to that in the cervix. It is similarly disrupted by diethylstilbestrol, leading to structural abnormalities of these components of the genital canal as well.[15]

DEVELOPMENT OF EXTERNAL GENITALIA

The external genitalia develop between the 4th and the 10th week of embryonic life[16] (Figure 2-11). Initially, two paired primordia of subepithelial mesenchyme form ventral to the cloacal membrane and fuse in the midline. These become the genital tubercle. From the posterior edge of each, subepithelial mesenchymal ridges extend dorsally around the edge of the cloacal membrane. These are termed the *cloacal folds*. Lateral to them, two parallel folds, the *labioscrotal folds*, extend ventrally beyond the genital tubercle to form the future mons veneris. If male development occurs, the cloacal folds will fuse from their posterior edge to their anterior or ventral end and thus form the posterior wall of the penile urethra. The labioscrotal folds will similarly fuse from posterior to anterior end, forming the scrotum. This fusion is normally complete by the end of the 10th or 12th embryonic week. In the case of female development the vestibule experiences great anteroposterior enlargement as differential growth occurs.

CLINICAL IMPLICATIONS

There are many clinical implications associated with this embryologic development. Perhaps the most significant one is that, from the hymenal ring up, the entire female genital canal is derived from one germ layer, the mesoderm. Many biologic properties are therefore shared, including responsiveness to the sex steroids. This property is, for the same reason, shared with all other mesodermal derivatives, although there are quantitative differences. In contrast, the vestibule lined by epithelium of endodermal origin reveals clinical differences. The epithelium does not respond to the sex steroids. It is uniquely sensitive to 5-fluorouracil. When this agent is placed in the vagina, it does not usually cause irritation. If it leaks into the vestibule, however, it may produce sloughing of the endodermal epithelium. The vestibular epithelium also possesses specific appendages, the minor and major vestibular glands.

Of particular importance to the histopathologist is the fact that all the upper genital tract is simply an evagination of the coelomic cavity. The histologic features of the vagina, cervix, endometrium, tubes, gonads, and peritoneum are the result of local differentiation in the wall of a continuous tube that is uniform in the undifferentiated state. Therefore, consistent with observed natural variation, one expects foci of heterotopic differentiation throughout this anatomic system. Perhaps the most important is the ubiquitous presence of endometrial-type foci at levels of the genital canal other than the endometrial cavity.

To the gynecologic oncologist the most significant result of this common embryologic background is that

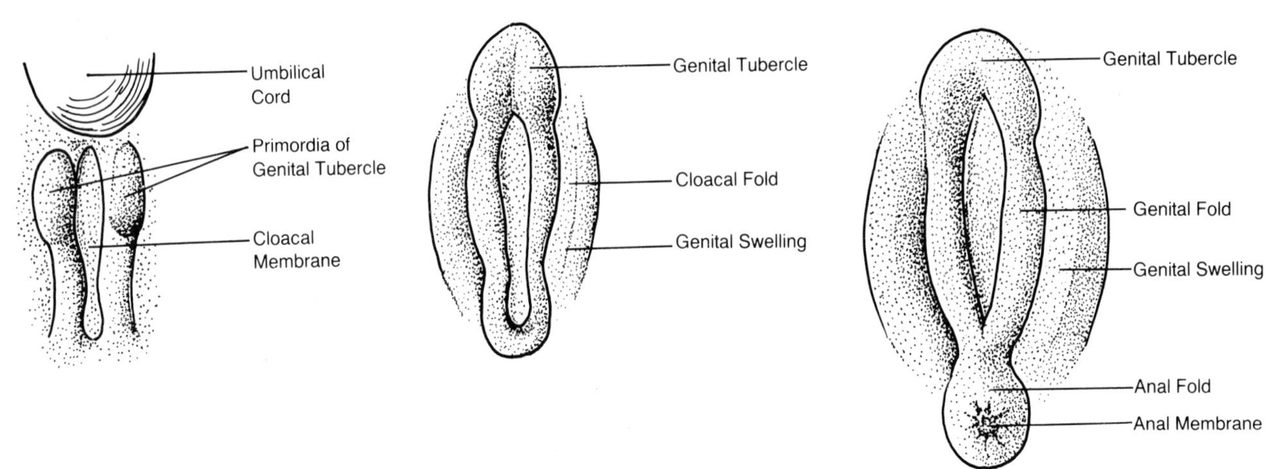

Figure 2-11 Paired primordia underlie paired structure of adult phallus. Development illustrated is female. If male development occurs, genital folds fuse posteriorly to anteriorly to form phallic urethra, and genital tubercle enlarges. Genital swelling then fuses posteriorly to anteriorly to form scrotum. *Source:* Reprinted from *Illustrated Human Embryology*, Vol 2 (p 98) by H Tuchmann-Duplessis and P Haegel with permission of Springer-Verlag, © 1974.

malignant tumors from one level of the genital canal share many properties with those of other levels. Also, in all likelihood they are only significantly different in their site of origin, rather than in any biologically fundamental way.

Gynecologists are classically taught that renal anomalies are highly associated with müllerian duct anomalies. In reviewing the preceding embryologic events, however, clearly the renal anomaly is primary.[17] If the wolffian duct is absent, or fails to enter the pelvis properly or produce a ureteral diverticulum, the definitive kidney may fail to develop. In turn, the müllerian duct lacks the proper scaffolding on which to descend into the pelvis. It may not develop at all, or it may fail to descend adequately enough to achieve fusion with the duct from the other side. If it fails to reach the urogenital sinus, it will not induce a vaginal plate on that side. A common result is a normally formed fallopian tube attached to a uterine horn that connects through a small cervix with a closed vaginal chamber that is separated from the complete vagina on the other side by a septum.[13] Findings with an intravenous urogram show no kidney is present on the side of the incomplete canal. Because the wolffian duct was defective on this side, the kidney did not develop. Also, without the wolffian duct, the müllerian duct did not descend into the pelvis adequately. Therefore it did not fuse with the müllerian duct from the other side. Because it did not reach the urogenital sinus, it did not induce a vaginal plate and never became connected with the external surface.

Routinely, only microscopic rudiments of the wolffian duct are found in the mesosalpinx of the adult woman, but remnants may persist as cysts all along its course. Low along the vaginal canal they may present as vulvar masses. Higher they occasionally present as formidable surgical problems that, when approached from below, are found to extend high into the broad ligament.[18] They may also persist as paraovarian or paratubal cysts. Even more rarely the entire mesonephric system may persist, in which case rudimentary glomeruli will be found high in the retroperitoneal space connected to a ''ureter'' that descends parallel to the normal ureter but extends beyond it to empty as an ectopic ureter in the vagina or the vestibule. Such structures may not be patent along their whole course and may be the source of recurrent abscesses.

REFERENCES

1. Hamilton WJ, Mossman HW. *Hamilton, Boyd, and Mossman's Human Embryology*. 4th ed. Baltimore, MD: Williams & Wilkins Co; 1972.

2. Slack JMW. *From Egg to Embryo*. New York: Cambridge University Press; 1983.

3. Slack JMW. Peptide regulatory factors in embryonic development. *Lancet*. 1989;1:1312–1315.

4. Johnston MC. Embryology of the pharyngeal and facial areas. In: Bosma JF and Showacre J, eds. *Development of Upper Respiratory Anatomy and Function*. Washington, DC: US Government Printing Office; 1976. Publication 617-046-00033-1.

5. Witschi E. Migration of the germ cells of human embryos from the yolk sac to the primitive gonadal folds. *Contrib Embryol*. 1948;32:67.

6. Hutchinson JB, ed. *Biological Determinants of Sexual Behavior*. New York: John Wiley & Sons, Inc; 1978.

7. Konishi I, Fujii S, Okamura H, Parmley T, Mori T. Development and regression of interstitial cells in the human fetal ovary: an ultrastructural study. *J Anat*. 1986;148:121–135.

8. Parmley TH. Embryology of the female genital tract. In: Kurman RJ, ed. *Blaustein's Pathology of the Female Genital Tract*. 3rd ed. Springer-Verlag; New York: 1987.

9. Gruenwald P. The relation of growing müllerian duct to the wolffian duct and its importance for the genesis of malformations. *Anat Rec*. 1941;81:1–19.

10. Cunha GR. The dual origin of vaginal epithelium. *Am J Anat*. 1975;143:387–392.

11. Terruhn V. A study of impression moulds of the genital tract of female fetuses. *Arch Gynecol*. 1980;229:207.

12. Forsberg JG. Cervicovaginal epithelium: its origin and development. *Am J Obstet Gynecol*. 1973;115:1025–1043.

13. Jones HW Jr, Rock JA. *Reparative and Constructive Surgery of the Female Genital Tract*. Baltimore, MD: Williams & Wilkins Co; 1983:167.

14. Robboy SJ. A hypothetic mechanism of diethylstilbestrol (DES)-induced anomalies in exposed progeny. *Hum Pathol*. 1983;14:831–833.

15. Kaufman RH, Adam E, Binder GL, Gerthoffer E. Upper genital tract changes and pregnancy outcome in offspring exposed in utero to diethylstilbestrol. *Am J Obstet Gynecol*. 1980;137:299–308.

16. England M. *Color Atlas of Life before Birth*. Chicago, IL: Year Book Medical Publishers, Inc; 1983:157–162.

17. Marshall FF, Beisel DS. The association of uterine and renal anomalies. *Obstet Gynecol*. 1978;51:559–562.

18. Muram D, Jerkins GR. Urinary retention secondary to a Gartner's duct cyst. *Obstet Gynecol*. 1988;72:510–511.

3

Anatomy of Genital Support

John O. L. DeLancey and A. Cullen Richardson

To perform surgery for genital prolapse with skill the gynecologic surgeon must

> have an exact knowledge of the anatomy and pathology of the pelvis and a correct comprehension of its physiology. His extensive mechanical knowledge must be instinctive as well as acquired, for no two cases present exactly the same conditions to be remedied by plastic work. . . . He must have an abiding sense that his aim is not to remove but always to restore. And finally he must love his work for the opportunity it affords him to restore a mutilated part almost to that perfection which it originally received from the Master Hand.[1]

It is with this quotation from J. Marion Sims' able assistant and chronicler J.D. Emmet, that James Ricci began his book on *The Cystocele in America*.[2] It remains as true today as it did a century ago and forms the justification for this chapter.

GENERAL PRINCIPLES OF SUPPORT

A description of the pelvic floor must start with its relation to the abdominopelvic cavity because it is the unique position of the pelvic floor at the bottom of this space that determines the role that it must play in supporting the abdominal and pelvic viscera (Figure 3-1). The abdominopelvic cavity extends from the thorax above to the bottom of the pelvis below and contains the abdominal and pelvic viscera. It is a boxlike space that takes a somewhat flattened cylindric shape. Its top is the dome-shaped respiratory diaphragm. The vertebral column and its attached muscles form the posterior wall, and the abdominal muscles constitute its sides and front. The pelvic bones surround the lower part of this box. The floor of the box comprises the soft tissue structures that close the space between the bony side walls of the pelvis, and these structures are collectively referred to as the *pelvic floor*. The pelvic floor extends from the peritoneum that covers the pelvic viscera to the skin of the vulva, the perineum, and the buttocks. It can be arbitrarily divided into several layers (Figure 3-2).

The first layer of the pelvic floor is the peritoneum, which covers the underlying viscera and the pelvic side walls. Immediately below the peritoneum are the pelvic viscera. These viscera are attached to the pelvic walls by the endopelvic fascia. The combination of these organs and their attachments to the pelvis through the endopelvic fascia forms the next layer of support. Below this network of viscera and endopelvic fascia are the striated muscles called the *levator ani*. They form a muscular diaphragm (referred to as the *pelvic diaphragm*) across

Portions of this chapter have been taken from recent reviews by the authors and are indicated by reference numbers in the section headings.

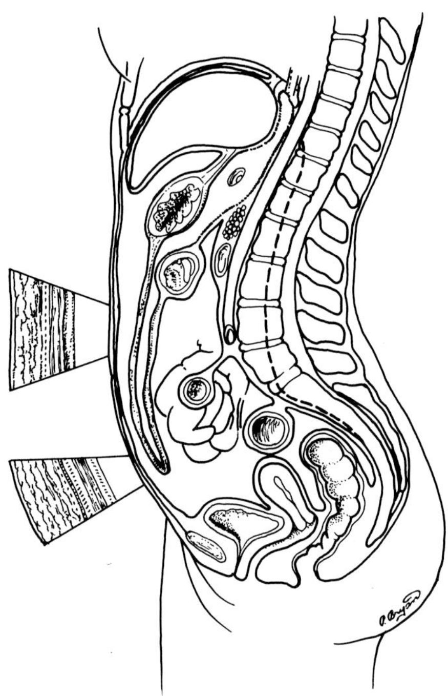

Figure 3-1 Sagittal view of the abdominopelvic cavity. Details of the layering of the abdominal wall are shown in the insets to the left. The dotted line indicates the extension of the peritoneal space lateral and dorsal to the spine. *Source*: Reprinted from *Hernia: Surgical Anatomy and Technique* (pp 244–250) by JE Skandalakis et al (eds) with permission of McGraw-Hill, © 1989.

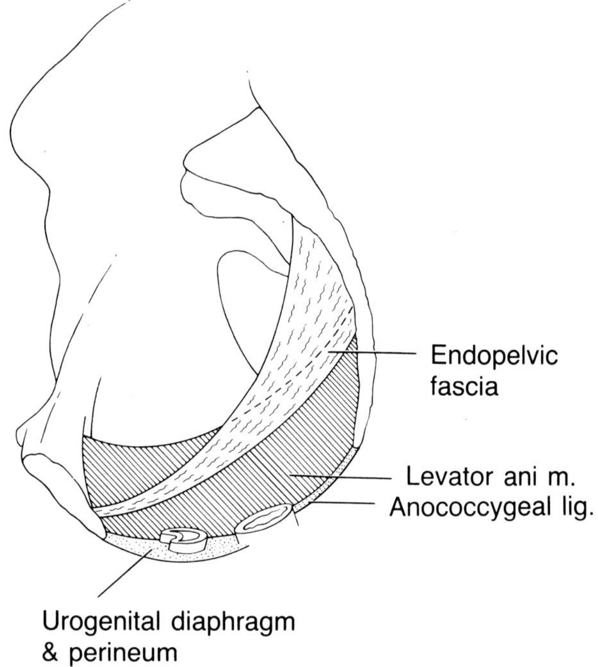

Figure 3-2 Layers of the pelvic floor. The levator ani muscles form an intermediate layer between the endopelvic fascia and the urogenital diaphragm. The endopelvic fascia lies on the inner surface of the levator ani muscles in their anterior portion. *Source*: Reprinted from *Hernia: Surgical Anatomy and Technique* (pp 244–250) by JE Skandalakis et al (eds) with permission of McGraw-Hill, © 1989.

the pelvic cavity with a cleft in its anterior portion through which the urethra, the lower aspect of the vagina, and the rectum pass.

Caudal to the levator ani muscles lie the structures that span the pelvic outlet. This space can be subdivided into anterior and posterior segments by a line drawn between the ischial tuberosities. The perineal membrane (also referred to as the *urogenital diaphragm*) with its attached external genital muscles fills the anterior segment of the outlet. It spans the space between the inferior ischiopubic rami. The urethra and the perineal body are fixed to the pelvic bones by this perineal membrane. Attached to and lying beneath the perineal membrane are the external genital muscles: bulbocavernosus, ischiocavernosus, and transversus perinei superficialis muscles. The anal sphincter is found under the skin of the posterior segment of the pelvic outlet and fuses posteriorly with the anococcygeal ligament, which attaches it to the coccyx and the sacrum.

Together these several layers form the pelvic floor. Rather than being an uninterrupted layer, like the layers of the abdominal wall above, the pelvic floor in women is traversed by the urethra, the vagina, and the rectum. It must not only support the visceral structures of the abdomen and pelvis but also allow for reproductive and excretory functions. In addition, it has to expand and stretch sufficiently for parturition to occur.

SUPPORT OF THE PELVIC ORGANS

All the pelvic viscera—urethra, bladder, vagina, uterus, and anorectum—rest on or are contained within the floor of this box-like cavity. If the support offered by the pelvic floor fails, certain of the pelvic viscera will be displaced outward by the pressure within the abdominopelvic cavity. It has been traditional to name any defect in pelvic support according to the displaced visceral structure (eg, cystocele or rectocele), as though the problem had to do with that structure (eg, bladder or rectum) itself. This has led to some confusion about the nature of prolapse and its cause. Much has been made of the descriptions of the anatomic supports of each viscus, as though they were in some way each suspended individually by a series of isolated ligaments. The various structures of the pelvic floor form a continuous unit that must work together and offer support from the symphysis in front to the sacrum in back and from ischial spine to ischial spine side to side. These many and various tissues act in continuity with one another to support the viscera of the abdomen and the pelvis.

Damage can occur at one location, or many individual locations, within this continuity of support. The location of the support defect (or defects) will determine what visceral structure prolapses. Nevertheless, in all support defects the primary problem is in the pelvic floor, not in the displaced organ.

Three fundamental principles are important in considering the mechanism by which prolapse develops.

1. The mechanism of prolapse is from the inside out. The viscera never fall out; they are pushed out by intra-abdominal pressure. Gravity alone will not account for any defect seen.
2. The problem that gives rise to prolapse is not in the displaced viscus but, rather, in the pelvic floor on which or within which the visceral structure lies.
3. Any major support problem implies some break in the uppermost layer, the *endopelvic fascia*, rather than a generalized stretching in this tissue as previously believed.

To understand its supporting function, the pelvic floor must be viewed as a unit. It comprises both contractile and noncontractile elements, and one must keep in mind that there is always a delicate interplay between the actions of the active muscles and the passive supporting connective tissue elements.

FAILURE OF THE SUPPORT SYSTEM

Much remains to be learned about the causes of prolapse. Total prolapse of the pelvic organs as an initial finding in a patient obviously represents end-stage disease with several defective supporting structures. What was the initial event that started the cascade of tissue damage that led to prolapse? This needs to be elucidated.

If the striated muscles that support the viscera and the endopelvic fascia are strong, there is less chance that the fascial and ligamentous elements will be stressed and less chance of their failure. Clearly, the striated muscle component is of paramount importance. Much work is being done on this element of the supporting mechanism, and it is apparent that the initial event in the development of prolapse might have been some weakness in support provided by the levator ani muscles.[3] In virtually all patients who initially present with major support problems such as a complete procidentia, the levator ani muscles, are found to be weak on simple palpation and the levator hiatus is both widened and lengthened.

Muscle weakness, however, is not always present in patients with prolapse. An occasional patient has a urethrocele, but examination shows that contraction of the levator ani muscles is excellent. Apparently, unusual stress on, or weakness within, the fascial supports can lead to isolated breaks within the supports of the urethra, yielding a urethrocele.

Operative procedures for correction of defective support must necessarily focus on work with connective tissues, the so-called ligaments and fascias, because these are the tissues with which the surgeon works. The defects in the fascial and ligamentous supports must be corrected. This, unfortunately, is all that can be done because, as yet, there is no good surgical correction for weakened muscles. Conceivably, implantation of fetal muscle cells or, possibly, injection of some medication directly into the levator ani muscles to stimulate muscle growth may be part of any reparative operation. That possibility awaits scientific progress.

ANATOMY OF SUPPORT

Pelvic Wall

All the structures in the pelvic floor are held in place by their attachments to the pelvic side walls. By the term, pelvic side wall, we refer to those muscles (eg, obturator internus and piriformis muscles) and fascial structures fixed firmly to the pelvic bones that do not undergo dilation during vaginal delivery.

If one looks at the pelvic side wall, the ischial spine is located approximately halfway between the pubic bones and the sacrum (Figures 3-3 and 3-4). Anterior to the spine lie the obturator internus muscles, whereas posterior to these structures lie the piriformis muscles and the sacrospinous ligaments and their overlying coccygeus muscles. The portion of the pelvic cavity dorsal to the spine is frequently referred to as the *posterior segment*, whereas the ventral portion is called the *anterior segment*.

Two bands of fibrous tissue exist on the pelvic wall between the spine and the pubic bones. They are referred to as *tendinous arches* (Figure 3-5): the arcus tendineus fasciae pelvis (*fascial arch*) and the arcus tendineus

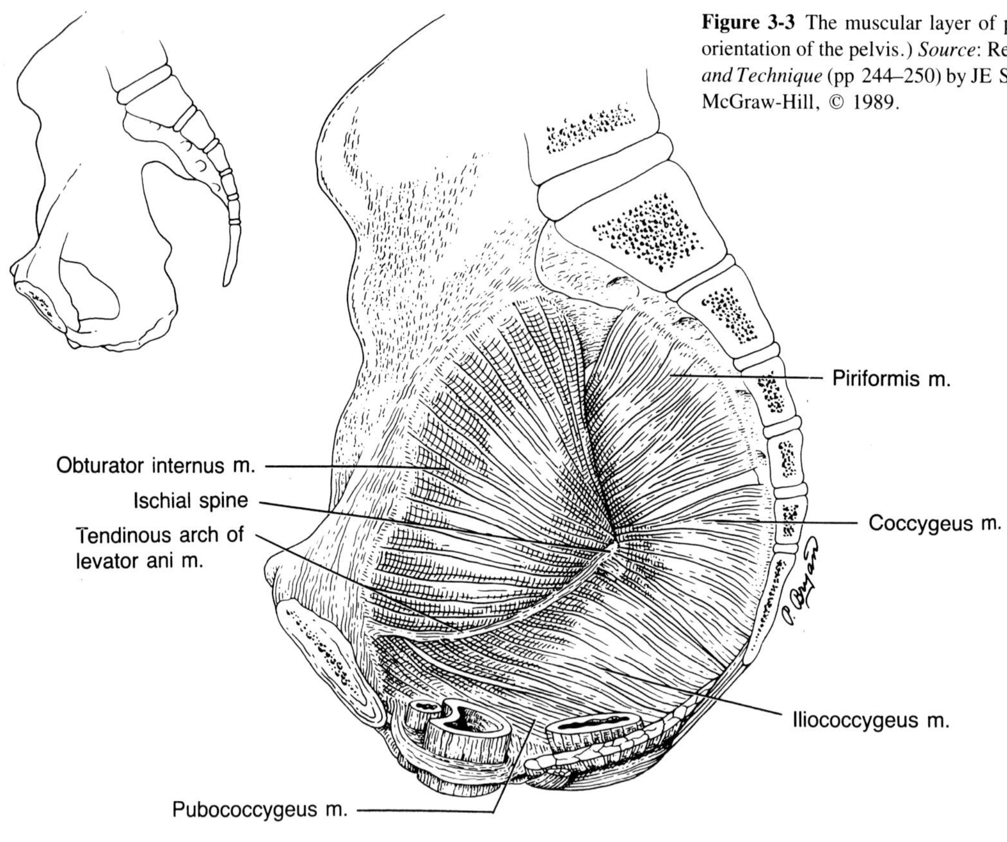

Figure 3-3 The muscular layer of pelvic floor. (The inset at left indicates orientation of the pelvis.) *Source*: Reprinted from *Hernia: Surgical Anatomy and Technique* (pp 244–250) by JE Skandalakis et al (eds) with permission of McGraw-Hill, © 1989.

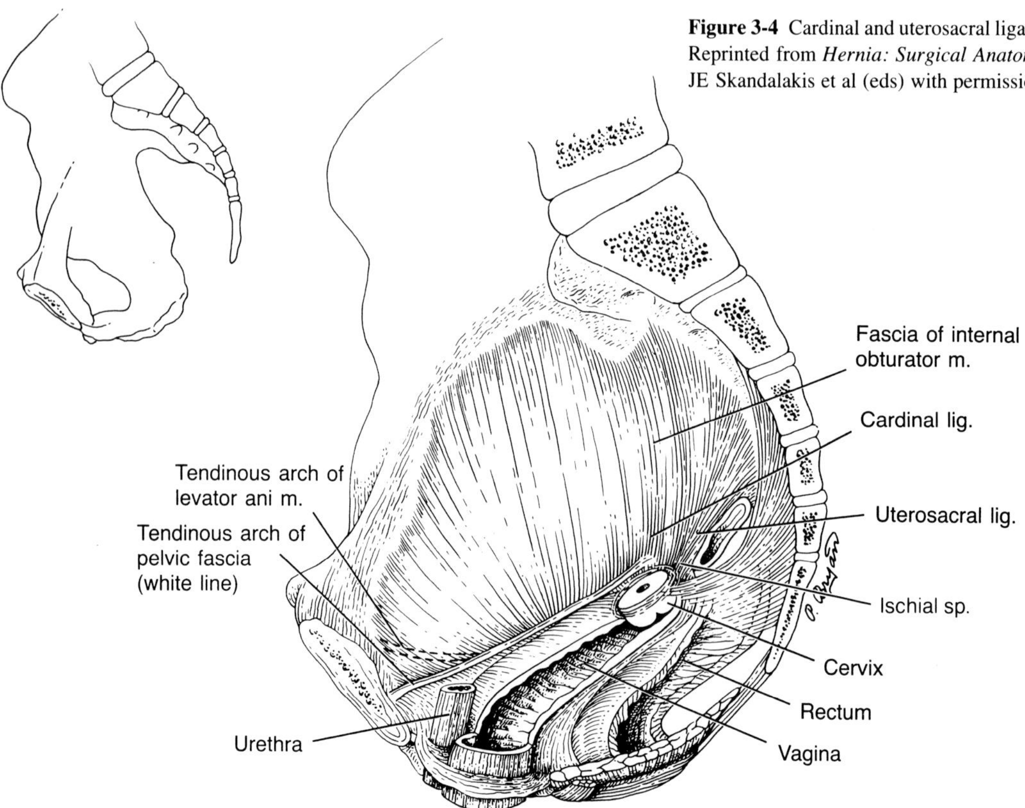

Figure 3-4 Cardinal and uterosacral ligaments and tendinous arches. *Source*: Reprinted from *Hernia: Surgical Anatomy and Technique* (pp 244–250) by JE Skandalakis et al (eds) with permission of McGraw-Hill, © 1989.

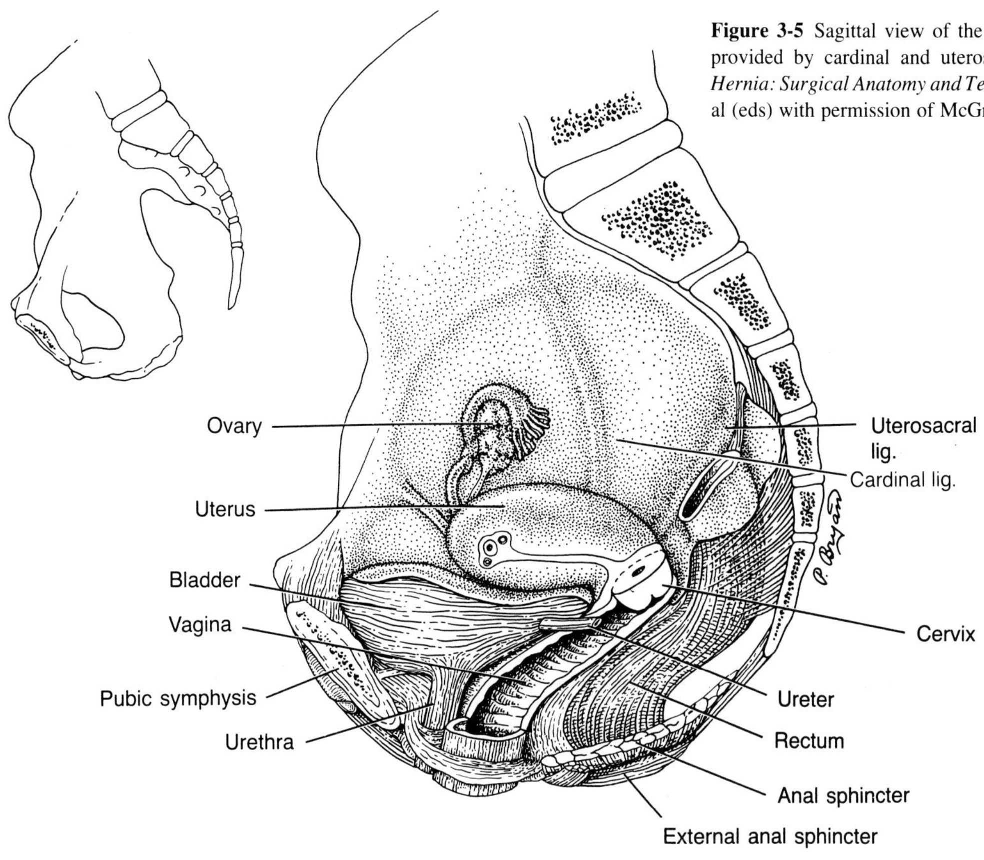

Figure 3-5 Sagittal view of the pelvic organs and the upward suspension provided by cardinal and uterosacral ligaments. *Source*: Reprinted from *Hernia: Surgical Anatomy and Technique* (pp 244–250) by JE Skandalakis et al (eds) with permission of McGraw-Hill, © 1989.

musculi levatoris ani (*levator arch*). Many of the pelvic floor structures attach to the pelvic wall at these structures. Although separate anteriorly, these two arches fuse near the ischial spine.

The levator arch is the semitendinous origin of the iliococcygeus muscle. It lies on the surface of the obturator internus muscle. The fascial arch is the lateral attachment of the pubocervical fascia to the pelvic wall. These two fascial arches fuse near the spine to form a single structure, whereas near the pubic bones they diverge.

Posterior to the spine is the sacrospinous ligament with its overlying coccygeus muscle. This structure marks the posterior limit of the pelvic diaphragm. The greater sciatic foramen is bounded by the sacrospinous ligament, the ischial bones, and the sacrum and is filled by the piriformis muscle, which inserts in the greater trochanter of the femur. Coursing over the surface of the piriformis muscle are the trunks of the sciatic nerve, which also emerge from the pelvis through this greater sciatic foramen. The lowermost trunk of the sciatic nerve lies immediately above and adjacent to the upper edge of the coccygeus tendon overlying the sacrospinous ligament.

Ligaments and Fasciae

Cardinal-Uterosacral Ligament Complex

The uppermost portion of the pelvic floor is composed of the pelvic viscera and their fibrous attachments to the pelvic walls: the cardinal and uterosacral ligaments and the pubocervical and rectovaginal fasciae. (See Figures 3-4 and 3-5.) The cardinal-uterosacral ligament complex is a single structure composed of an admixture of smooth muscle and connective tissue. The cardinal ligament portion is primarily perivascular connective tissue that runs along the uterine vessels,[4] whereas the uterosacral ligaments are predominantly smooth muscle, fibrous tissue, and nerves.[5] The uterosacral ligaments form the medial borders of the cardinal-uterosacral ligament complex and as such form a distinct boundary as they pass posteriorly toward the sacrum. It is this edge that appears as a sharp, well-defined line when seen at laparotomy or laparoscopy or felt on pelvic examination. The cardinal ligaments arise from the area of the greater sciatic foramen, whereas the uterosacral ligaments extend to originate from the second, third, and fourth sacral vertebrae. These ligaments encircle the cervix, forming a pericervical ring (see Figure 3-6), and extend downward to envelop and suspend the upper portion of the vagina. The ligaments suspend the cervix to the pelvic walls through their attachments to the pericervical ring. It is therefore a combination of these suspensory ligaments and the cervix that forms the first layer of the pelvic floor.

As these fibrous tissues extend along the vagina, they surround it in a way similar to how they surround the cervix. In their cephalic portion, the attachments suspend the viscera upward, as is true of the cardinal ligaments, and gradually begin to attach the vagina laterally to the tendinous arch of the pelvic fascia in the more caudal part (Figure 3-6). This is the transition from the cardinal-uterosacral ligaments to the pubocervical fascia that is formed by the lateral connection of the pubocervical fascia at the tendinous arch to the pelvic side wall.

In addition to their attachments to the vagina and the cervix, these suspensory ligaments have a portion that envelops the base of the bladder as the cardinal ligaments of the bladder. When the bladder is separated from the cervix and the vagina, this band can be made visible, and it is called the *bladder pillar*.

Pubocervical Fascia

The midportion of the vagina comes into closer contact with the pelvic walls than does its upper portion, which is suspended by the cardinal-uterosacral ligament complex. This portion of the vagina forms a transverse flattened oval attached at each side to the pelvic wall (Figure 3-7). On its anterior surface lies the pubocervical fascia, and on its posterior surface is the rectovaginal fascia. The pubocervical fascia is bounded dorsally where it blends with the cardinal ligaments. Laterally and anteriorly it attaches to the fascial arch.[6] The urethra pierces the pubocervical fascia in its anterior portion to exit the pelvis. Within the pubocervical fascia there is abundant smooth muscle, whose thickness varies from one region to another. (The details of this anatomy as they relate to urinary incontinence are discussed in more detail later in the chapter.)

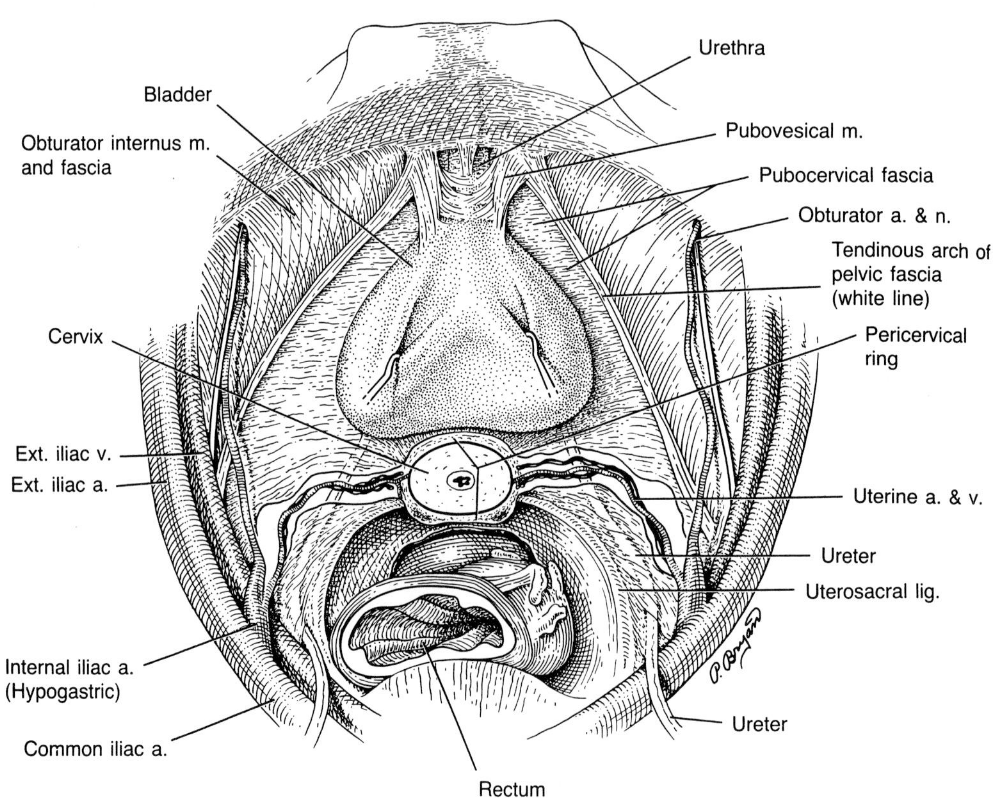

Figure 3-6 Attachment of the cardinal and uterosacral ligaments to the pericervical ring of connective tissue that supports the cervix. Also note the attachment of the pubocervical fascia at the tendinous arch of the pelvic fascia. *Source*: Reprinted from *Hernia: Surgical Anatomy and Technique* (pp 244–250) by JE Skandalakis et al (eds) with permission of McGraw-Hill, © 1989.

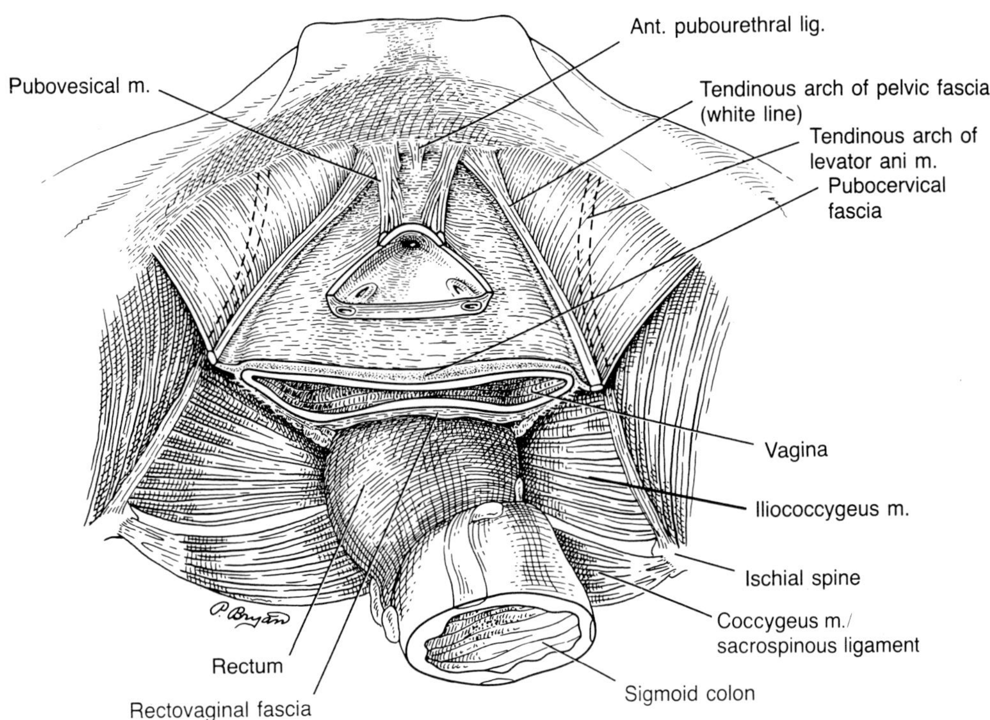

Figure 3-7 Relationships of the pubocervical and rectovaginal fasciae to the levator ani muscles and to the tendinous arches of the pelvic wall. *Source*: Reprinted from *Hernia: Surgical Anatomy and Technique* (pp 244–250) by JE Skandalakis et al (eds) with permission of McGraw-Hill, © 1989.

Rectovaginal Fascia

Posteriorly, the rectovaginal fascia (Figure 3-7) is a sheet of fibromuscular tissue that lies adjacent to the vagina.[7] It is found ventral to the rectovaginal space. Superiorly it blends with the cardinal-uterosacral ligament complex, which suspends its upper portions, whereas inferiorly it fuses with the perineal body. Laterally it attaches to the superior fascia of the pelvic diaphragm.

Endopelvic Fascia

A few words are necessary at this point about the use of the terms *fascia* and *ligament*. The ligaments and fasciae that suspend the pelvic organs are not ligaments, like those in the knee, or fasciae, like the rectus sheath covering the rectus abdominis muscles. Each of these latter structures is composed of dense regular collagen that is organized in parallel fibers aligned along lines of force. The ligaments of the pelvic organs are visceral ligaments and are a feltlike meshwork of fibrous tissue that contains considerable quantities of smooth muscle. Although their fibers generally lie along lines of tension, they are far less regular than the fibers of true skeletal ligaments. The endopelvic fascia is one continuous body of connective tissue. Innumerable regional names have been applied to various portions of this tissue, and often they are more confusing than useful. We have restricted our comments to the functionally important aspects of this tissue.

Muscles of the Pelvic Floor

The pubococcygeus and iliococcygeus are the muscles that support the pelvic viscera (see Figure 3-3). A preferable term for the pubococcygeus muscle would be the *pubovisceral muscle*[8] because this muscle attaches the pelvic organs to the pubic bones. The individual parts of the pubovisceral muscle are referred to individually as *pubovaginalis* and *puborectalis*, as well as *pubococcygeus*, but the latter term is in such wide use that we will not abandon it here. The pubococcygeus muscles begin on the inner surface of the pubic bones and pass laterally to the urethra, the vagina, and the rectum to insert on the inner surface of the sacrum. The puborectalis shares a common origin with the pubococcygeus but inserts between the internal and external anal sphincters and also forms a sling around the dorsal aspect of the anorectal junction. The medial portion of these muscles is attached to the vagina, and it is this portion of the levator ani muscle, between the vagina and the pubic bone, that is known as the pubovaginalis. There is no direct attachment of the levator ani muscles to the urethra as has sometimes been reported.[9]

The flat iliococcygeus muscle arises from the tendinous arch of the levator ani muscle on each side of the pelvis. The two sheets of muscle are joined in a midline raphe just above the anococcygeal ligament and between the anus and the coccyx. The coccygeus muscle takes origin from the ischial spine and inserts into the lateral aspect of the sacrum. Because its origin and insertion are fixed, it has little mobility. In the midline, between the coccyx and the rectum, the two iliococcygeal muscles form a shelf-like portion of the pelvic floor along with the dorsal extension of the pubococcygeus. This area has been referred to clinically as the *levator plate*,[10] and its angle of inclination reflects the activity of both the pubococcygeus muscles and the iliococcygeal muscles. This is the ''shelf'' upon which the pelvic viscera rest.

Physiologic study findings have clearly demonstrated that the levator ani group of muscles is similar to the external anal sphincter in its constant activity.[11] This contraction is present even at rest, in contrast to the usual voluntary muscles that are active primarily when willfully contracted. The activity of these muscles provides a resilient and functional shelf on which the other viscera may rest.

Support of the Pelvic Outlet

The support structures of the pelvic outlet are shown in Figure 3-8. Lying below the level of the levator ani muscles is the perineal membrane (urogenital diaphragm). Previous descriptions of the urogenital diaphragm, which indicate that it is a trilaminar structure with two layers of fascia separated by the deep transverse perineal muscle, are incorrect.[12] This layer is a single sheet of tissue that spans the area between the ischiopubic rami and has therefore been renamed the *perineal membrane*. The striated muscle that is associated with it is the compressor urethrae and urethrovaginal sphincter muscles that are part of the striated urogenital sphincter (described later). They lie just cephalad to the perineal membrane and are continuous with the striated urethral sphincter.

In men, the perineal membrane is a continuous sheet from side to side on which the prostate and the viscera may rest. In women, it has a large opening for the vagina. Therefore its support results from the attachments of this membrane to the vagina and the perineal body. In this way two sheets of tissue extend from the ischiopubic ramus to the perineal body on either side. At rest, these fibers are probably stressed little because of the support in this area provided by the tonic activity of the levator ani muscles. During increases in intra-abdominal pressure or with relaxation of the levator ani muscles, however, this sheet supports the perineal body and introitus.

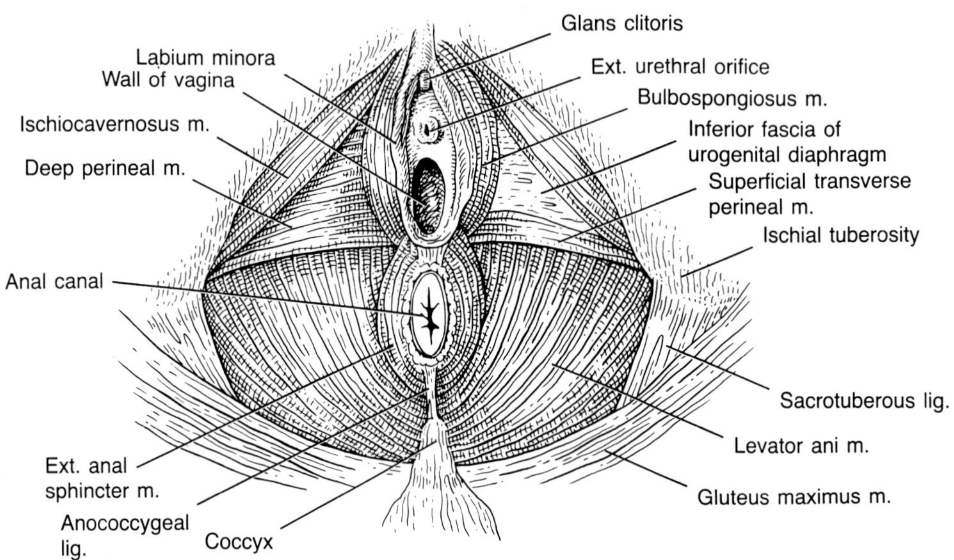

Figure 3-8 External genital muscles and urogenital diaphragm (perineal membrane) seen from the perineum. *Source*: Reprinted from *Hernia: Surgical Anatomy and Technique* (pp 244–250) by JE Skandalakis et al (eds) with permission of McGraw-Hill, © 1989.

Lying caudal to the level of the perineal membrane is a group of muscles that can be referred to as the *external genital muscles*. These include the ischiocavernosus, bulbocavernosus, and transversus perinei superficialis muscles. The first two of these muscles probably have little supportive role and are primarily involved in sexual function.

The external anal sphincter is a teardrop-shaped muscle with its apex anchored at the coccyx. It exerts some dorsal traction on the anus that opposes the ventral traction of the puborectalis muscle. This attachment to the coccyx probably has some influence in supporting the perineal body in which the anterior portion of the muscle is embedded.

LOWER URINARY TRACT AND PELVIC FLOOR

The portion of the pelvic floor that includes and surrounds the lower urinary tract is important to urinary continence and deserves special consideration. Although the mechanism of continence is poorly understood, its structure can be determined with some accuracy and is summarized here.

Subdivisions of the Continence Mechanism[13]

The structures that might influence continence are listed in Table 3-1. In addition to separating these structures according to whether they are intrinsic or extrinsic to the lower urinary tract, clinical observations suggest that these structures can be grouped into two different systems: one pertaining to normal lower urinary tract support and one pertaining to urethral closure. Problems with closure of the urethra can be further divided into (1) those that involve the proximal or internal sphincter (in the vesical neck) and (2) those that involve the external sphincter in the urethra. A functional classification would therefore divide these structures as follows:

- Urethral supports
- Sphincteric mechanism
  —Internal sphincter (vesical neck)
  —External sphincter

The internal sphincter lies at the level of the vesical neck. In patients with myelodysplasia or who have undergone surgery, it can be open, resulting in the occurrence of stress incontinence despite normal support. The distal urethral sphincter lies below the vesical neck and is capable of voluntary contraction. When urine gets past the vesical neck, as it does in some continent women,[14] this mechanism acts as a backup mechanism to ensure continence. The external sphincter is not strong enough in women to provide continence, as it can in men, but it may help minimize incontinence in patients with imperfect support.[15]

Table 3-1 Structures Potentially Involved in Continence

Intrinsic to Lower Urinary Tract
Detrusor loop of bladder base musculature
Trigonal ring
Circular smooth muscle of urethra
Striated urogenital sphincter (sphincter urethrae)
Urethral connective tissue
Urethral submucosal vascular plexus
Urethral mucosa
Extrinsic to Lower Urinary Tract
Connective tissue supports (endopelvic fasciae)
Muscular supports (levator ani muscles)
Striated urogenital sphincter (compressor urethrae and urethrovaginal sphincter)

Location of Structures Involved in Continence[13]

The spatial relations of the elements in the sphincteric mechanism are illustrated in Figure 3-9. The internal sphincteric mechanism lies in the region where the

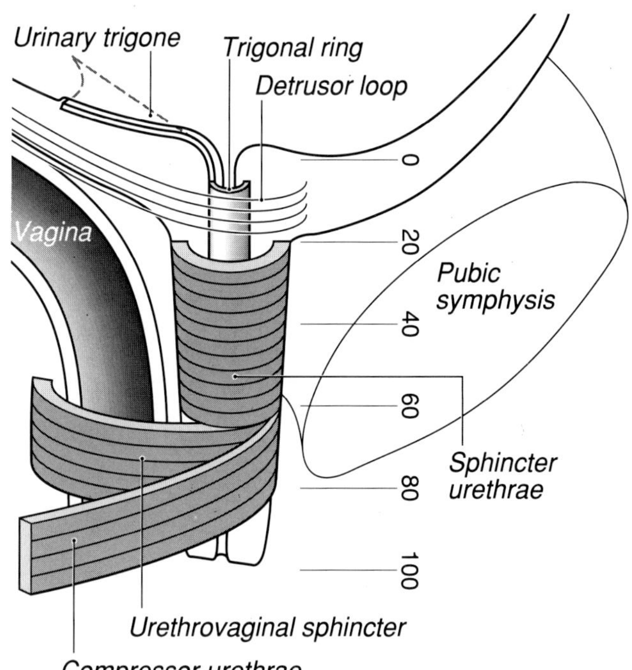

Figure 3-9 Diagrammatic representation showing component parts of internal and external sphincteric mechanisms and their locations. Sphincter urethrae, urethrovaginal sphincter, and compressor urethrae are all parts of striated urogenital sphincter muscle. *Source*: © 1989, University of Michigan.

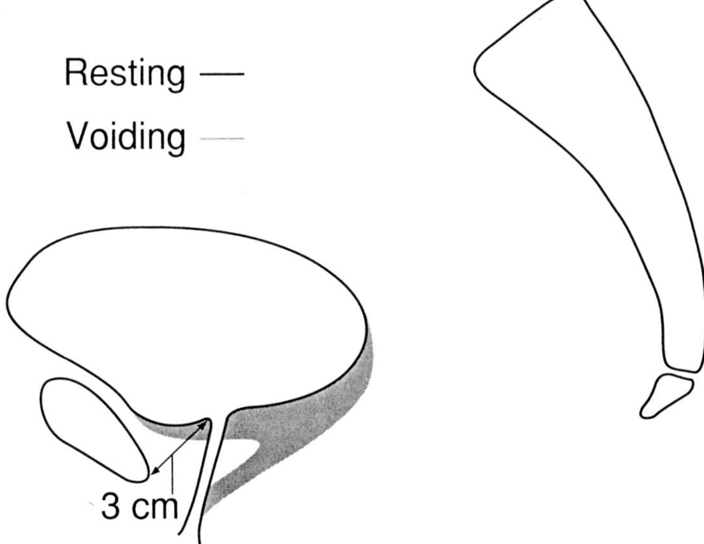

Figure 3-10 Topography and mobility of normal proximal aspect of urethra and vesical neck on basis of resting and voiding in normal women.[18,20] *Source*: © 1989, University of Michigan.

urethral lumen traverses the bladder wall. This region is often referred to as the *vesical neck*. It extends for approximately the first 20% of the urethral lumen. The distal sphincteric mechanism extends from 20% to 80% of the luminal length. Its bulkiest component is the striated urogenital sphincter.

The important structures that support the urethra and the vesical neck have their attachments to the paraurethral tissues in the area from approximately 20% to 60% of the urethral length, but they may influence the urethra and the vesical neck beyond this region.

Support of the Urethra[16]

Nature of Support

Poor support of the proximal segment of the urethra and the vesical neck is by far the most common cause of stress incontinence. Early clinical studies of this region were done with the use of static bead-chain cystourethrograms, and investigators described the relation between the urethra and the pubic bones on the basis of their results. It was initially believed that this support was provided by bands of connective tissue, called the pubourethral ligaments, which went from the urethra to the pubic bones.[17] It is now apparent that vesical neck support comes from the pubocervical fascia and its attachment to the fascial arch.[6] Careful dissection of this area fails to reveal a direct fibrous connection from the urethra to the pubis, which would be called the pubourethral ligament.

The importance of recognizing that the urethra is not firmly attached to the pubic bones by pubourethral ligaments is illustrated by the following examples:

- Normally, in a woman in the standing position the vesical neck lies above the attachment of pubourethral ligaments to the pubic bones.[18]
- The positions of the proximal segment of the urethra and the vesical neck are mobile and under voluntary control.[19]

Fluoroscopic studies of the bladder and the vesical neck show that contraction of the levator ani muscles can elevate the vesical neck[20] and that relaxation of these muscles at the time of urination may obliterate the posterior urethrovesical angle[20] (Figure 3-10). These findings indicate that the levator ani muscles play a role in controlling vesical neck support. Furthermore, the normal location of the vesical neck at a level 2 to 3 cm above the insertion of the pubourethral ligaments[18] can be explained by the origin and the insertion of the levator ani muscles. Clinically, the junction of this mobile upper portion of the urethra, which is influenced by these muscles, and the lower fixed portion of the urethra occurs at 56% of the urethral length and has been termed the *knee of the urethra*.[21] This is the region where the urethra enters the perineal membrane[22] and reflects the firm fixation of the urethra to the pubic bones by this structure.

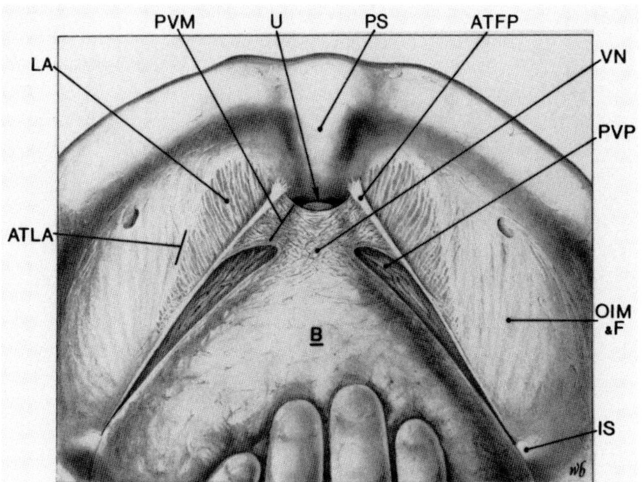

Figure 3-11 Retzius space (drawn from cadaver dissection). Pubovesical muscle (PVM) can be seen going from vesical neck (VN) to arcus tendineus fasciae pelvis (ATFP) and running over paraurethral vascular plexus (PVP). ATLA, Arcus tendineus levator ani; B, bladder; IS, ischial spine; LA, levator ani muscles; OIM&F, obturator internus muscle and fascia; PS, pubic symphysis; U, urethra. *Source*: Reprinted with permission from JOL DeLancey, Pubovesical ligament: a separate structure from the urethral supports (pubo-urethro ligaments), *Neurourology and Urodynamics* (1989;8:53–61), Copyright © 1989, Alan R Liss Inc.

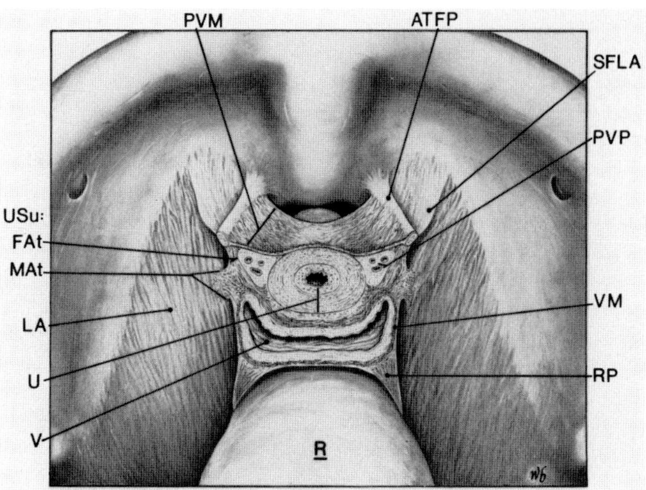

Figure 3-12 Cross-section of urethra (U), vagina (V), arcus tendineus fasciae pelvis (ATFP), and superior fascia of levator ani (SFLA) just below vesical neck (drawn from cadaver dissection). Pubovesical muscles (PVM) lie anterior to urethra and anterior and superior to paraurethral vascular plexus (PVP). Urethral supports (USu) (pubourethral ligaments) attach vagina and vaginal surface of urethra to levator ani muscles (LA) (MAt, muscular attachment) and to superior fascia of levator ani (FAt, fascial attachment). R, rectum; RP, rectal pillar; VM, vaginal wall muscularis. *Source*: Reprinted with permission from JOL DeLancey, Pubovesical ligament: a separate structure from the urethral supports (pubo-urethro ligaments), *Neurourology and Urodynamics* (1989;8:53–61), Copyright © 1989, Alan R Liss Inc.

Structure of the Supportive Mechanism

The previously described observations indicate that the support of the urethra involves both voluntary muscle and connective tissue. The anterior wall of the vagina and the urethra arise from the urogenital sinus and are intimately connected. The support of the urethra depends not on attachments of the urethra to adjacent structures but on the connection of the vagina and the endopelvic fascia to the muscles and the fasciae of the pelvic wall (Figure 3-11).

The tissues that provide urethral support have two lateral attachments: a fascial attachment and a muscular attachment (Figures 3-12 and 3-13). The fascial attachment connects the periurethral tissues and the anterior wall of the vagina to the arcus tendineus fasciae pelvis

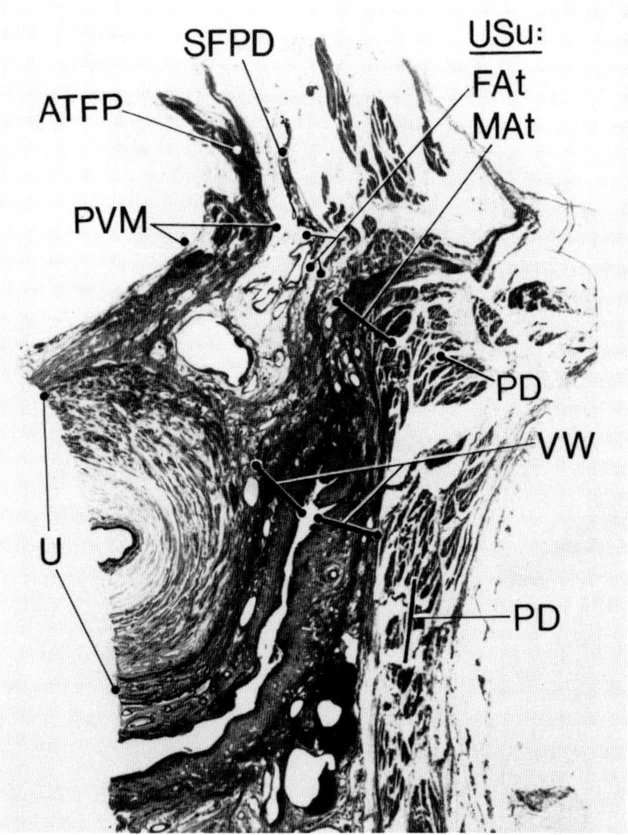

Figure 3-13 Cross-section of urethra (U), vaginal wall (VW), and pelvic diaphragm (PD) (levator ani muscles) from right half of pelvis taken just below vesical neck at approximately same level as shown in Figure 3-12. Pubovesical muscles (PVM) can be seen anterior to urethra and attach to arcus tendineus fasciae pelvis (ATFP). Urethral supports (USu) run underneath (dorsal to) urethra and vessels. Some of its fibers (MAt) attach to muscle of levator ani (LA), whereas others (FAt) are derived from vaginal wall (VW) and vaginal surface of urethra (U) and attach to superior fascia of levator ani (SFLA). *Source*: Reprinted with permission from Pubovesical ligament: a separate structure from the urethral supports (pubo-urethro ligaments), *Neurourology and Urodynamics* (1989;8:53–61), Copyright © 1989, Alan R Liss Inc.

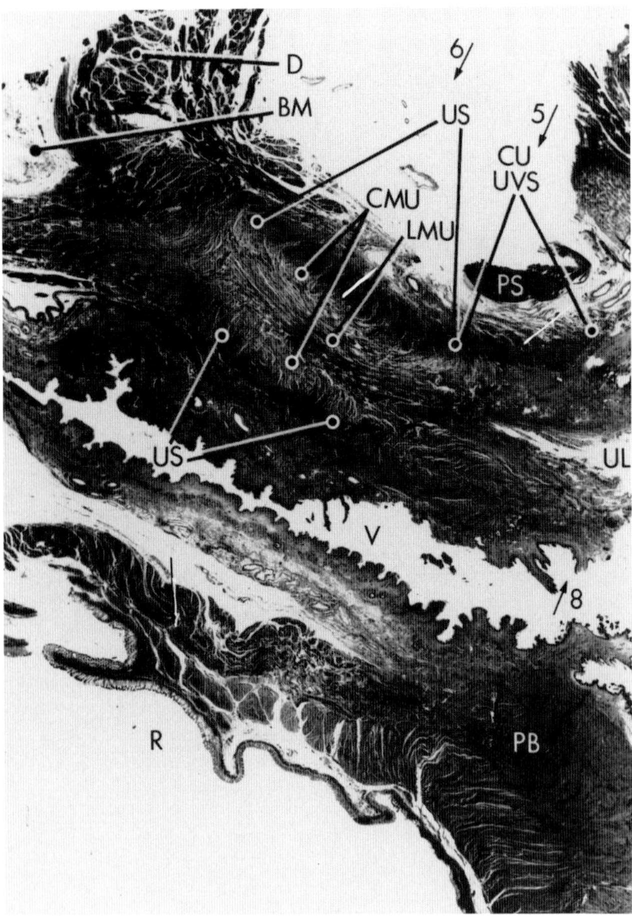

Figure 3-14 Sagittal section from 29-year-old cadaver. Section is cut just lateral to midline and not quite parallel to it. It contains tissue nearer midline in distal aspect of urethra, where lumen can be seen, than at vesical neck. BM, Bladder mucosa; CMU, circular smooth muscle of urethra; CU, compressor urethrae; D, detrusor muscle; LMU, longitudinal smooth muscles of urethra; PB, perineal body; PS, pubic symphysis; R, rectum; TR, trigonal ring; UL, urethral lumen; US, urethral sphincter; UVS, urethrovaginal sphincter; V, vagina. *Source*: Reprinted with permission from *Obstetrics and Gynecology* (1986;68:91), Copyright © 1986, American College of Obstetricians and Gynecologists.

and are called the *paravaginal fascial attachments*.[6] The muscular attachment connects these same periurethral tissues to the medial border of the levator ani muscle.[9,23] These attachments allow the normal resting tone of the levator ani muscle,[11] along with the fascial attachments, to maintain the position of the vesical neck. When the muscle relaxes at the onset of micturition, the vesical neck is able to rotate downward to the limit of the elasticity of the fascial attachments, and contraction at the end of urination allows it to resume its normal position.

The relation between urethral support and sphincteric function is a complex one. Miniaturized pressure transducers have permitted investigators to record the rapid sequence of events that occur during a cough, and the study findings reveal a significant increase in intraurethral pressure during a cough.[24] These urethral pressure changes have been ascribed to the "transmission" of abdominal pressure to the "intra-abdominal" portion of the urethra. Anatomically, it is not clear what separates the abdominal from the extra-abdominal urethra. There is no single structure that the urethra pierces to exit the abdomen (Figure 3-14), and the entire length of the urethra is separated from the lumen of the vagina only by the vaginal wall and the endopelvic fascia. Rather than the urethra piercing a single specific layer between the pelvic and the extra-pelvic cavities, it is incorporated into the pelvic floor. The series of events that occur during a cough suggests that several pelvic floor structures are involved in maintaining continence. If passive pressure transmission were the only factor involved in continence, pressures during a cough would be maximum in the proximal segment of the urethra. Measurements taken in patients, however, reveal that the distal portion of the urethra has the highest pressure elevations.[25,26] This occurs from 60% to 80% of the urethral length in the region where the compressor urethra and urethrovaginal sphincter are found, suggesting that these muscles augment urethral pressure in this region.

The pressures seen in the urethra during a cough frequently exceed the increase that occurs in intravesical pressure in normal women, revealing a contribution of factors other than the influence of abdominal pressure. In addition, these pressure rises precede the rise in abdominal pressure,[25] an observation that suggests contraction of the pelvic floor muscles in preparation for the cough. This indicates that abdominal pressure is not the only factor important in increasing urethral pressure during a cough. The fact that some patients persist in having stress incontinence despite adequate suspension of the urethra further indicates the need to expand the concept of the urethra's response during a cough. Recent study results have demonstrated the importance of denervation of the pelvic floor to the problem of stress urinary incontinence and genital prolapse.[3,27] This new area of investigation may prove helpful in further understanding the relation of structure and function in the mechanism of urinary continence.

Sphincteric Structures[28]

Internal Sphincter Mechanism

Kelly[29] observed an open vesical neck in patients with stress incontinence in his original description of this condition. McGuire[30] documented the clinical importance of this phenomenon and differentiated this condition from other types of stress incontinence caused by poor support. He termed it type III stress incontinence. In persons with type III stress incontinence the proximal centimeter of the urethral lumen has poor intrinsic closure. This can occur as a result of defective innervation to the region or surgical trauma.

Two tissues surround the proximal centimeter of the urethra: the detrusor loop and the trigonal ring. The former is a defined band of detrusor muscle that forms a U-shaped loop open posteriorly that runs anterior to the vesical neck. A separate innervation of the base of the bladder may allow this region to function in a different way than the muscle of the dome[31] and may be isolated to a structure known as the trigonal ring.[32] Woodburne[33] has further reported a high concentration of elastin here, which may contribute to closure. Finally, as discussed previously, mechanical factors may favor compression of the vesical neck here.

External Sphincter

Urethral support and the proximal sphincter both act to prevent urine from entering the proximal segment of the urethra. In healthy women, this is the level of continence, but this may not be true for all women. In fact, 50% of women proved to be continent have urine enter the urethra during a cough.[14] In these persons, the function of the distal segment of the urethra would be the difference between continence and incontinence. The importance of this mechanism is illustrated by the occurrence of stress incontinence in patients in whom the distal segment of the urethra is excised during radical vulvectomy. Incontinence develops in these patients even though they have no change in urethral support or resting sphincteric function.[15] As previously mentioned, the external sphincter is not capable of maintaining continence on its own, contrary to the situation in men. It is an auxiliary mechanism of continence.

Misconceptions about the role of the extrinsic continence mechanism in continence have come from its inaccurate descriptions in the older anatomic literature. This is a difficult area to dissect, and microscopic examination of the urethra in situ has been hampered by difficulties in sectioning the pubic bones. Most investigators have removed the urethra to study it microscopically and have missed the extensions of its striated muscle outside its walls. Recent descriptions by Oelrich,[12] however, have corrected much of this confusion and correlate well with functional observations.

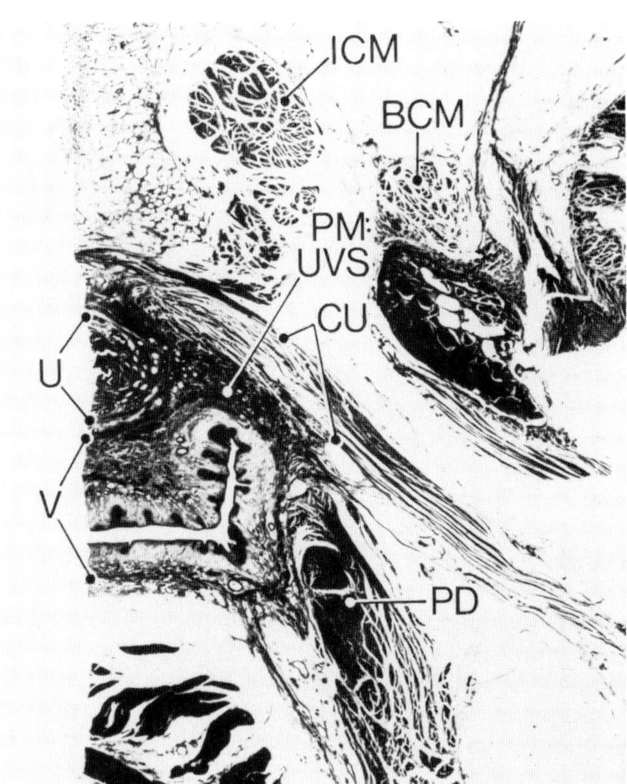

Figure 3-15 Cross-section taken just above level of perineal membrane (PM) showing compressor urethrae (CU) and urethrovaginal sphincter (UVS) portions of striated urogenital sphincter. BCM, Bulbocavernosus muscle; ICM, ischiocavernosus muscle; PD, pelvic diaphragm (levator ani); U, urethra; V, vagina. *Source*: Reprinted with permission from *Obstetrics and Gynecology* (1988;72:296–301), Copyright © 1988, American College of Obstetricians and Gynecologists.

Closure of the urethra comes from a number of different tissue elements. Smooth muscle, striated muscle, and vascular elements each contribute between one quarter and one third of the urethra's closing pressure at rest, as determined by blocking the activity of each of these elements.[34] The outer layer of the urethra is formed by the muscle of the striated urogenital sphincter, which is located from about 20% to 80% of the urethral luminal length,[22] and has previously been called the *rhabdosphincter*. In its upper two thirds the sphincter fibers lie in a circular orientation, whereas distally they leave the confines of the urethra and insert either into the vaginal wall, as the urethrovaginal sphincter, or into the region just above the perineal membrane, as the compressor urethrae[12] (Figure 3-15). (See also Figure 3-9.) This muscle is composed largely of slow-twitch muscle fibers[35] that are well suited to maintaining the constant tone this muscle exhibits. In addition, it allows for voluntary increases in activity as a backup continence mechanism during times when the need for increased closure pressure arises. In the distal segment of the urethra, this striated muscle compresses the urethra from above, whereas proximally it constricts the lumen. It is also possible that the striated urogenital sphincter muscle plays a role in stress continence beyond its resting and conscious voluntary contraction. As previously mentioned, measurements of urethral pressure during a cough have shown that the rise in pressure is highest in the distal area of the urethra, around 60% of the urethral length,[27] in the region where the considerable bulk of muscle of the compressor urethrae and urethrovaginal sphincter are found.[22]

The smooth muscle of the urethra has an inner longitudinal layer and a thin outer circular layer. The former is by far the more prominent of the two. The urethral smooth muscle lies inside the striated urogenital sphincter muscle and is present throughout the upper four fifths of the urethra. The configuration of the circular muscle suggests a role in constricting the lumen. This layer, however, is thin and much less prominent than the striated urogenital sphincter muscle. The longitudinal smooth muscle contracts during micturition, assisting in funneling the urethra and shortening it.

In addition to the contractile and vascular tissue of the urethra, a considerable amount of connective tissue is interspersed within the muscle and the submucosa. This tissue has both collagenous and elastin fibers. It is difficult, however, to study the function of these tissues specifically, because there is no specific way to block their action pharmacologically or surgically. Table 3-2 lists the hypotheses concerning the function of elements of the urinary continence mechanism and summarizes many of the preceding points.

Table 3-2 Hypotheses Concerning the Function of Elements of the Urinary Continence Mechanism

Structure	*Hypothetical Function*
Levator ani muscles (through muscular attachment of urethral supports)	Tonic contraction helps maintain high position of vesical neck, and these muscles may contract during cough to support vesical neck. They relax to change position of vesical neck relative to pubovesical muscles to facilitate micturition.
Connection to arcus tendineus (through fascial attachment of urethral supports)	It assists levator ani muscles in support and limits downward excursion of vesical neck when these muscles are relaxed, or overcome, during cough.
Pubovesical muscles and ligaments	They may facilitate vesical neck opening by pulling on vesical neck when levator ani muscles relax and may contribute to closure when they are contracted.
Internal sphincteric mechanism	It maintains vesical neck closure at rest and is necessary, in addition to normal support, for continence during cough.
External sphincteric mechanism	Resting tone contributes to resting urethral pressure, and contraction prevents incontinence when marginally compensated proximal mechanism leaks.

CONCLUSION

In the past, descriptions of the pelvic floor support and urinary continence have attempted to isolate the one factor that provides pelvic support or urinary continence. These have never provided satisfactory explanations for the diversity of defects that are seen in patients with prolapse,[36] as well as for the objective observations of pelvic floor damage after childbirth.

Each portion of the support and continence mechanism has a characteristic structure that has evolved in response to a structural need. Understanding the mechanism of pelvic support is similar to understanding the way in which any mechanical device works. To understand how a watch works one must understand not only the dynamics of the spring and flywheel but also how the escape and gear mechanisms work. It is no more correct to say that the ligamentous supports of the urethra are responsible for urinary continence than it is to say that the watch spring is what makes a watch work. Without the pelvic floor musculature the ligaments would ultimately fail, and without the gears and escape mechanism the watch could not keep its orderly mechanism functioning.

As investigators begin to study the role that each of these elements plays in normal support and continence, a better understanding of the mechanism of prolapse will begin to emerge. This is a new and challenging era of surgical gynecology and one that should greatly improve the functional results of operative procedures. Furthering the understanding of pelvic floor function will improve treatments, and, thereby, patients will be better served.

REFERENCES

1. Emmet JD. *Am Gynecol Obstet J*. 1899;15:155.

2. Ricci JV. *The Cystocele in America*. Philadelphia, Pa: Blakiston Co; 1950:xi.

3. Smith ARB, Hosker GL, Warrell DW. The role of partial denervation of the pelvic floor in the etiology of genitourinary prolapse and stress incontinence of urine: a neurophysiological study. *Br J Obstet Gynaecol*. 1989;96:24–28.

4. Range RL, Woodburne RT. The gross and microscopic anatomy of the transverse cervical ligaments. *Am J Obstet Gynecol*. 1964; 90:460–467.

5. Campbell RM. The anatomy and histology of the sacrouterine ligaments. *Am J Obstet Gynecol.* 1950;59:1–12.

6. Richardson AC, Edmonds PB, Williams NL. Treatment of stress urinary incontinence due to paravaginal fascial defect. *Obstet Gynecol.* 1981;57:357–362.

7. Nichols DH, Milley PS. Surgical significance of the rectovaginal septum. *Am J Obstet Gynecol.* 1970;108:215–220.

8. Lawson JON. Pelvic anatomy: pelvic floor muscles. *Ann R Coll Surg Engl.* 1984;54:244–252.

9. DeLancey JOL, Starr RA. The histology of the connection between the vagina and levator ani muscles. *J Reprod Med.* 1990; 35:765–771.

10. Nichols DH, Milley PS, Randall CL. Significance of restoration of normal vaginal depth and axis. *Obstet Gynecol.* 1970; 36:251–256.

11. Parks AG, Porter NH, Melzak J. Experimental study of the reflex mechanism controlling muscles of the pelvic floor. *Dis Colon Rectum.* 1962;5:407–414.

12. Oelrich TM. The striated urogenital sphincter muscle in the female. *Anat Rec.* 1983;205:223–232.

13. DeLancey JOL. Anatomy of the urethral sphincters and supports. In: *Micturition: Proceedings of the Royal College of Obstetricians and Gynaecologists Study Group.* Drife JO, Hilton P, Stanton SL, eds. London: Springer-Verlag; 1990.

14. Versi E, Cardozo LD, Studd JWW, Brincat M, O'Dowd TM, Cooper DJ. Internal urinary sphincter in maintenance of female continence. *Br Med J.* 1986;292:166–167.

15. Reid GC, DeLancey JOL, Hopkins MP, Roberts JA, Morley GW. Urinary incontinence following radical vulvectomy. *Obstet Gynecol.* 1990;75:852–858.

16. DeLancey JOL. Anatomy and embryology of the lower urinary tract. *Obstet Gynecol Clin N A.* 1989;16:717–732.

17. Zaccharin RF. The anatomic supports of the female urethra. *Obstet Gynecol.* 1968;21:754–759.

18. Noll LE, Hutch JA. The SCIPP line—an aid in interpreting the voiding lateral cystourethrogram. *Obstet Gynecol.* 1969;33: 680–689.

19. Muellner SR. Physiology of micturition. *J Urol.* 1951; 65:805–810.

20. Jeffcoate TNA, Roberts H. Observations on stress incontinence of urine. *Am J Obstet Gynecol.* 1952;64:721–738.

21. Westby M, Asmussen M, Ulmsten U. Location of maximum intraurethral pressure related to urogenital diaphragm in the female subject as studied by simultaneous urethrocystometry and voiding urethrocystography. *Am J Obstet Gynecol.* 1982;144:408–412.

22. DeLancey JOL. Correlative study of paraurethral anatomy. *Obstet Gynecol.* 1986;68:91–97.

23. DeLancey JOL. Structural aspects of the extrinsic continence mechanism. *Obstet Gynecol.* 1988;72:296–301.

24. Enhörning G. Simultaneous recording of the intravesical and intra-urethral pressures. *Acta Obstet Gynecol Scand (Suppl).* 1961; 276:1–68.

25. Constantinou CE. Resting and stress urethral pressures as a clinical guide to the mechanism of continence in the female patient. *Urol Clin North Am.* 1985;12:247–258.

26. Hilton P, Stanton SL. Urethral pressure measurement by microtransducer: the results in symptom-free women and in those with genuine stress incontinence. *Br J Obstet Gynaecol.* 1983; 90:919–933.

27. Snooks SJ, Badenoch DF, Tiptaft RC, et al. Perineal nerve damage in genuine stress urinary incontinence: an electrophysiological study. *Br J Urol.* 1985;57:422–426.

28. DeLancey JOL. Functional anatomy of the female lower urinary tract and pelvic floor. In: *Neurobiology of Continence.* Sussex, England: John Wiley & Sons, Inc; 1990:57–68.

29. Kelly HA. Incontinence of urine in women. *Urol Cutan Rev.* 1913;1:291–293.

30. McGuire EJ. Urodynamic findings in patients after failure of stress incontinence operations. *Prog Clin Biol Res.* 1981;78: 351–360.

31. Elbadawi A. Neuromuscular mechanisms of micturition. In: Yalla SV, McGuire EJ, Elbadawi A, Blaivas JG, eds. *Neurourology and Urodynamics.* New York: Macmillan, Inc; 1988:3–35.

32. Huisman AB. Aspects on the anatomy of the female urethra with special relation to urinary continence. *Contrib Gynecol Obstet.* 1983;10:1–31.

33. Woodburne RT. Anatomy of the bladder and bladder outlet. *J Urol.* 1968;100:474–487.

34. Rud T, Anderson KE, Asmussen M, Hunting A, Ulmsten U. Factors maintaining the intraurethral pressure in women. *Invest Urol.* 1980;17:343–347.

35. Gosling JA, Dixon JS, Critchley HOD, Thompson SA. A comparative study of the human external sphincter and periurethral levator ani muscles. *Br J Urol.* 1981;53:35–41.

36. Richardson AC, Lyons JB, Williams NL. A new look at pelvic relaxation. *Am J Obstet Gynecol.* 1976;126:568–573.

4

Evaluation of Urinary Incontinence

Alfred E. Bent

In women, *urinary incontinence* is the demonstrable involuntary loss of urine that is (1) socially or hygienically unacceptable to the patient or (2) detrimental to her physical well-being. The differential diagnoses are shown in Table 4-1. The most frequent causes of incontinence are genuine stress incontinence (GSI), detrusor instability (DI), and mixed incontinence (combined GSI and DI). Other entities compose only 5% to 10% of the total causes.

NEED FOR EVALUATION

Urinary symptoms and pelvic examination do not accurately define the causes of incontinence.[1] In one study, case histories of 494 women referred with the symptom of stress incontinence were reviewed.[2] Symptoms of DI were present in 417 of these patients. Stress loss of urine was observed in only 168 patients, but it was not a reliable guide to the final diagnosis of GSI. Urodynamic studies were required in 488 patients to obtain an accurate diagnosis.

In another study,[3] the symptoms and urodynamic diagnoses in 218 women were compared. In detecting GSI the symptom of stress incontinence had 100% sensitivity but only 65.2% specificity. Urgency and urge incontinence had 77.9% sensitivity and 38.7% specificity in detecting DI. Patients thought to have isolated stress incontinence had DI 34.9% of the time. Three percent of patients complaining of urinary incontinence had no objective evidence of incontinence on urodynamic investigation.

The diagnosis of GSI must be precisely made before surgical intervention. Although DI is not an absolute contraindication to surgery for GSI, its presence needs to be documented to assess the contribution of each condition to the incontinence problem. The presence of DI usually merits a trial of nonsurgical therapy. If surgery is performed, the patient needs to be aware that the DI component may or may not be cured and that incontinence related to DI can persist after GSI is corrected. In most of these situations the DI will persist in a form similar to that observed before surgery, and a few cases

Table 4-1 Causes of Urinary Incontinence

Genuine Stress Incontinence (GSI)
Detrusor Instability (DI)
Mixed Incontinence (Combined GSI and DI)
Overflow Incontinence
Bypass of Continence Mechanism
- Fistula
- Urethral diverticulum
- Congenital anomaly

Functional Disorders

will worsen. Of equal importance is the de novo development of DI in 5% to 18% of patients after surgery for isolated GSI.[4,5] Medical management may be indicated as primary therapy for combined GSI and DI.

TESTS AND EVALUATIVE PROCEDURES

1. History and Physical Examination

The medical history is facilitated by having the patient complete a questionnaire detailing current complaints, past medical and surgical history, medications, allergies, social history, and functional inquiry. The current urinary problem is reviewed, including duration of problem, aggravating or relieving factors, severity, and current and past treatments. Specific questions help in screening the patient for the kind of incontinence she experiences and may help formulate a complete evaluation so no pertinent tests are omitted (Table 4-2).

Physical examination must include an assessment of the nerve supply to the urethra and the bladder, that is, the sympathetic (T-11 to L-2), parasympathetic (S-2 to S-4), and pudendal (S-2 to S-4) nerves. Asymmetry of findings is most important. Major neurologic involvement can be partly screened by reviewing the history, observing the patient's gait and movement, and listening as the patient talks. The legs are evaluated for sensation, tendon reflexes, and strength. The bulbocavernosus reflex, elicited by stroking lateral to the labia minora, and the clitoral reflex, elicited by applying pressure to (tapping) the clitoris, both cause contraction of the anal sphincter. Assessment of anal sphincter tone during the rectal examination completes the local neurologic evaluation.

The vulva is assessed for irritation related to urinary leakage, or from protective pads, and the vagina is observed for estrogen effect. The gynecologic examination includes a demonstration of pelvic relaxation with the use of a Sims speculum or the posterior half of a Graves speculum. While the posterior wall of the vagina is depressed by the speculum, the anterior vaginal wall is observed during forceful straining and coughing. Urinary leakage may be observed. The urethra and the anterior wall of the vagina are palpated to detect a bulge from a urethral diverticulum, as well as tenderness along the urethra, and to assess mobility (lack of scarring or fixation). The anterior wall of the vagina is supported by the speculum while the posterior wall and the vaginal vault are observed. A rectal examination helps delineate rectocele and enterocele. The patient is examined in the standing position for complete evaluation of pelvic floor support defects. Rectal tone and strength of voluntary contractions of the pelvic floor musculature (Kegel exercises) are also assessed.

Table 4-2 Questions To Ask Patients with Urinary Incontinence

Do you lose urine by spurts during coughing, sneezing, or lifting?
Do you ever have a very strong urge to void, so that if you do not reach the bathroom in time, you will leak?
Have you actually leaked urine because you could not reach the bathroom in time?
How many times a day do you urinate?
How many times do you get up from sleep to urinate?
Have you wet the bed in the past year?
When you are passing urine, can you stop the flow?
Do you wear protection (pads) to protect your clothing from the loss of urine?
How severe a problem do you consider your urinary leakage to be?
Do you leak urine with intercourse?

2. Voiding Diary

The patient should bring a 24-hour voiding diary (urolog summary) to the office. The appropriate forms (Figure 4-1) can be mailed to her ahead of time. The record serves as a clinical cystometrogram and summarizes voiding times and amounts, leak episodes, and fluid intake. Normally a person voids seven or eight times per day and does not get up to void, or voids only once at night; total urinary volume is 1000 to 3000 mL per day. Frequent voiding and leak episodes may be associated with DI, and DI must be differentiated from GSI.

3. Urine Culture

A urine culture is obtained before or during the initial visit, because many lower urinary tract symptoms are caused or aggravated by urinary infection. Urinary tract infection must be treated prior to urodynamic testing.

4. Uroflowmetry

Uroflowmetry is a timed measure of voided urine volume. Normally, at least 200 mL of urine is voided in 20 seconds, and the residual urine is less than 100 mL. The major problems discovered with this test are prolonged voiding, intermittent voiding, and high residual urine. Conditions characterized by voiding dysfunction include detrusor sphincter dyssynergia, which may be a result of multiple sclerosis. Abnormal residual urine may

The voiding diary (urolog) is a record of your voiding (urinating) and leakage (incontinence) of urine. Please complete the record according to the following instructions before you visit our office. Choose a *24-hour* period to keep this record when you can conveniently measure every voiding, and begin your record with the first voiding on arising, as shown in the example below.

EXAMPLE:

Time[1]	*Voided*[2]	*Activity*[3]	*Leak Volume*[4]	*Urge*[5]	*Intake (Amount/Type)*[6]
6:45 AM	550 mL	Awakening			
7:00		Turned on water	2 oz	Yes	2 cups coffee 6 oz orange juice

EXPLANATORY NOTES:

[1]Record time of all voidings, leakage, and intake of liquids.
[2]Measure output in *milliliters* (mL) or *ounces* (oz).
[3]Describe activity you were performing at time of leakage. If you were not actively doing anything, record whether you were sitting, standing, or lying down.
[4]Estimate amount of leakage according to the following scale:
1 = damp; few drops only
2 = wet underwear or pad
3 = soaked or emptied bladder
[5]Write Yes if urge to urinate accompanied (or preceded) urine leakage. Write No if you felt no urge when leakage occurred.
[6]Record amount and type of *all liquid* intake by using either milliliters (mL) or ounces (oz) (1 cup = 8 oz = 240 mL).

Time	*Voided*	*Activity*	*Leak Volume*	*Urge*	*Intake (Amount/Type)*

Figure 4-1 Voiding diary (urolog). Patient instructions and take-home record of voiding and fluid intake. *Source*: Adapted from *Danforth's Obstetrics and Gynecology*, ed 6 (p 912) by JR Scott et al (eds) with permission of JB Lippincott, © 1982.

be associated with overflow incontinence. This may be caused by bladder hypotonia related to diabetes mellitus, hypothyroidism, or recurrent overdistention. Electronic uroflow equipment is relatively expensive, and adequate information may be obtained by using a stopwatch to measure voiding time and manually measuring the voided volume. The postvoid residual urine is measured by catheterizing the patient's bladder using sterile technique.

5. Visualization of Urine Loss with Stress (Sign of Stress Incontinence)

The stress test is performed with a full bladder (confirmed by a subjective feeling of fullness by the patient or accomplished by instilling 300 to 350 mL of fluid into the bladder). The patient is asked to cough and strain vigorously, first in the lithotomy position and then in the standing position if necessary. The examiner observes for fluid loss from the urethra. The Bonney stress test, or any of its modifications that elevate the urethrovesical junction (UVJ) to predict the results of surgery, is not performed, because invariably direct pressure is placed on the urethra and the UVJ, causing occlusion.[6]

Although patients may complain of intolerable urine loss with stress or coughing during their normal or stressful activities, stress loss may not be demonstrated in the office setting in 5% to 10% of cases. A 20-minute or 1-hour pad test may be performed in the office setting to demonstrate urine loss, although the exact cause of the loss (GSI or DI) cannot be determined for certain. The patient is given a 500 mL oral fluid load to promote diuresis, or the bladder is filled retrograde to subjective fullness. A preweighed sanitary pad is worn and the patient performs a series of exercises (Table 4-3) with a full bladder. Fluid loss in excess of 2 g is considered significant, because it exceeds the amount of fluid which may be lost through perspiration or secretion. Small amounts of fluid loss are thought to occur as a result of GSI, whereas large amounts are assumed to be related to DI.[7]

A 12- or 24-hour pad test may be performed to help demonstrate or quantitate urine loss.[8] Phenazopyridine hydrochloride (Pyridium) tablets may be administered orally to the patient to aid in visualizing very small amounts of urine loss. The patient is given 12 sanitary napkins (preweighed and numbered), each sealed in an interlocking storage bag (Ziploc bag). Each pad is worn for 2 hours during waking hours, unless wetness necessitates that it be changed earlier. Pads are changed at night only if needed. With each change, the used pad is replaced in the appropriately numbered storage bag, and the bag is sealed and stored in the refrigerator. The pads are returned to the physician for weighing the next day. It is important for the patient to keep a voiding diary (urolog) (see Figure 4-1) in conjunction with the pad test, as well as a record of her activities before each pad change. Patients with a mild degree of GSI may have a few damp pads, whereas those with DI usually have at least one or two soaked pads.

Table 4-3 Exercises for 20-Minute or 1-Hour Pad Test

Walk briskly for 3 minutes.
Sit and then stand 10 times.
Walk up and down stairs for 1 minute.
Pick up objects on the floor five times.
Cough 12 times.
Run in place for 1 minute.

6. Tests for Detrusor Instability

The simplest test to evaluate DI is performed after a postvoid residual urine determination. A large syringe (60 mL) is attached to the same straight red rubber catheter used in determining the residual urine. The bladder is gradually filled with fluid with the syringe and the catheter supported upright. The bladder capacity (normal, 350 to 550 mL) is determined. An abnormal rise in bladder pressure is visualized by fluid flowing back up the catheter and the syringe. This has been called *eyeball urodynamics*.

A *cystometrogram* (CMG) is an observation and/or recording of the volume:pressure relation during bladder filling, and is used to rule out DI. The simplest CMG is the screening CMG described earlier with the use of a catheter and attached syringe. A slightly more sophisticated method consists of a Foley catheter, a three-way stopcock, surgical tubing (taped alongside a meter stick on an intravenous pole), and an infusion source (Figure 4-2). The patient stands, and the zero mark on the meter stick is placed opposite the upper border of her symphysis pubis. The stopcock is turned, so that the flow from the patient's bladder is directed to the vertical column. The fluid column should rest at 10 to 15 centimeters of water (cm H_2O). The bladder is filled in increments of 50 to 100 mL. After each increment, the height of the fluid column is compared to that in its starting position. The patient reports first sensation of bladder filling, fullness, and maximum bladder capacity when no further filling can be tolerated (Table 4-4). The pressure should not rise higher than 15 cm H_2O during

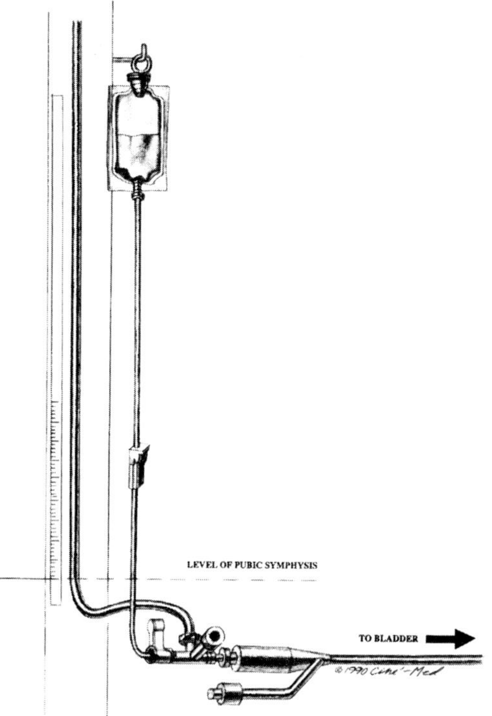

Figure 4-2 Simple cystometrogram technique used in office setting. Foley catheter is in place, and zero mark of meter stick is aligned with upper border of patient's symphysis pubis. *Source*: The American College of Obstetricians and Gynecologists. *Urogynecologic Evaluation, Endoscopy, and Urodynamic Testing in the Symptomatic Female* by Alfred E Bent. ACOG Audiovisual Library, Washington DC, © 1990.

Table 4-4 Normal Values for Cystometry

	Fluid (mL)	*Carbon Dioxide (mL)*
First Sensation of Bladder Filling	50 to 100	50
Fullness	250 to 400	100 to 200
Maximum Bladder Capacity	350 to 550	200 to 300

bladder filling. There should be no involuntary contractions. These are observed as the fluid stops flowing into the bladder or when the fluid rise is greater than 15 cm above the baseline value.

In another CMG technique a Foley catheter is attached to an infusion source and a pressure transducer, which is connected to a single-channel chart recorder (eg, fetal monitor). A continuous hard copy of pressure measurements is generated during bladder filling, and the volume of fluid infused can be marked on the paper chart (Figure 4-3). Carbon dioxide can also be used as a filling medium, and it can be delivered either with the urethroscope during endoscopy or through connecting tubing leading to the bladder. (See Table 4-4 for the normal CMG values with carbon dioxide as a filling medium.) The single-channel CMG has been criticized because intra-abdominal pressure is not measured simultaneously, and increased bladder pressure may be due to abdominal straining. Measures, such as palpating the

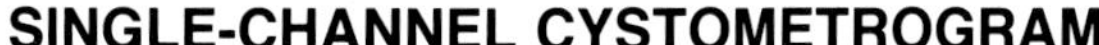

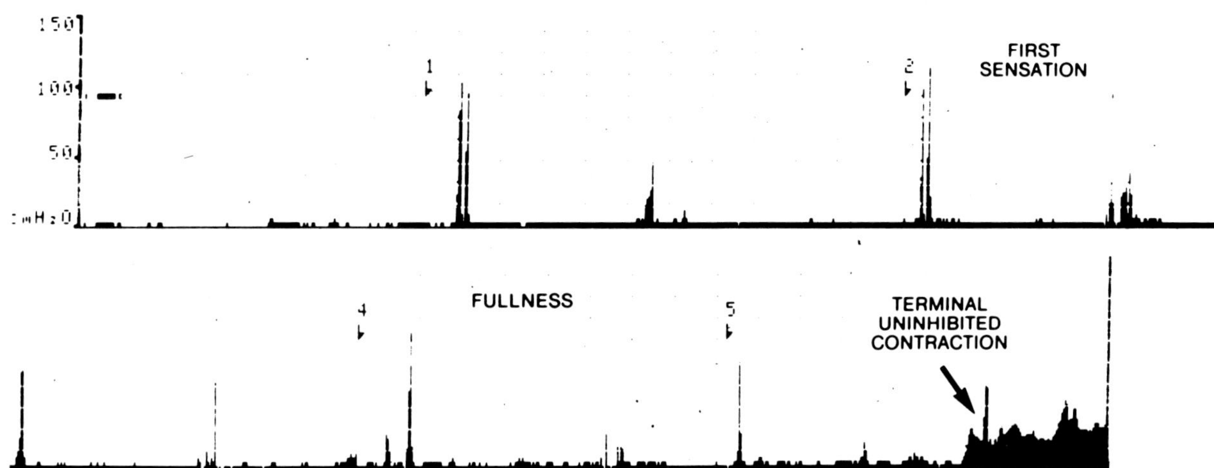

Figure 4-4 Detrusor instability. Patient thought her surgery for genuine stress incontinence was a failure. Cystometrogram (CMG) shows detrusor contraction (*) after cough (↓). Pressure increase in detrusor pressure recording (*top graph*) is accompanied by corresponding drop in urethral pressure (*bottom graph*). During cough (Cough UCPP; *bottom graph*), there is no pressure equalization, indicating success of operation for stress incontinence. UCPP, Urethral closure pressure profile; RPU, retro pubic urethropexy.

patient's abdomen and asking her to inhale during pressure rises, should help exclude increased intra-abdominal pressure. In a study of elderly patients[9] simple cystometry demonstrated good correlation with multichannel methods, with a sensitivity of 75% and a specificity of 79%.

The most accurate method for performing a CMG includes measurements of three pressures: intra-abdominal (vaginal or rectal), urethral, and bladder pressure. The true detrusor pressure is calculated by subtracting intra-abdominal pressure from bladder pressure. The test is best performed with the patient in the standing position with provocative maneuvers, such as having the patient cough, listen to running water, and perform heel bounces. Simultaneously measured intraurethral pressure should decline when detrusor contractions occur. If a detrusor contraction is perceived, the patient is asked to inhibit the contraction. The true detrusor pressure reading is very sensitive, and small changes in pressure can be determined. Detrusor instability is diagnosed if true detrusor pressure rises occur during filling or provocative maneuvers that the patient cannot suppress (Figure 4-4). The contractions are pressure rises of 15 cm H_2O or greater, or less than 15 cm H_2O in the presence of urgency symptoms, urethral pressure decline, or fluid loss from the bladder. The indications for a CMG are shown in Table 4-5.

All the previously described testing methods may fail to detect DI in approximately 10% of patients. One option is to have the patient return at a later date, especially when symptoms have been occurring regularly. Her medications should be reviewed for possible

Table 4-5 Indications for Cystometrogram

Irritative Voiding Symptoms
Urgency
Frequency
Nocturia
Urge Incontinence
Evaluation before Any Surgery for Genuine Stress Incontinence
Sudden, Unexplained Incontinent Episodes
Small Capacity Bladder
Recurrent Incontinence after Surgery
Incontinence after Age 50 Years

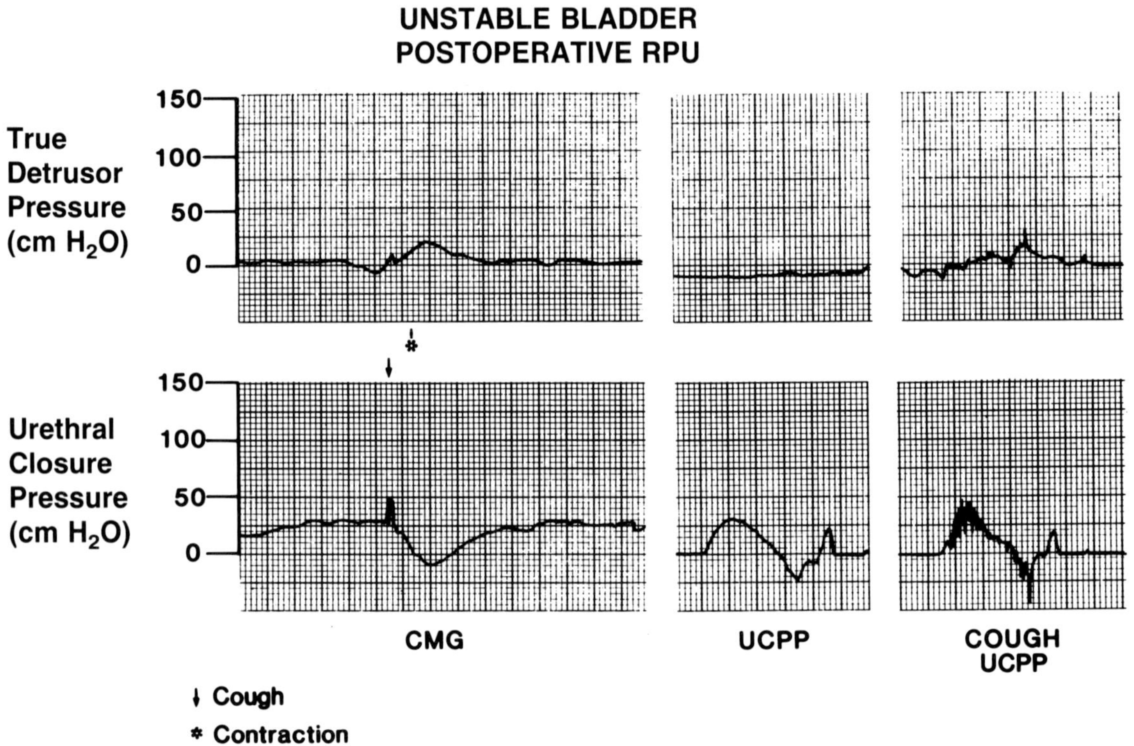

Figure 4-4 Detrusor instability. Patient thought her surgery for genuine stress incontinence was a failure. Cystometrogram (CMG) shows detrusor contraction (*) after cough (↓). Pressure increase in detrusor pressure recording (*top graph*) is accompanied by corresponding drop in urethral pressure (*bottom graph*). During cough (Cough UCPP; *botton graph*), there is no pressure equalization, indicating success of operation for stress incontinence. UCPP, Urethral closure pressure profile; RPU, retro pubic urethropexy.

bladder relaxant effects. Another option is to perform ambulatory urodynamic monitoring. A small (4F) catheter is placed in the bladder to measure intravesical and intraurethral pressures. A second catheter of similar size is placed in the vagina to measure intra-abdominal pressure. The catheters are taped securely in place and attached to pressure trandsducers leading to a portable recorder. The signals are monitored continuously (usually for 6 hours) while the patient performs her usual activities. The catheters are removed, and the information is transferred to a computer for analysis. This method allows a much higher recovery rate for diagnosing DI than even dual-channel cystometry in the urodynamic laboratory.[10]

7. Demonstration of Anatomic Defect

If GSI has been diagnosed and surgery is being contemplated, the UVJ mobility or anatomy must be assessed. The simplest test consists of placing a lubricated cotton-tipped applicator (Q-tip) through the urethra and pulling it back against the UVJ. The angle of the applicator at rest is measured by comparing the end of the applicator with the horizontal plane (Figure 4-5). The patient strains and coughs vigorously, and the applicator end deflects upward according to the severity of the anatomic defect. A positive finding is a straining angle greater than 30 degrees from the horizontal plane. This indicates that an anatomic defect exists, and the defect should be surgically correctable. The test findings cannot be used to diagnose GSI.[11]

The UVJ anatomy and mobility also can be assessed endoscopically during urethroscopy. While the operator views the UVJ in a partially open state, the patient is asked to perform the following maneuvers: "hold your urine," "squeeze your rectum," "strain down," and "cough." The UVJ normally should close during these activities. In a patient with GSI, however, the UVJ opens with straining and coughing. Because the interpretation of the maneuvers is so affected by movement of the urethroscope, an exact diagnosis is virtually impossible. By visualizing movement of the UVJ with the various commands, however, one can determine that the patient is unlikely to have a scarred, fibrotic urethra. Additional information is obtained by observing the entire urethra in a panoramic view, as well as by palpating through the vaginal tissue with a finger placed beyond the end of the scope. A short, flaccid urethra that is open from the meatus to the UVJ is obviously damaged. Palpation may reveal scarring and immobility of the UVJ. Genuine stress incontinence and an associated defect in the urethra or urethral sphincteric mechanism (or both) are very difficult to treat with the use of standard surgical techniques. Additional studies of anatomic and physiologic function of the urethra and the UVJ are required in these instances.[12]

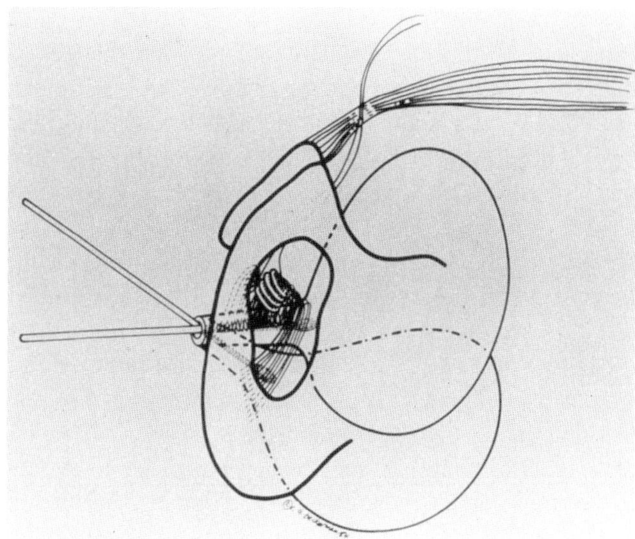

Figure 4-5 Applicator (Q-tip) test. Resting angle and straining angle (cough) are measured by comparing external portion of applicator with horizontal plane. *Source*: Reprinted from *Gynecologic Urology and Urodynamics: Theory and Practice*, ed 2 (p 535) by DR Ostergard (editor) with permission of Williams & Wilkins Company, © 1985.

8. Imaging Techniques

Hodgkinson[13] described a method for observing UVJ anatomy that became known as a bead-chain cystogram. A modified version, called a stress cystogram, may be performed with contrast medium (instilled in the bladder), barium paste (instilled in the bladder base to outline the UVJ), and a pediatric feeding tube (8F) to outline the urethra. Anteroposterior and lateral views of the UVJ are taken with the patient standing both at rest and with vigorous straining. In addition, a video recording can be obtained with fluoroscopy of the UVJ during straining and coughing. Normal anatomy at the UVJ includes a supported position opposite the lower border of the symphysis pubis, absence of funneling, nondependent bladder neck, and minimal descent with stress.

A further extension of the cystogram has been described by Blaivas and Olsson.[14] Of particular significance is the finding of an immobile open bladder neck at rest (type III stress incontinence), which, in all likelihood, will not be corrected with standard surgical approaches for GSI. Advances with ultrasound have now made it possible to evaluate the bladder and UVJ effectively with this technique. Approaches have included transabdominal,[15] transvaginal, transrectal,[16,17] perineal, and introital sonography.[18] A dynamic evaluation is made during bladder filling and with maneuvers to provoke increased intra-abdominal pressure or opening of the bladder neck with contractions. Imaging studies may be performed in incontinent patients for whom incontinence surgery is contemplated. Baseline study results ensure that an anatomic defect exists and that it is one that can potentially be corrected by surgery and be reassessed for adequacy of repair after surgery. Of particular importance is the information obtained regarding patients with recurrent incontinence. Type III stress incontinence has a strong potential for operative failure, unless the correct surgery is performed well.

9. Endoscopy

Urethroscopy is indicated for patients with recurrent incontinence after surgery to assess visually the urethra and the UVJ, as described earlier.[12] It also can help to evaluate for urethral diverticulum, urinary tract fistula, and urethral integrity. Cystoscopy should be performed in patients with recurrent incontinence to assess bladder and urethral integrity. It has many other indications, including the presence of irritative voiding symptoms, hematuria, and fistula.[19,20]

10. Urodynamic Studies

Multichannel urodynamic testing is most easily performed by using microtip transducer catheters to measure pressures simultaneously in the urethra, the bladder, and the vagina (intra-abdominal pressure). The catheters are connected to a recording device that prints out pressure readings and subtracted pressures for urethral closure pressure (urethra pressure minus bladder pressure) and true detrusor pressure (bladder pressure minus intra-abdominal pressure).[21] The *urethral pressure profile* is a record of pressure along the urethral lumen as the pressure sensor on the catheter is slowly withdrawn from the bladder through the full length of the urethra. *Urethral closure pressure* is the urethral pressure in excess of simultaneously measured bladder pressure. As long as it maintains a positive value, urine cannot pass from the bladder through the urethra (Figure 4-6). The *urethral functional length* is that length of urethra over which the urethral pressure exceeds the bladder pressure. Normal values for urethral closure pressure range from 40 to 60 cm H_2O; those for urethral functional length are 2.5 to 3.5 cm. Profiles are performed at rest and during stress (coughing). This latter test is very important, because its results form the urodynamic basis for assessing GSI.[22] When bladder pressure exceeds urethral pressure during coughing and other stress maneuvers, the urethral closure pressure is zero (pressure equalization), and urine is generally visualized escaping from the urethra (Figure 4-7).

Indications for a urethral closure pressure profile (UCPP) are outlined in Table 4-6. This type of sophisticated test is not required to make the diagnosis of GSI in all patients. In some problem cases discrepancies in other test findings may exist or symptoms may make diagnosis incomplete without UCPP. One of the greatest concerns, especially in patients with recurrent GSI, is that the urethra is scarred and nonfunctional. This type of urethra, even when in normal anatomic position, will function poorly and cannot prevent urine escaping with stress. The only reason to perform UCPP in all patients would be to determine whether poor urethral sphincteric function is present in low-risk patients. Up to the present time this has been determined by measuring urethral closure pressure in the sitting position with a full bladder. Low urethral closure pressure, a value less than 20 cm H_2O,[23] is a strong indicator of altered urethral sphincteric function and, at the least, should merit further evaluation of UVJ mobility, vaginal scarring, and urethral fibrosis.

11. Tests for Fistulas

Continuous urinary leakage after gynecologic surgery or obstetrical deliveries strongly suggests a urinary fistula. Historically, leakage related to hysterectomy becomes clinically apparent as the patient is being discharged from the hospital or during the next 2 weeks, because the formation of a defect requires breakdown of sutures or necrotic tissue. Fistulas occurring after obstetrical injury usually become apparent almost immediately. When a patient presents with the foregoing history, the details of the surgery or delivery should be carefully reviewed by obtaining records of the hospital stay and the procedure. Physical examination shows vulvar irritation from urine, and placement of a vaginal speculum usually causes pooling of urine. Smaller

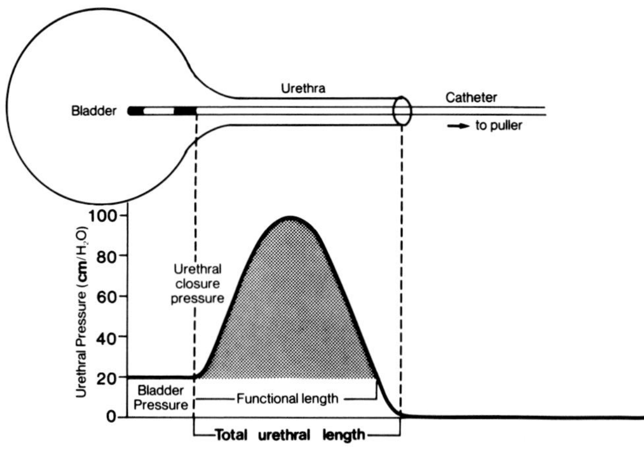

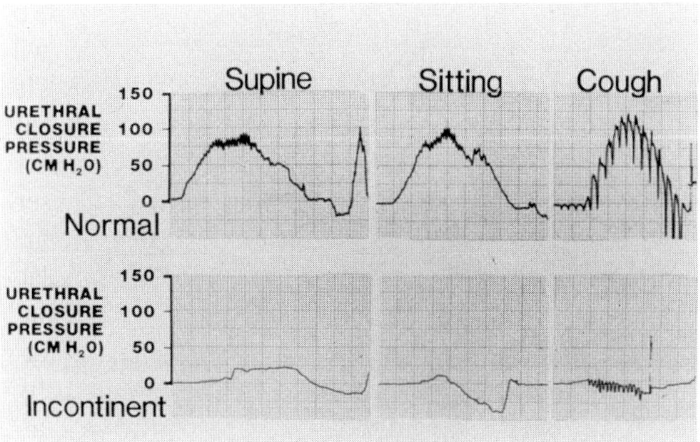

Figure 4-7 Genuine stress incontinence: Patient with normal findings (*top graph*) and patient with genuine stress incontinence (*bottom graph*). Closure pressures are lower in incontinent patient, and there is pressure equalization during cough profile of this patient. *Source*: The American College of Obstetricians and Gynecologists. *Urogynecologic Evaluation, Endoscopy, and Urodynamic Testing in the Symptomatic Female* by Alfred E Bent. ACOG Audiovisual Library, Washington DC, © 1990.

Table 4-6 Indications for Urethral Closure Pressure Profile

Prior Surgical Failure
Continuous Incontinence (Exclusive of Fistula)
Severe Genuine Stress Incontinence (GSI)
GSI after Age 65 Years or before Age 25 Years
Genital Vault Prolapse (To Rule Out Potential Incontinence)
Urethral Diverticula
Mixed Incontinence (Combined GSI and Detrusor Instability)
Symptomatic Patient with No Demonstrable Urine Loss
Possibly All Patients with GSI

amounts of leakage may be detected by having the patient take phenazopyridine hydrochloride the day before examination. The speculum has to be manipulated to visualize a defect, which, for vesicovaginal fistula after hysterectomy, occurs just anterior to the vault scar.

Vesicovaginal fistula is determined clinically by instilling 200 to 300 mL of a dilute solution of methylene blue or indigo carmine into the patient's bladder and placing a tampon in the vagina. The patient walks for 10 to 15 minutes, and the tampon is carefully removed. If there is staining on the end at the vaginal vault, a vesicovaginal fistula is almost certainly present. The vagina can be examined again after tampon removal if the vaginal defect has not been previously viewed. The test for ureterovaginal fistula is performed after the methylene blue test has resulted in a negative test. The patient is asked to drink two glasses of water, and 1 mL of indigo carmine solution is injected intravenously. A tampon is placed in the vagina, and the patient is asked to walk for 10 to 15 minutes. The tampon is carefully removed and examined for the presence of dye. Again, the vagina may be examined directly for a defect.

Once the presence of a vesicovaginal fistula is determined, it is localized with endoscopy of the bladder and the vagina. Similarly, a urethrovaginal fistula (which may occur after urethral diverticulum repair or anterior colporrhaphy) is localized with urethroscopy of the urethra and the vagina while the examiner palpates along the urethra. Ureterovaginal fistulas require intravenous pyelography with or without anterograde ureteral catheterization.

If a recent vesicovaginal fistula is found, bladder drainage is instituted for 2 weeks, and the patient is reassessed for possible spontaneous closure.

12. Tests for Urethral Diverticulum

A urethral diverticulum presents most often with recurrent urinary tract infection, periurethral pain, palpable mass, or postmicturition dribbling (or a combination of these signs and symptoms). Physical examination is assisted with a Sims speculum or the posterior half of a Graves speculum retracting the posterior wall of the vagina. The urethra is palpated and massaged firmly. Pus may be seen at the urethral meatus. A mass is more readily palpated with a urethral sound in place in the urethra. Urethroscopy is performed next, and this is one of few instances in which one can still recommend the use of carbon dioxide to fill the bladder and then distend the urethra by palpating firmly just beyond the end of the urethroscope to obstruct the proximal portion of the urethra while the gas distends the urethral diverticula opening.[11] Pus may be seen exiting from the diverticular orifice, or the duct may be wide open with the diverticulum visible.

Voiding cystourethrograms will demonstrate most communicating urethral diverticula. As an alternative, a Davis or Trattner urethrogram catheter may be used to perform positive pressure urethrography. This study is helpful in documenting the location and number of diverticula.[24] The Davis and Trattner catheters have three channels: The first channel inflates the balloon with air to maintain the catheter in the bladder. The second one leads to a large balloon, which slides along the catheter and is inflated with 30 to 50 mL of air to hold it firmly against the urethral meatus. The third channel leads to a small opening between the two balloons, which allows dye to be injected under pressure into the urethra. Positive pressure urethrography has a diagnostic accuracy of 90%.

SEQUENCE OF TESTS FOR GENUINE STRESS INCONTINENCE

During the initial visit, the complete history and physical examination, 24-hour voiding diary, and basic evaluation (ie, urine culture, residual urine determination, Q-tip test, and stress test) are completed. In the patient diagnosed with GSI who has had no prior surgery for incontinence, and in whom there are no features in the voiding diary (urolog), history, or screening test to suggest DI, voiding dysfunction, or other abnormality, the evaluation may be complete.

The suggested sequence of testing in the office setting is to have the patient bring a completed history form and voiding diary with her and then complete the office tests in the following order: history and physical examination, postvoid residual urine, culture of residual urine, determination of bladder capacity, stress test, and Q-tip test. If only these tests are performed, the voiding diary must be studied carefully to detect voiding frequency and amount. Uroflowmetry could be done if desired just before assessing the residual urine or after the stress test. Determination of bladder capacity may help rule out DI, especially if the patient readily holds 500 to 600 mL. A CMG with the patient in standing position is strongly recommended in all patients before surgery because, as mentioned earlier, 5% to 18% of patients may develop DI de novo after surgery for GSI.[4] In contrast, of patients with mixed incontinence (combined GSI and DI), 33% to 50% have resolution of the DI component after surgery for GSI.[25,26]

Patients with primary GSI at risk for urethral sphincteric dysfunction (see Table 4-6) should have a UCPP. They may also require endoscopy and imaging studies of the UVJ. The patient with recurrent GSI after surgery presents a complex problem, which must be fully assessed.[27,28] After the initial visit and preliminary tests, the patient should have endoscopy, a UCPP, and UVJ imaging studies to complete the work-up. The UCPP provides a physiologic basis for investigation of the UVJ and the urethral function. Similar information is obtained with imaging studies, but only an anatomic description of an abnormality is obtained. Although both studies may be done, many clinicians rely primarily on one or the other, rather than both.

DIAGNOSTIC CRITERIA FOR SPECIFIC CONDITIONS

1. Genuine Stress Incontinence

The diagnosis of GSI is not made with just one or two specific tests. It is a condition diagnosed when all the appropriate information and results from the history, physical examination, and tests have been assembled. The patient by definition has urine loss with stress or activity. The incontinence is socially disruptive and occurs in the absence of detrusor activity. The most helpful signs are positive stress tests and mobility of the UVJ with stress. The other important indicator is a negative CMG. The physiologic gold standard for diagnosis of GSI is the UCPP, which shows pressure equalization along with urine loss during coughing (see Figure 4-7). The anatomic gold standard is the observation of opening of the bladder neck during coughing, with loss of urine, or contrast medium, into the urethra.

a. Genuine Stress Incontinence with Damaged Urethral Sphincteric Mechanism

Damage to the urethral sphincteric mechanism in the patient with GSI is determined physiologically when there is a urethral closure pressure of less than 20 cm H_2O with the patient in sitting position and the patient's bladder is full. Anatomically, it is demonstrated by imaging studies of the UVJ, which show an open, immobile bladder neck. Endoscopically, the UVJ appears open and pale, and it does not move with maneuvers such as holding urine, straining, or coughing. The urethra looks (and is) very short.

b. Potential Genuine Stress Incontinence

Potential GSI is the demonstration of urine loss during a stress test, or pressure equalization during a UCPP, when pelvic relaxation (severe cystocele, vault prolapse, or procidentia) is reduced and the prolapsed tissue is held in position to simulate the effects of surgery in correcting the disorder. This maneuver is performed by using one of three methods: (1) insertion of a Sims speculum held at the vaginal apex; (2) placement of a pessary for 1 week to determine the effects on the patient; or (3) placement of a pessary with manual stabilization, if needed, during testing. If potential GSI is demonstrated and surgery is performed to correct the pelvic relaxation, the procedure should also include repair for GSI.

2. Detrusor Instability

The diagnosis of DI is made by using CMG (provocative standing cystometry) in which detrusor contractions are demonstrated. The contractions usually are greater than 15 cm H_2O in amplitude, but may be less than 15 cm H_2O in the presence of clinical symptoms or with the observation of concomitant urethral relaxation with or without urine loss.

3. Mixed Incontinence

Mixed incontinence is the presence of two types of incontinence in the same person and, by convention, usually refers to combined GSI and DI. Either condition may be the dominant one. If DI is dominant, exhaustive medical treatment is undertaken. Only if GSI remains a significant problem, should surgery for incontinence be performed.

4. Overflow Incontinence

Overflow incontinence presents with frequent voiding and small amounts of incontinence usually occurring with stressful activity. Diagnosis is made during the first office visit with determination of postvoid residual urine.

5. Bypass of Continence Mechanism

Diagnosis of fistula and of urethral diverticulum has been described earlier. Because as much information as possible is desired, endoscopy and intravenous pyelography are performed for fistula, and endoscopy or positive pressure urethrography and UCPP are required for urethral diverticulum. The position of the urethral diverticulum in relation to peak urethral pressure is important to determine during the UCPP. Diverticula in the proximal segment of the urethra must be excised, whereas those in the distal segment can be treated by marsupialization.

Although a congenitally ectopic ureter may present after childhood, it is quite uncommon. Constant leakage is not always the initial finding. At times, the leakage may be intermittent and even related to stress. Diagnosis is by ultrasound and intravenous pyelography findings, which show a duplicated system and spilling of contrast medium outside the bladder into the vagina or the urethra.

6. Functional Disorders

Urine loss may not be demonstrable, and all other test results may be normal. In these cases, review of the history and test results is indicated. Sometimes ambulatory urodynamic monitoring or prolonged (3 to 5 day) pad tests may be indicated. Further questioning of the patient may reveal circumstances that have culminated in a functional disorder. These patients require a great deal of help and understanding. Referral for counseling may be required.

CONCLUSION

Any patient who complains of urinary incontinence deserves an evaluation to diagnose precisely the cause of leakage and to determine therapy. Initial evaluation of the history and physical examination, voiding diary, urine culture, residual urine determination, stress test, and Q-tip test will direct the investigator in the proper direction and sequence of testing. Further studies, including endoscopy, imaging, cystometry, and UCPP, will help resolve the difficult problem. A few specialized tests may be required for diagnosis of fistula and urethral diverticulum. It is of utmost importance to determine the presence or absence of DI, as well as to clarify whether the urethral sphincteric mechanism in patients with GSI is normal.

REFERENCES

1. Thiede HA, Saini VD. Urogynecology, comments and caveats. *Am J Obstet Gynecol*. 1987;157:563–568.

2. Haylan BT, Sutherst JR, Frazer MI. Is the investigation of most stress incontinence really necessary? *Br J Urol*. 1989; 64:147–149.

3. Sand PK, Hill RC, Ostergard DR. Incontinence history as a predictor of detrusor stability. *Obstet Gynecol*. 1988;71:257–260.

4. Cardozo LD, Stanton SL, Williams JE. Detrusor instability following surgery for genuine stress incontinence. *Br J Urol*. 1979;51:204–207.

5. Langer R, Ron-El R, Newman M, Herman A, Casti E. Detrusor instability following colposuspension for urinary stress incontinence. *Br J Obstet Gynaecol*. 1988;95:607–610.

6. Bergman A, Bhatia NN. Urodynamic appraisal of the Marshall-Marchetti test in women with stress urinary incontinence. *Urology*. 1987;29:458–462.

7. Mouritsen L, Berild G, Hertz J. Comparison of different methods for quantification of urinary leakage in incontinent women. *Neurourol Urodyn*. 1989;8:579–587.

8. Wilson PD, Mason MV, Herbison GP, Sutherst JR. Evaluation of the home pad test for quantifying incontinence. *Br J Urol*. 1989;64:155–157.

9. Ouslander J, Leach G, Abelson S, Staskin D, Blaustein J, Raz S. Simple versus multichannel cystometry in the evaluation of bladder function in an incontinent geriatric population. *J Urol*. 1988; 140:1482–1486.

10. Griffiths CJ, Assi MS, Styles RA, Ramsden PD, Neal DE. Ambulatory monitoring of bladder and detrusor pressure during natural filling. *J Urol*. 1989;142:780–784.

11. Walters MD. The diagnostic value of history, physical examination, and the Q-tip cotton swab test in women with urinary incontinence. *Am J Obstet Gynecol*. 1988;159:145–149.

12. Robertson JR. Urethroscopy. In: Ostergard DR, Bent AE, eds. *Urogynecology and Urodynamics: Theory and Practice*. 3rd ed. Baltimore, MD: Williams & Wilkins Co; 1991:chap 10, 115–121.

13. Hodgkinson CP. Metallic bead chain urethrocystography in preoperative and postoperative evaluation of gynecologic urologic problems. *Clin Obstet Gynecol*. 1978;21:725–735.

14. Blaivas JG, Olsson CA. Stress incontinence: classification of surgical approach. *J Urol*. 1988;139:727–731.

15. Bhatia NN, Ostergard DR, McQuown D. Ultrasonography in urinary incontinence. *Urology*. 1987;29:90–94.

16. Fellows GJ. Dynamic ultrasonography for voiding dysfunction. *Urol Clin North Am*. 1989;16:809–814.

17. Gordon D, Pearce M, Norton P, Stanton SL. Comparison of ultrasound and lateral chain urethrocystography in the determination of bladder neck descent. *Am J Obstet Gynecol*. 1989;160:182–185.

18. Koelbl H, Bernaschek G, Deutinger J. Assessment of female urinary incontinence by introital sonography. *JCU*. 1990; 18:370–374.

19. Worth PHL. Cystourethroscopy. In: Stanton SL, ed. *Clinical Gynecologic Urology*. St Louis, MO: CV Mosby Co; 1984:136–140.

20. Bent AE, Ostergard DR. Urethrocystoscopy. In: San Filippo JS, Levine RL, eds. *Operative Gynecologic Endoscopy*. New York: Springer-Verlag; 1989;20:272–280.

21. Asmussen M, Ulmsten U. A new technique for measurement of the urethra pressure profile. *Acta Obstet Gynecol Scand* (Suppl). 1976;55:167–173.

22. Bump RC, Copeland WE, Hurt WG, Fantl JA. Dynamic urethral pressure profilometry pressure transmission ratio determinations in stress incontinent and stress continent subjects. *Am J Obstet Gynecol*. 1988;159:749–755.

23. Sand PK, Bowen LW, Panganiban R, et al. The low pressure urethra as a factor in failed retropubic urethropexy. *Obstet Gynecol*. 1987;69:399–402.

24. Robertson JR. Urethral diverticula. In: Ostergard DR, Bent AE, eds. *Urogynecology and Urodynamics: Theory and Practice*. Baltimore, MD: Williams & Wilkins Co; 1991:chap 25, 283–291.

25. Bent AE. Concurrent genuine stress incontinence and detrusor instability. *Int Urogynecol J*. 1990;1:128–131.

26. Sand PK, Bowen LW, Ostergard DR. The effect of retropubic urethropexy on detrusor stability. *Obstet Gynecol*. 1988;71:818–822.

27. Bent AE, Ostergard DR. Recurrent stress incontinence. Causes and treatment in the female patient. *Postgrad Med*. 1988; 83:113–117.

28. Bent AE. Management of recurrent genuine stress incontinence. *Clin Obstet Gynecol*. 1990;33:358–366.

5

Stress Urinary Incontinence—Corrective Approaches

5-1

Anterior Colporrhaphy

R. Peter Beck

EVOLUTION OF THE PROCEDURE

In 1913, Kelly described an operation to correct stress incontinence of urine, which consisted of a vertical incision in the anterior wall of the vagina and a horizontal mattress suture of fine silk or linen "to suture together the torn or relaxed tissues at the neck of the bladder."[1] He then placed one or two more superficial but similar sutures to buttress the first stitch. Kelly stated there should be "a little jump to it [a mushroom catheter] as it clears the reconstructed sphincter at the neck of the bladder." After placing the "Kelly" sutures, he trimmed the vaginal wall flaps and closed the vaginal wall with one or two layers of continuous fine catgut.

In 1924, Watson and, in 1928, Miller described an inverted T incision in the anterior wall of the vagina (with the transverse bar at the cervix) for anterior colporrhaphy.[2,3] Watson used an interrupted Lembert type inverting chromic catgut to plicate the fascia under the urethra and the bladder and interrupted horizontal mattress sutures of chromic catgut to close the trimmed vaginal skin edge. Miller used a continuous chromic catgut suture "to pleat" the fascia under the urethra and the bladder base, starting the suture at the external meatus and extending it down to the cervix. He then used the same suture to run back to the external meatus, further "pleating" the fascia. He finished by closing the trimmed vaginal wall with a continuous chromic catgut suture. Watson and Miller seemed to perform anterior colporrhaphy in a nonspecific manner with respect to the urethra and the bladder, simply plicating the fascia under the urethra and the bladder in the same way.

In 1937, Kennedy described an operation for anterior vaginal wall repair that, like the Kelly procedure, restored a focus on the urethra.[4] He made a vertical incision in the anterior wall of the vagina and used two layers of interrupted vertical mattress chromic catgut sutures to plicate the fascia under, and to some extent lateral to, the urethra. Like Miller, Kennedy started the fascial plication at the external meatus. He then placed two horizontal Lembert sutures of silver wire under the proximal segment of the urethra close to the bladder neck, superficial to the two layers of chromic catgut. He used a single layer of vertical mattress sutures to plicate the fascia under the bladder base and interrupted chromic catgut sutures to close the vaginal wall. He removed the silver wire sutures 5 days after surgery.

In 1955 Kennedy described a retropubic approach for treating stress incontinence, entering the space of Retzius and placing two rings of silver wire snugly around the proximal aspect of the urethra.[6]

In 1940, Heaney described a technique for vaginal hysterectomy including anterior colporrhaphy. Although his name is frequently applied to the inverted T incision, it is likely that Watson, and then Miller, described the same incision earlier.[5]

In 1963, Ball and Hoffman and, in the same year, Zacharin and Gleadall reported an improvement in their correction of stress urinary incontinence (SUI) by using a combined anterior colporrhaphy–retropubic procedure.[7,8] Interest in the combined approach seemed to be limited and brief.

In 1969, Barnett emphasized that the "usual Kelly [Kennedy] operation produces a mere platform under the urethra and bladder" and that the proximal segment of the urethra should be elevated with a series of vertical mattress sutures ("one on top of the other") plicating the fascia at the bladder neck and recreating the posterior urethrovesical angle.[9] He then used a single layer of horizontal interrupted chromic catgut sutures to buttress the entire length of the urethra, as well as the bladder base if necessary, with similar sutures. He emphasized that the bladder base should not be elevated excessively to preserve the posterior urethrovesical angle.

In 1981, Powell described "a vaginal Marshall-Marchetti-Krantz type procedure."[10] He mobilized the paraurethral and vaginal tissues, so that the posterior surface of the symphysis pubis could be easily palpated. While holding the bladder neck area to the back of the symphysis pubis, he sutured the pubocervical fascia on each side of the urethra at the bladder neck to the periosteum.

In 1982, Beck and McCormick described 4 years of experience with a modified anterior colporrhaphy, which produced a 91% cure rate in treating genuine stress incontinence (GSI).[11] The focus of the operation was to create differentially better support to the urethra than to the bladder base by elevating the proximal aspect of the urethra to a level higher than the bladder base. This was accomplished by using delayed-absorption sutures placed at right angles to the vaginal fascial plane under the urethra, scratching the back of the symphysis pubis; more rapidly absorbed sutures were placed parallel to the vaginal fascial plane under the base of the bladder. The foregoing measures were designed to produce a mechanical kinking effect in the urethra at the instant of cough and an increased cough-pressure spike transmission ratio between the urethra and the bladder.[11,12] An effort was also made to tighten the urethra to increase the resting urethral closure pressure. In 1984, Mattingly and Davis described a similar procedure.[13] They emphasized that "high plication of the urethra behind the symphysis pubis is an essential component of this procedure. This is done by means of suturing the para-urethral fascia of the posterior [aspect of the] urethra to the posterior pubourethral ligaments, using a delayed absorbable suture material similar to the technique of Beck."[13] Mattingly and Davis' technique differed from Beck's only in that they used two diagonal sutures that crossed in the midline to plicate the fascia, instead of a continuous figure-of-eight suture to elevate and support the urethra.[11,13]

In 1988, Nichols and Ponchak described a vaginal operation that involved a plication of tissue from the urogenital diaphragm and the pubourethral ligaments under the urethrovesical junction. It was designed to elevate the proximal aspect of the urethra behind the symphysis pubis.[14]

ANTERIOR COLPORRHAPHY WITH AND WITHOUT THE PRESENCE OF GENUINE STRESS INCONTINENCE

Anterior colporrhaphy may be used to treat anterior vaginal wall prolapse with or without GSI. The latter condition is the result of equalization of pressure between the urethra and the bladder at the instant of stress (eg, cough). This unphysiologic condition is usually associated anatomically with a slight to moderate cystourethrocele. If the cystourethrocele becomes more marked, the patient often spontaneously regains continence as a result of an accentuated mechanical kinking effect in the urethra (discussed later). If the marked cystourethrocele is repaired without creating differentially better support to the urethra than to the bladder base, GSI may recur as a complication of the prolapse surgery.[15] Therefore anterior colporrhaphy should be performed with the same technique whether GSI is or is not present, in the first instance to cure the incontinence and in the second instance to prevent the new development of GSI.

MECHANISMS IN THE SURGICAL CORRECTION OF GENUINE STRESS INCONTINENCE

Any operation that corrects GSI enhances one or both components of the urethral resistance that maintains continence with stress: (1) the resting urethral closure pressure and, more important, (2) the urethral cough-pressure spike (Figure 5-1.1).

Surgery that cures GSI is usually associated with an increase in resting urethral closure pressures.[12,16–18] Indeed, the latter may be the primary mechanism of surgical cure in a minority of cases.[12] Surgical cure of GSI, however, may not be associated with increased

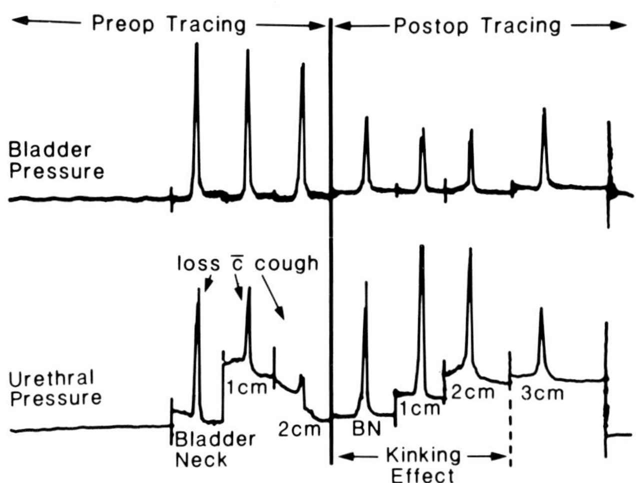

Figure 5-1.1 Normal pressure gradient on the right and pressure equalization on the left. Simultaneous intraurethral and intravesical pressure tracing (bladder pressure at top and urethral pressure at bottom) in a patient with GSI before and after an anterior colporrhaphy which cured the problem. The tracing on the left shows pressure equalization due to a scar tissue effect, bladder base descent, and urethral laxity. The patient lost urine with cough due to an ineffective urethral pressure spiking (kinking) mechanism. The postoperative tracing, on the right, of the same patient cured of incontinence shows the cough-pressure transmission in the proximal urethra is >100% of the pressure transmission to the bladder and slightly less than 100% in the distal centimeter of the urethra. The mechanism of cure in this case was due to an improved urethral pressure spiking (kinking) mechanism. Usually when there is an improved pressure spiking mechanism, there is an improvement in maximal resting intraurethral pressure at some point(s) in the urethra but not so in this case, although the total urethral closing pressure was increased due to urethral lengthening. *Source*: Reprinted with permission from *Obstetrics and Gynecology* (1982;59:269), Copyright © 1982, American College of Obstetricians and Gynecologists.

intraurethral closure pressures when the mechanism of cure is an increase in the cough-pressure spike transmission ratio between the urethra and the bladder.[19] Increase in the resting closure pressures along the urethra is accomplished (1) by tightening the urethra through increasing the tension in the support tissue (pubocervical fascia and pubourethral ligaments) laterally and above or laterally and under the urethra or (2) by applying a direct tensile force to the urethra (eg, with a sling).

An increase in the urethral cough-pressure spike (absolute and/or relative to the bladder pressure spike) is the most frequent main mechanism whereby surgery cures GSI.[12,18–20] An increase in the cough-spike transmission ratio between the urethra and the bladder, however, is not always the mechanism of surgical cure.[12,18] Increase in the urethral cough-pressure spikes, absolute and/or relative to the bladder-pressure spike, is accomplished (1) by restoring the urethrovesical junction to its normal position (1.5 to 2.0 cm behind and 1.5 to 2.0 cm above the inferior edge of the symphysis pubis) and (2) by providing the entire length of the urethra (or a portion of the urethra, as with a sling procedure) with differentially more rigid and fixed support than that provided to the bladder base (Figures 5-1.2 and 5-1.4). As a result, there is some descent of the urethra when the patient coughs. The descent of the bladder base is greater, however, and a mechanical kinking effect is created along the entire length of the urethra (or a portion of the urethra, as with a sling procedure) (Figures 5-1.3 and 5-1.4). The mechanical kinking effect in the urethra at the instant of cough produces urethral cough-pressure spikes along the entire length (or portion) of the urethra.[11] (See Figure 5-1.1.) Restoration of the urethrovesical junction to proper position not only enhances the urethral kinking mechanism with cough, but also reduces the magnitude of the intravesical cough-pressure spike, thus increasing the numerator and decreasing the denominator of the urethral–vesical cough-pressure ratio.[12] (See Figure 5-1.1.) Usually, an increase in the resting intraurethral pressure is associated with an increase in the transmission ratio, and vice versa, but this is not always true.

I believe that a patient is surgically cured of GSI by increasing the cough-pressure transmission ratio between the urethra and the bladder or by increasing the resting urethral closure pressures (or by both mechanisms). These concepts are discussed further in the description of the operative technique for anterior colporrhaphy.

Various operations and variations thereof, such as the Marshall-Marchetti-Krantz procedure, Burch pro-

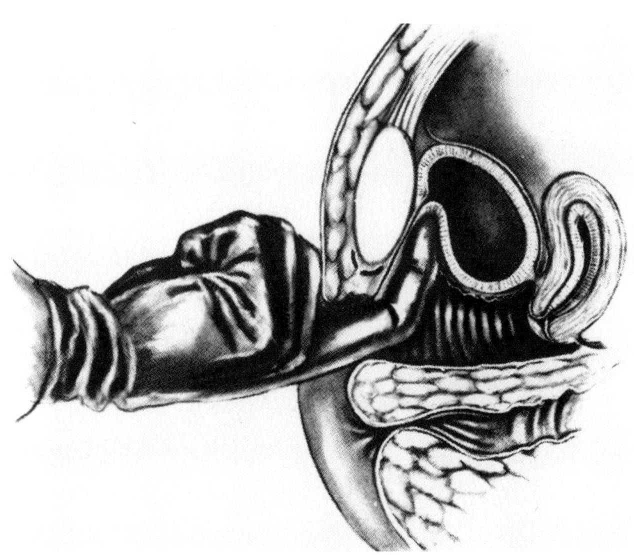

Figure 5-1.2 In sagittal section, placement of peri-urethral sutures with the Marshall-Marchetti-Krantz procedure accomplishing the same effect as anterior colporrhaphy. *Source*: Reprinted with permission from *American Journal of Obstetrics and Gynecology* (1976;122:220), Copyright © 1976, Mosby-Year Book.

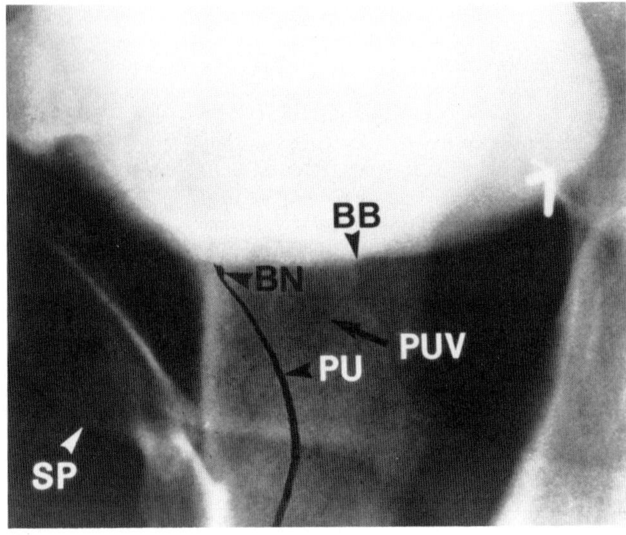

A

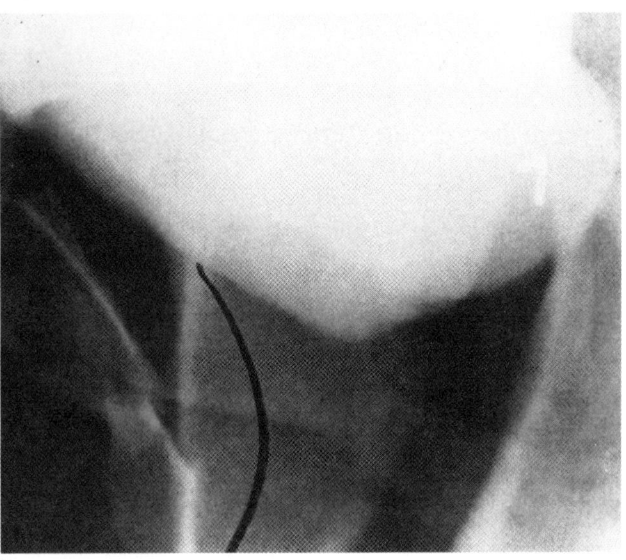
B

Figure 5-1.3 Cine-cystourethrogram, after a fascia lata sling procedure, at rest (**A**) and with the stress of cough (**B**). Note the excellent location behind the symphysis pubis (SP) of the bladder neck (BN) and the good posterior urethrovesical angle (PUV) at rest (**A**). Note, in **B**, the fixed position of the proximal urethra (PU) and the urethral kinking effect at the sling site as the bladder base (BB) descends with hard cough, reducing the posterior urethrovesical angle and producing the urethral pressure spikes seen in Fig 5-1.1. *Source*: Reprinted with permission from *Obstetrics and Gynecology* (1988;72:302), Copyright © 1988, American College of Obstetricians and Gynecologists.

cedure, sling procedures, needle suspension procedures, and anterior colporrhaphy, when properly performed, can accomplish one or both of the aforementioned surgical objectives with equal effectiveness. Like many other operations for treating GSI, the success of an anterior colporrhaphy depends on the quality of the local support tissue, in addition to other considerations. I favor anterior colporrhaphy for the initial treatment of

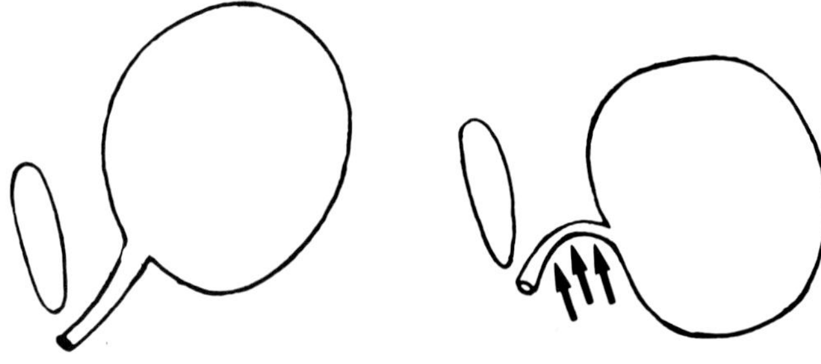

Figure 5-1.4 The diagram on the left shows the normal anatomic relationship at the bladder neck and its relationship to the symphysis pubis in the resting state. The diagram on the right shows greater descent of the bladder base than the urethra with cough in the normal woman as a result of differentially better support to the urethra than to the bladder base (see Figs. 5-1.3 and 5-1.8), resulting in a mechanical kinking effect in the urethra at the instant of cough, etc. *Source*: Reprinted with permission from *Canadian Journal of Obstetrics and Gynecology* (1989;1:24), Copyright © 1989, Rodar Publishing Company.

GSI, because not only is it associated with a very competitive cure rate (91%) but also the frequently coexistent vaginal prolapse can be corrected in the same operative field with minimal operating time. Also, there is minimal morbidity relative to other procedures used to treat GSI.[15,21] I have obtained better results in treating GSI with the fascia lata sling procedure, as compared with anterior colporrhaphy, in a more difficult group of patients with recurrent incontinence.[16] I do not use the fascia lata sling procedure as the initial operation (with one exception in 198 sling procedures), however, because of greater morbidity with the sling procedure than with anterior colporrhaphy. In selecting a procedure for treating GSI the choice should be made on the basis of achievable cure rates, as well as on comparative morbidity and other considerations such as quality of local support tissues, coexistent genital prolapse, chronic pulmonary disease, obesity, and need for abdominal surgery. I believe the only contraindication to an anterior colporrhaphy for treating GSI is the presence of local support tissues that are considered to be irreparably poor, in which case a fascia lata sling procedure should be done.[16]

PROCEDURE OF ANTERIOR COLPORRHAPHY: A MODIFIED TECHNIQUE

The standard Kelly-Kennedy type of anterior colporrhaphy was designed to correct the bulge (prolapse) of the anterior wall of the vagina by creating a shelf-like support for the anterior vaginal wall without overcorrecting the cystocele. If the anterior vaginal wall prolapse was associated with concomitant SUI, it was anticipated that plication of the support tissue under the urethra and bladder would also correct SUI. The results in treating SUI were not as good as those achieved by retropubic procedures.

The standard anterior colporrhaphy was revised so as to include a vaginal retropubic urethropexy plus a ''standard'' cystocele repair, ie, the modification relates to the urethral part of the anterior colporrhaphy. The modification has three objectives: (1) tightening the urethra; (2) elevating the proximal urethra so that the urethrovesical junction is higher than the lowest point of the bladder base (reducing the pubourethral angle to less than 45 degrees and the posterior urethrovesical angle to less than 120 degrees); and (3) creating more fixed and rigid support for the urethra than for the bladder base (including less angle change on Q-tip testing). The first objective increases the resting intraurethral pressure and the other two increase the intraurethral cough-pressure transmission through a urethral kinking mechanism with cough. These objectives are achieved by two basic changes in surgical technique. The first is a directional and depth change in needle (suture) placement under and around the urethra (Figures 5-1.12–5-1.16). Formerly, needle (suture) placement in the pubocervical fascia under the urethra and bladder base was done with the long axis of the needle inserted superficially into the pubocervical fascia and parallel to the fascial surface and that of the anterior vaginal wall. The direction of needle placement is changed so that the long axis of the needle is inserted deeper and at right angles into the fascia below, lateral, and above the urethra (Figures 5-1.12–5-1.16). The depth and direction of needle (suture) placement in the fascia under the bladder base has not been changed (Figures 5-1.12–5-1.14). The second change in technique is the use of delayed absorption polyglycolic suture material in the urethrocele repair (urethropexy) instead of more rapidly absorbed chromic catgut. The use of chromic catgut to plicate the fascia in the cystocele part of the repair has been continued. This change was designed to enhance the differentially better support to the urethra than to the bladder base, an anatomic relation required for urethral kinking.

The procedure is begun by inserting a suprapubic Foley catheter (20F) with a 30-mL balloon into the bladder. An inverted V-shaped incision (Figure 5-1.5) is made through the vaginal wall down to the underlying pubocervical fascia. The apex of the inverted V is at the external meatus of the urethra. The inverted V-shaped incision is designed to trim the vaginal wall edges. It is calculated so that the cut edges of the vaginal wall can be brought together in the midline with plicating vertical

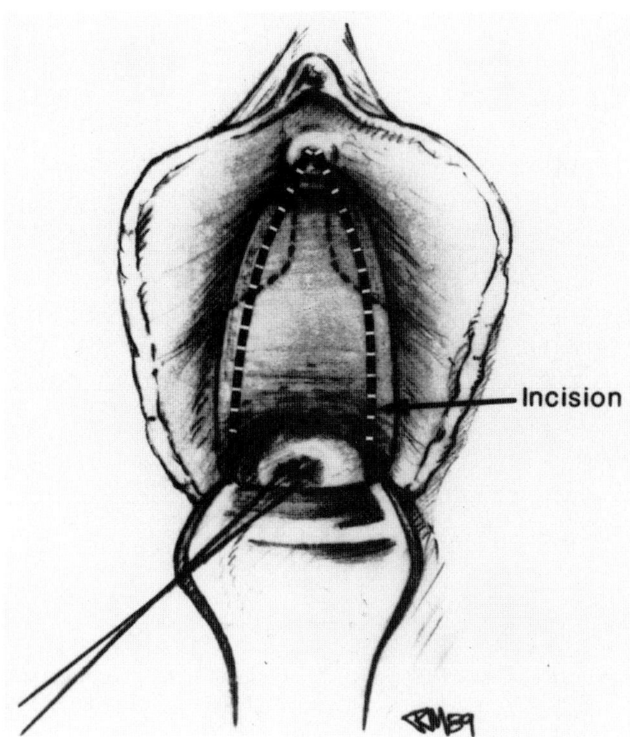

Figure 5-1.5 Shows vaginal wall ''inverted V'' incision for anterior colporrhaphy. *Source*: Reprinted with permission from *Canadian Journal of Obstetrics and Gynecology* (1989;1:26), Copyright © 1989, Rodar Publishing Company.

mattress sutures in the pubocervical fascia. These sutures are placed under and slightly lateral to each of the vaginal wall incisions.

If the base of the triangle created by the incisional arms of the inverted V is too wide, two important problems can occur. The first problem is overcorrection of the cystocele. This overcorrection would increase the posterior urethrovesical angle (which should be less than 120 degrees) to one approaching 180 degrees, causing the angle to disappear and negating the effect of subsequent elevation of the proximal aspect of the urethra later in the operation (Figure 5-1.6). (See also Figure 5-1.4.) The posterior urethrovesical angle is made up of a urethral arm and a bladder base arm. The objectives of surgery are to elevate the urethral arm, especially at the vertex of the angle, and to prevent excessive elevation of the bladder base arm, which would increase the angle to more than 120 degrees. (See Figure 5-1.2.) A proper posterior urethrovesical angle (<120 degrees), with differentially better support to the urethra than to the bladder, promotes an effective urethral kinking mechanism (and a further reduction in the posterior urethrovesical angle) at the instant of cough, producing an effective intraurethral cough-pressure spike that will ensure continence of urine. (See Figures 5-1.1–5-1.4.)

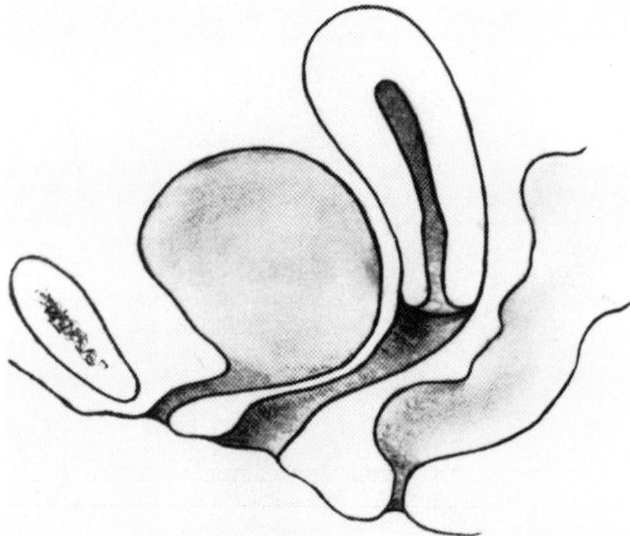

Figure 5-1.6 This drawing demonstrates a mild cystourethrocele. A mild to moderate cystourethrocele is the classic anatomic defect associated with genuine stress incontinence of urine, contrasted by the usual state of continence with stress, associated with a marked cystourethrocele. *Source*: Reprinted with permission from *Canadian Journal of Obstetrics and Gynecology* (1989;1:25), Copyright © 1989, Rodar Publishing Company.

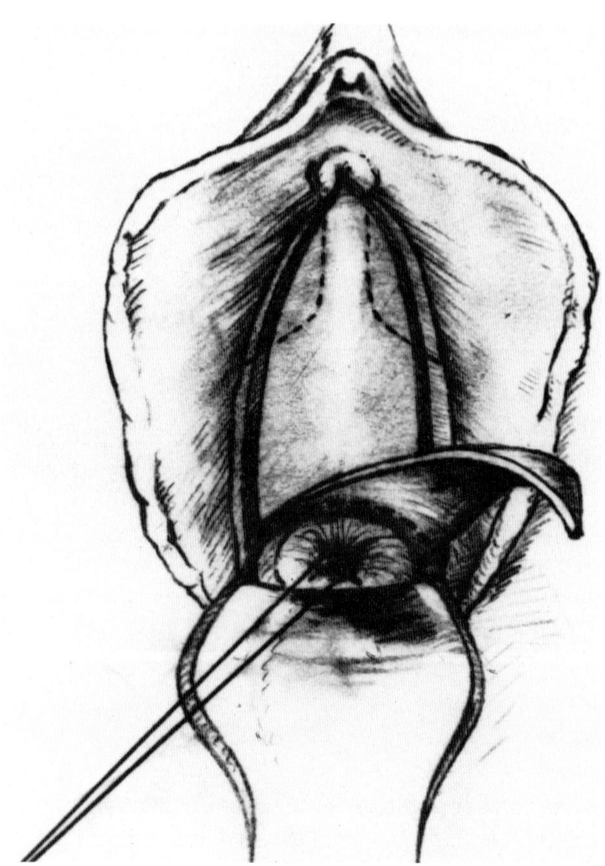

Figure 5-1.7 Shows vaginal wall flap being peeled from underlying pubocervical fascia. Dotted line at base of triangle indicates incision that completes removal of triangular vaginal wall flap. *Source*: Reprinted with permission from *Canadian Journal of Obstetrics and Gynecology* (1989;1:26), Copyright © 1989, Rodar Publishing Company.

The second problem related to the incisional arms being too far apart is that the plicating sutures in the pubocervical fascia, when tied, would be under too much tension. This would violate one of the most important principles in any hernia repair. With too much tension, the fascia, especially under the bladder base, will tear, leading to defective wound healing.

When the inverted V incision is placed properly and the underlying fascial sutures are tied, the vaginal wall edges come into apposition for easy subsequent closure without tension. Unless there is gross miscalculation, the fascia and the vaginal skin edges can be brought together in the midline, but sometimes under too much tension. With practice and experience, the inverted V incision can be made so as to prevent overcorrection of the cystocele and undue tissue tension and tearing. The medial cut edges of the incision are freed from the underlying pubocervical fascia with sharp dissection. The triangular skin flap is then separated from the underlying pubocervical fascia by means of thumb and gauze dissection, as indicated in Figure 5-1.7.

The advantages of the triangular incision and technique, first described by Archibald Campbell, M.D., at the Montreal General Hospital, are as follows:

1. The vaginal wall edges are trimmed.
2. The pubocervical fascia is left intact with minimal damage to the local nerve supply to the urethra and the bladder and to the blood supply of the pubocervical fascia.
3. The vaginal wall flap can be used as a tractor to pull the operative field into better view in separating the vaginal skin from the underlying pubocervical fascia.
4. The traction on the triangular flap can be used to extend the incisions in the vaginal wall up to the cervix or the vaginal vault.

The chief support to the urethra and the bladder is the pubocervical fascia, as shown diagrammatically in Figure 5-1.8. The pubocervical fascia is thicker (and tougher) under the urethra than under the bladder base, as shown in Figures 5-1.9 and 5-1.10. (See also Figure 5-1.8.) The pubocervical fascia under the urethra is also thicker (and tougher) in the midline than more laterally (Figure 5-1.10). Condensations of this fascia superior to the urethra have been described as the pubourethral ligaments by Zacharin and Gleadall[8] (Figure 5-1.11). It is this midline condensation of fascia, rather than the lateral thinner (weaker) fascia, that is most useful for tightening and elevating the urethra.

Unless the urethra is fixed by scar tissue and requires mobilization, there is no point in dissecting the vaginal

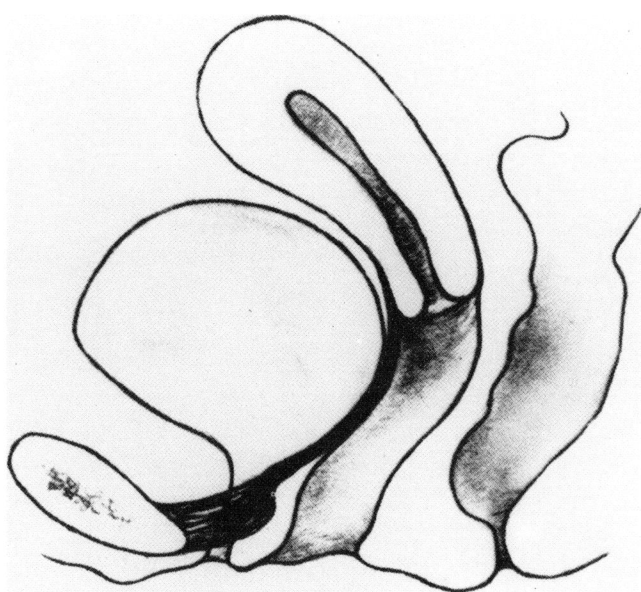

Figure 5-1.8 Shows pubocervical fascia is thicker and more dense under and around urethra than under bladder base, creating differentially better support to urethra than to the bladder base (see also Figures 5-1.9 and 5-1.10). *Source*: Reprinted with permission from *Canadian Journal of Obstetrics and Gynecology* (1989;1:24), Copyright © 1989, Rodar Publishing Company.

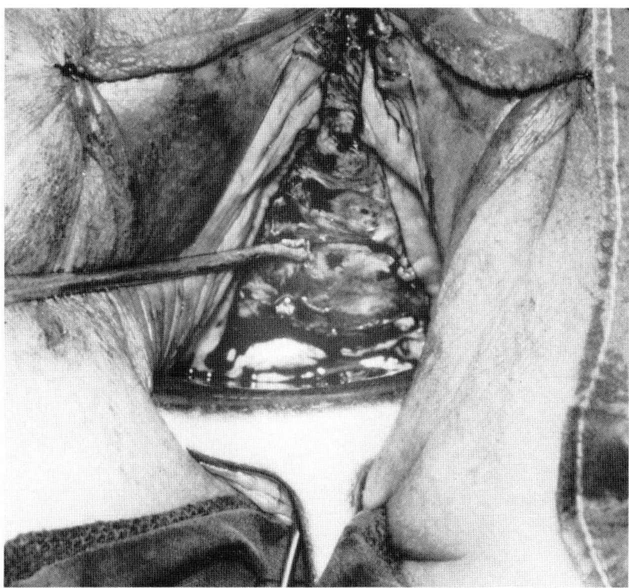

Figure 5-1.9 This photograph taken at anterior colporrhaphy demonstrates the thicker, more dense, pubocervical fascia under the urethra relative to the less dense fascia under the bladder base. The uterine sound points to the urethrovesical junction.

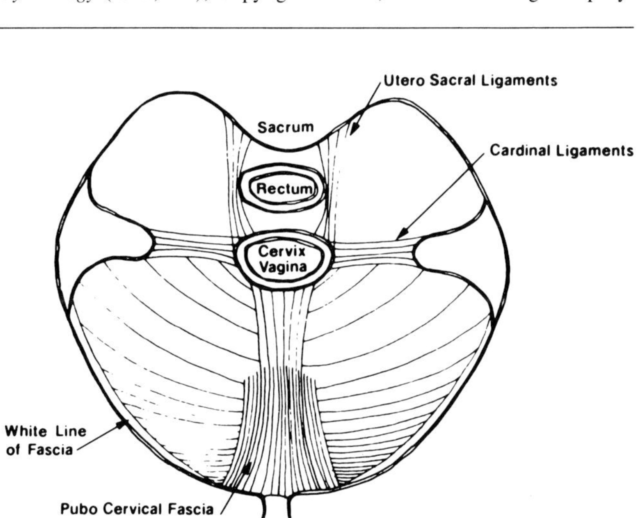

Figure 5-1.10 This diagram, at the plane of the midpelvis, shows the fascial supports of the cervix and vaginal vault, suspending those structures in the midpelvis. The pubocervical fascia is thicker and more dense under urethra and in midline. *Source*: Reprinted from *Principles and Practice of Clinical Gynecology* (p 679) by NG Kase and AB Weingold, eds, with permission of Churchill Livingstone, © 1983.

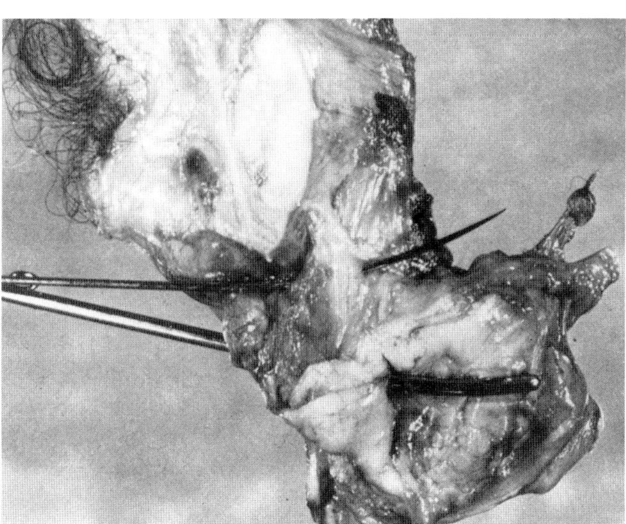

Figure 5-1.11 Specimen cut in the sagittal plane through the symphysis and urethra. The needle passes through the broad paraurethral attachment of the right posterior pubourethral ligament. *Source*: Reprinted with permission from *American Journal of Obstetrics and Gynecology* (1963;86:989), Copyright © 1963, Mosby-Year Book.

wall from the underlying pubocervical fascia lateral to the inverted V incision (Figure 5-1.12). (See also Figure 5-1.5.) Such lateral dissection creates unnecessary bleeding. Also, the use of fascia lateral to the midline fascial condensation is unwise because this tissue is not as tough and strong as the midline fascia. It is impossible to pull the white line of fascia on the side wall of the pelvis under the bladder base. Leaving the vaginal wall applied to the pubocervical fascia lateral to the inverted V incision (see Figures 5-1.7 and 5-1.12) prevents unnecessary bleeding at surgery and subsequent hematoma formation and maintains the blood supply to the fascial support tissues in the operative field, thus maximizing subsequent wound healing.

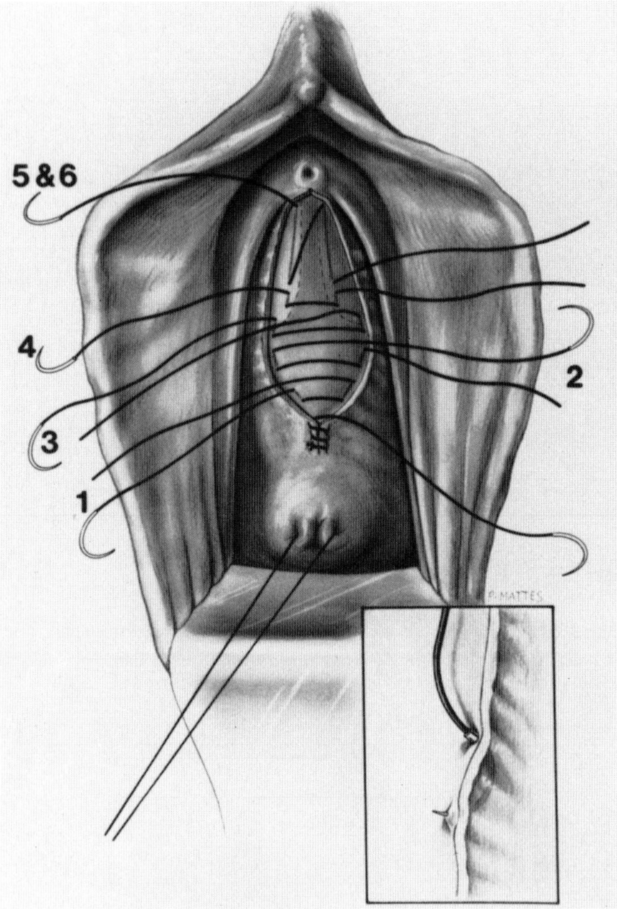

Figure 5-1.12 Placement of no. 1 chromic catgut, vertical mattress sutures (1, 2, and 3) plicating the fascia under the bladder base with long axis of the needle parallel to the fascial surface (*also bottom insert*). Number 1 polyglycolic suture (4) is inserted into fascia at the bladder neck with long axis of the needle at right angles to the fascial surface (*also top insert*). Figure-of-eight no. 1 polyglycolic sutures (5 and 6) are inserted into the pubocervical fascia, scratching the back of the symphysis pubis with long axis of the needle held at right angles to the fascial surface (*also top insert*). *Source*: Reprinted with permission from *Obstetrics and Gynecology* (1991;78:1013), Copyright © 1991, American College of Obstetricians and Gynecologists.

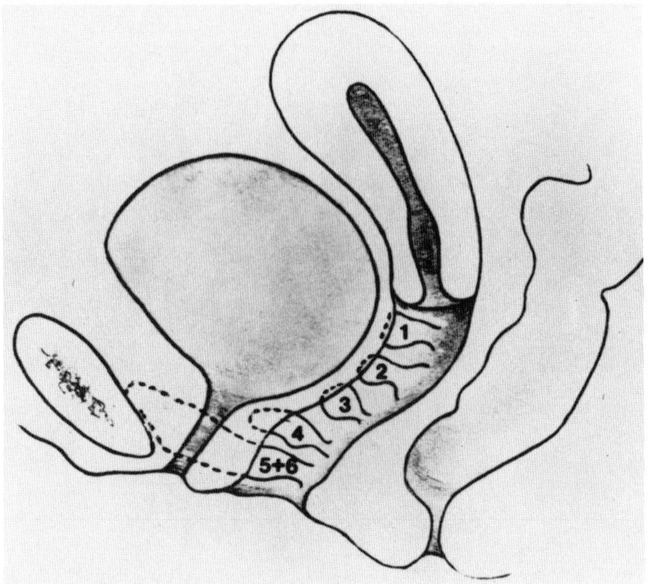

Figure 5-1.13 Shows placement of sutures in Figure 5-1.12 in sagittal view. When tied, the fascia under the bladder base is plicated. Overcorrection of the cystocele is avoided. When sutures 5 and 6, in the fascia under and around the urethra are tied, the urethra is elevated more than bladder base (and is tightened). *Source*: Reprinted with permission from *Canadian Journal of Obstetrics and Gynecology* (1989;1:27), Copyright © 1989, Rodar Publishing Company.

The base of the triangular skin flap is now cut to remove the flap. (See Figure 5-1.7.) A continuous suture is placed in the base angles of the triangular defect in the vaginal skin, as indicated in Figure 5-1.12 (lowest, unnumbered suture). This suture brings the skin edges together over the fascial repair without tension. It is important to delay closure of the vaginal wall until the vertical mattress sutures in the pubocervical fascia under the base of the bladder have been inserted (Figure 5-1.13; see also Figure 5-1.12) and tied. Usually three chromic no. 1 catgut sutures (sutures 1, 2, and 3) are necessary to plicate the pubocervical fascia under the base of the bladder to correct the cystocele. Chromic catgut is used to plicate the fascia here to minimize tearing of this tissue. More sutures are required for a larger cystocele. When placing these mattress sutures, a large bite of pubocervical fascia is taken immediately lateral to the edge of the incision in the vaginal wall, while the long axis of a Mayo (no. 3) needle is held parallel to the surface of the vaginal wall (Figure 5-1.14; see also Figures 5-1.12 and 5-1.13). It is important to keep this large bite of pubocervical fascia superficial to prevent problems with the ureter and the bladder. These sutures are tied in succession toward the bladder neck, plicating the underlying pubocervical fascia in the midline and bringing the vaginal wall edges together in the midline. The continuous chromic no. 1 catgut suture that is used to close the vaginal skin over the fascial plication is continued at appropriate times throughout the procedure.

The bladder neck is identified endoscopically or by observing the transverse crease in the pubocervical fascia (the latter can be accentuated by pushing in a cephalad manner on the distal aspect of the urethra and external meatus). A ''Kelly''-type, no. 1 polyglycolic suture (1 Dexon on a DT-12 needle) is inserted in the pubocervical fascia at the bladder neck, as shown previously in Figures 5-1.12 and 5-1.13 (suture 4). Instead of the classic horizontal mattress suture described by Kelly,[1] I use a vertical mattress suture. This suture is designed specifically to correct funneling of the proximal aspect of the urethra. Failure to correct funneling of this structure can predispose to postoperative detrusor

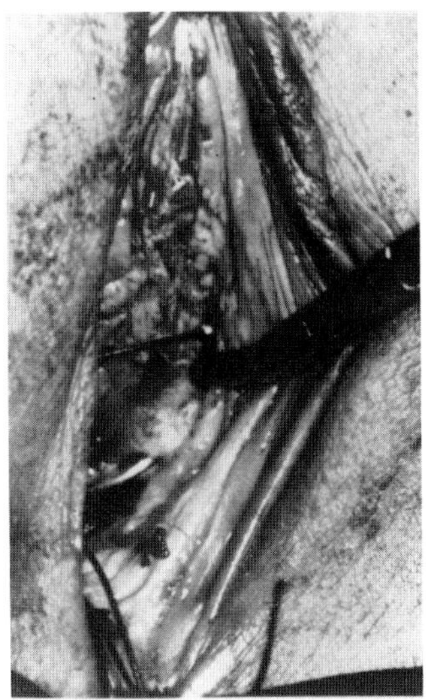

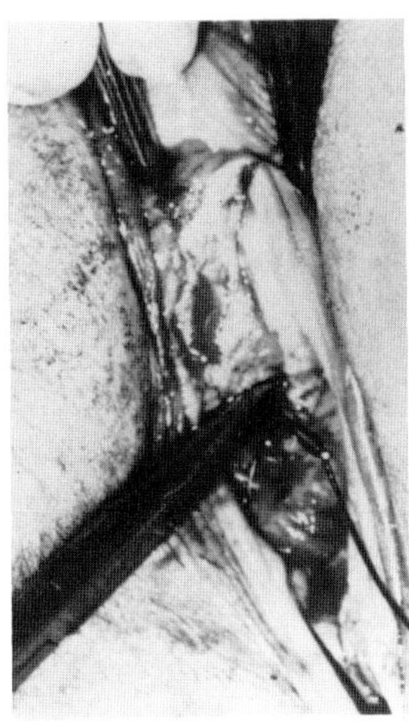

Figure 5-1.14 Needle placement at anterior colporrhaphy. Photograph at left shows #3 Mayo needle parallel to the surface of the vaginal wall taking a substantial bite in pubocervical fascia lateral to the incision in the vaginal wall. A similar bite on the other side creates a vertical mattress suture plicating fascia under bladder base (see also Figure 5-1.12). Usually 3 to 5 similar sutures are required to correct the cystocele. Photograph on right shows #3 Mayo needle placed at right angles to the surface of the vaginal wall, close but lateral to metal catheter in urethra (see also Figures 5-1.12, 5-1.15, and 5-1.16) scratching the symphysis pubis. A similar bite with the same suture on the other side creates a figure-of-eight suture which plicates the pubocervical fascia under and around the urethra. *Source*: Courtesy of the University of Alberta, Edmonton, Canada.

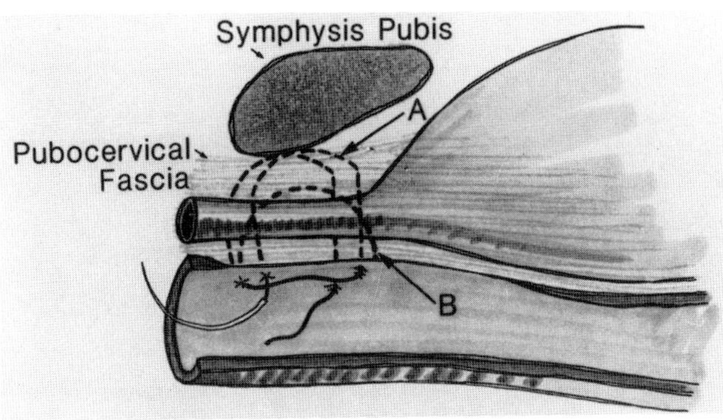

Figure 5-1.15 Technique for anterior colporrhaphy. The suture with the needle (Dexon with DT-12 needle) shows the proper placement (A) of the figure-of-eight suture in the pubocervical fascia lateral to and close to the urethra. When tied, the suture plicates the fascia lateral to and under the urethra and elevates the urethra. Arrow B points to improper placement of the suture with respect to depth and direction. *Source*: Reprinted with permission from *Obstetrics and Gynecology* (1982;59:269), Copyright © 1982, American College of Obstetricians and Gynecologists.

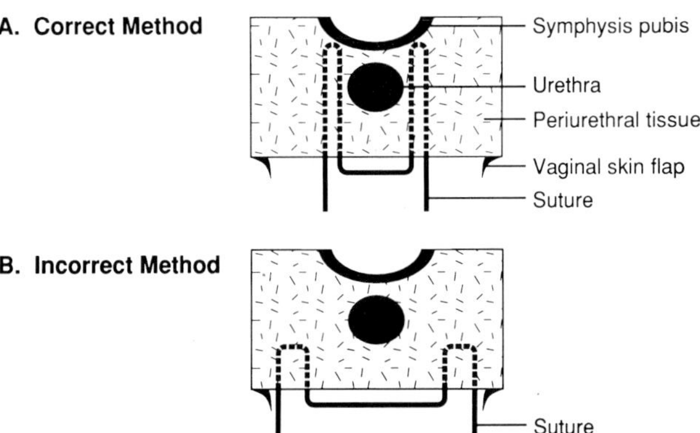

Figure 5-1.16 This diagram illustrates the correct and incorrect placement of sutures under and around the urethra. Correct placement of deep sutures close to the urethra tightens and elevates the urethra whereas incorrect placement (too shallow and too remote from the urethra) produces mimimal urethral tightening and elevation. Placement of suture, as in diagram B, may correct the urethrocele component of anterior vaginal wall prolapse but will likely result in a poor functional result in maintaining urinary continence with stress. *Source*: Reprinted with permission from *Obstetrics and Gynecology* (1991;78:1014), Copyright © 1991, American College of Obstetricians and Gynecologists.

instability and breakdown of more distal support of the urethra (creating decreased urethral closure pressures) as a wedge of urine is driven into the funneled area when the patient coughs. This suture should not be tied until sutures 5 and 6 have been placed under and around the urethra. (See Figures 5-1.12 and 5-1.13.) If the bladder neck suture is tied prematurely, it is difficult to gain mechanical access for placement of the subsequent sutures under and around the urethra. Polyglycolic suture material is used for the "Kelly"-type stitch, as well as for subsequent sutures under and around the urethra, because the pubocervical fascia in this area is much tougher than it is under the bladder base and is less likely to tear. The delayed-absorption suture material also provides prolonged stabilization of tissue during the critical first 3 weeks of healing and most of the subsequent 3 weeks. By using polyglycolic suture under and around the urethra and the more rapidly absorbed chromic catgut under the bladder base, further more rigid and fixed support is promoted differentially to the urethra than to the bladder base.

A straight metal catheter (14F) is then inserted into the bladder, so that the exact location of the urethra can be identified. (See Figure 5-1.14.) With the use of a no. 1 polyglycolic suture (1 Dexon on a DT-12 needle), which has the curvature of a 25-cent piece or a Mayo (no. 3) needle, the needle tip is inserted close to the urethra at the bladder neck on one side. The curvature of the needle is held at right angles to the surface of the vaginal wall. A deep bite of fascia is taken in a vertical manner. The tip of the needle is brought out close to the external urethral meatus, as shown in Figures 5-1.15 and 5-1.16. (See also Figures 5-1.12, 5-1.13, and 5-1.14.) As shown in Figures 5-1.13, 5-1.15, and 5-1.16, this suture (suture 5 in Figure 5-1.12) scratches the back of the symphysis pubis to ensure that it is of adequate depth. With the use of the same polyglycolic strand, this suture is then inserted in a similar manner on the other side of the urethra, as shown in Figures 5-1.12, 5-1.15, and 5-1.16. Thus, when this suture is tied, a figure-of-eight hammock is created under and around the urethra. Because these sutures are placed on either side of the urethra at right angles to the vaginal wall, the urethra is elevated more than is the base of the bladder. (The plicating sutures, under the bladder base, were placed superficially into the fascia with the long axis of the needle held parallel to the vaginal skin surface.) A second no. 1 polyglycolic suture (suture 6 in Figure 5-1.12) is placed in an identical manner as suture 5, buttressing the latter suture. These sutures go through the dense midline condensation of fascia under the urethra and through the pubourethral ligaments superior to the urethra, plicating the fascia under and along both sides of the urethra. (See Figures 5-1.8–5-1.15.) The bladder neck suture (suture 4) is then tied, and sutures 5 and 6 are tied in succession after the metal catheter has been removed. (See Figures 5-1.12 and 5-1.13.)

Some surgeons have questioned whether sutures 5 and 6 ever occlude the urethra. This is impossible, because only three sides of the urethra (the pubocervical fascia under and lateral to the urethra) are plicated and tightened. Before completing the closure of the vaginal wall with a continuous suture over the fascial repair at the bladder neck and under the urethra, urethral resistance is measured to determine whether suture placement under and around the urethra has been effective. The ligature of properly placed sutures will produce urethral closure pressures of 50 to 80 centimeters of water (cm H_2O) along the entire urethra. If urodynamic studies are not available, a catheter pull-through test can be performed. For this test, a pediatric Foley catheter (12F), with centimeter markings commencing at the balloon of the catheter, is inserted into the bladder, and the balloon is inflated with 0.5 mL of normal saline. By knowing the length of the urethra and by using the centimeter markings on the catheter (a marking pencil can be used for this purpose), the surgeon can determine the location of the catheter balloon in the urethra as it is withdrawn at 1-cm intervals. If the inflated balloon can be pulled through any given centimeter of the urethra, the resting intraurethral pressure at that point is less than 50 cm of H_2O, and the sutures should be replaced or augmented with another better placed suture under and around the urethra. If good resting urethral pressures are created, this resistance contributes significantly to the urethral–vesical pressure gradient. Good resting intraurethral closing pressures are often an indication that differentially better support has been created for the urethra, as compared to that for the bladder base. As discussed earlier, the latter anatomic relation promotes effective urethral kinking and pressure spiking with the stress of cough.

When the sutures (nos. 5 and 6) under and around the urethra have been placed properly and tied, the surgeon can also see that the proximal aspect of the urethra has been elevated effectively behind the symphysis pubis and that overcorrection of a cystocele has not occurred. As mentioned earlier, the bladder neck is normally situated 1.5 to 2 cm behind and 1.5 to 2 cm above the inferior edge of the symphysis pubis, and the bladder base should be distinctly lower than the proximal aspect of the urethra, as confirmed by transvaginal or endoscopic visual assessment. (See Figures 5-1.2–5-1.4.) After good urethral pressures (tightening of the urethra) and elevation of the proximal aspect of the urethra have been satisfactorily accomplished, closure of the vaginal skin over the fascial repair is completed with the continuous chromic catgut suture.

COMPLICATIONS AND RESULTS

In a recently reported series of 519 anterior colporrhaphies, we (Beck, McCormick, and Nordstrom) encountered a 1.2% significant complication rate (exclusive of the recurrence of incontinence or prolapse).[15] Peters and Thornton also reported a very low complication rate of 3% in 294 anterior colporrhaphies.[21] In contrast, Peters and Thornton reported a 13% significant complication rate in 127 retropubic procedures used to treat GSI, consistent with the experience of others.[21]

Using our modified technique for anterior colporrhaphy, we found a 93.5% cure rate for GSI and an 84% cure rate for selected patients with mixed incontinence.[15] We have reported a better cure rate (98.2%) for GSI using a sling procedure in a group of 170 patients with recurrent GSI.[16] However, 85% of those patients had significant problems after surgery (especially delayed voiding).[16]

In a series of 242 patients who had an anterior colporrhaphy procedure for prolapse without preoperative GSI, the incidence of new GSI following surgery was 5%.[15]

CONCLUSION

The modified anterior colporrhaphy (vaginal retropubic urethropexy plus standard cystocele repair) described in this chapter produces a cure rate that is competitive with all other procedures in treating GSI except for the sling procedure. The morbidity for the procedure is five to ten times less than the morbidity with retropubic procedures for GSI and much less than the morbidity with a sling procedure.

Parenthetically, the author uses this modified anterior colporrhaphy technique for treating patients with prolapse of the anterior vaginal wall without GSI in order to minimize the incidence of new GSI after surgery.

REFERENCES

1. Kelly HA. Incontinence of urine in women. *Urolog Cutane Rev*. 1913;17:291–293.
2. Watson BP. Imperfect urinary control following childbirth, and its surgical treatment. *Brit Med J*. 1924;2:566–568.
3. Miller NF. End-results from correction of cystocele by the simple fascia pleating method. *Surg Gynecol Obstet*. 1928;46: 403–410.
4. Kennedy WT. Incontinence of urine in the female: the urethral sphincter mechanism, damage of function and restoration of control. *Am J Obstet Gynecol*. 1937;34:576–589.
5. Heaney NS. Vaginal hysterectomy—its indications and technique. *Am J Surg*. 1940;48:284–288.
6. Kennedy WT. Incontinence of urine in the female: effective restoration and maintenance of sphincter control. *Am J Obstet Gynecol*. 1955;69:338–346.
7. Ball TL, Hoffman C Jr. Urinary stress incontinence. *Am J Obstet Gynecol*. 1963;85:96–101.
8. Zacharin RF, Gleadall LW. A modified technique for abdominal perineal urethral suspension. *Am J Obstet Gynecol*. 1963;86: 981–994.
9. Barnett RM. The modern Kelly plication. *Obstet Gynecol*. 1969;34:667–669.
10. Powell LC. Retropubic urethrocystopexy: vaginal approach. *Am J Obstet Gynecol*. 1981;140:91–97.
11. Beck RP, McCormick S. Treatment of urinary stress incontinence with anterior colporrhaphy. *Obstet Gynecol*. 1982;59: 269–274.
12. Beck RP, McCormick S, Nordstrom L. Intraurethral–intravesical cough-pressure spike differences in 267 patients surgically cured of genuine stress incontinence of urine. *Obstet Gynecol*. 1988;72:302–306.
13. Mattingly RF, Davis LE. Urinary incontinence: primary treatment of anatomic stress. *Clin Obstet Gynecol*. 1984;27:445–456.
14. Nichols DH, Ponchak SF. Treating incontinence transvaginally. *Contemp Ob/Gyn, Spec Issues*. 1988;109–115.
15. Beck RP, McCormick S, Nordstrom L. Experience with 519 anterior colporrhaphy procedures (1965–1990). *Obstet Gynecol*. 1991;78(6):1011–1018.
16. Beck RP, McCormick S, Nordstrom L. The fascia lata sling procedure for treating recurrent genuine stress incontinence of urine. *Obstet Gynecol*. 1988;72:699–703.
17. Bowen LW, Sand PK, Ostergard DR, Franti CE. Unsuccessful Burch retropubic urethropexy: a case controlled urodynamic study. *Am J Obstet Gynecol*. 1989;160:452–458.
18. Rydhstrom H, Iosif CS. Urodynamic studies before and after retropubic colpourethropexy in fertile women with stress urinary incontinence. *Arch Gynecol Obstet*. 1988;241:201–204.
19. van Geelan JM, Theeuwes AGM, Eskes AB, Martin CB. The clinical and urodynamic effects of anterior vaginal repair and Burch colposuspension. *Am J Obstet Gynecol*. 1988;159:137–144.
20. Bump RC, Fantl JA, Hurt WG. Dynamic urethral pressure profilometry pressure transmission ratio determinations after continence surgery: understanding the mechanism, failure and complications. *Obstet Gynecol*. 1988;72:870–874.
21. Peters WA, Thornton WN. Selection of the primary operative procedure for stress urinary incontinence. *Am J Obstet Gynecol*. 1980;137:923–930.

5-2

Transvaginal Needle Suspension

Mickey M. Karram

EVOLUTION OF THE PROCEDURE

In 1959, Pereyra described the first transvaginal bladder neck suspension for stress incontinence using a long needle to suspend sutures from the vagina to the anterior abdominal fascia.[1] The aim of the procedure was to combine a high cure rate with a low operative morbidity. When compared to retropubic procedures, needle procedures were quicker and did not require splitting of the anterior abdominal fascia, thus reducing perioperative and postoperative morbidity. The transvaginal approach also permitted the simultaneous correction of other pathologic findings, such as cystocele, rectocele, and enterocele.

More than 30 years later, at least 15 modifications of the original Pereyra procedure have been described. Whether stress incontinence is treated efficiently with these operations is an unresolved issue.[2] Increasing popularity of these various modifications has led to confusion among gynecologists and urologists with regard to nomenclature and procedural details.

SURGICAL ANATOMY AND TERMS

In the numerous modifications described, many different supportive tissues are used as anchoring tissue to elevate the bladder neck. Lack of a clear understanding of anatomic relations, as well as inconsistency in the terms used to describe these various tissues, has contributed to the confusion surrounding these procedures. With the exception of a few studies,[3–5] only rarely is periurethral and perivesical anatomy relative to function discussed. Tissues that have been used to anchor vaginally placed sutures have included the vaginal wall, the pubocervical fascia, the pubourethral ligaments, and the periurethral attachment to the inferior ramus of the pubic bone.

The bladder rests on the pubocervical fascia, which incorporates the entire vagina whose anterolateral sulci is attached to the tendinous arch of the pelvic fascia (the white line). The integrity of this tissue may be affected by the plane of dissection of the vaginal wall off the proximal segment of the urethra and the bladder neck. The pubocervical fascia is the anchoring tissue for sutures, or a vaginal buffer in the Stamey modification.[6]

The periurethral attachment to the pubic bone has more commonly been referred to as *endopelvic fascia*. To obtain this tissue, there must be either blunt or sharp dissection into the retropubic space to free this attachment from the pubic bone. When the retropubic space is entered sharply, the tips of the scissors are most likely to enter the space medial to the arcus tendineus fasciae pelvis and lateral to the vaginal veins. The medial aspect of this incision is the desired location for placement of transvaginal sutures for the modified Pereyra procedure.[7] This tissue is the medial condensation of endopelvic fascia that is densely adherent to the urogenital diaphragm lying immediately beneath it.[8]

The pubourethral ligaments are composed of an anterior and a posterior band. The posterior pubourethral ligament is believed to be an important structure with regard to urethral support and, thus, the development of stress incontinence. It has recently been identified as a dense band of connective tissue, which can be seen beside the urethra arising primarily from the vagina and the periurethral tissue to attach laterally to the pelvic wall. There are two components of this lateral attachment: the fascial attachment to the arcus tendineus fasciae pelvis and a muscular attachment to the medial edge of the levator ani muscle.[9] In Pereyra's final modification, he included these structures in his helical suture of endopelvic fascia and claimed that, when elevated retropubically, the suture held the posterior ligament firmly against the pubic bone.[7]

Finally, some modifications have included the use of the vaginal wall either in its full thickness[10] or excluding the epithelium.[11]

INDICATIONS

Transvaginal needle suspension procedures are performed to correct anatomic stress incontinence. The goal of these operations is to elevate and support the proximal urethra and bladder neck, thus achieving continence by improving pressure transmission to the proximal urethra during increased intra-abdominal pressure. Although various modifications of needle suspension procedures have been advocated for the correction of what has been termed a *type III urethra*[6] (poorly functioning urethral sphincteric mechanism at rest with or without urethral mobility), other procedures, such as placement of suburethral slings, and artificial sphincters, or periurethral injections, probably yield better results.

To diagnose GSI, the urethra is shown to be incompetent by demonstrating observable loss of urine during increases in intra-abdominal pressure by means of clinical observation or urodynamic techniques. Detrusor instability can coexist with urethral sphincteric incompetence up to 30% of the time,[12,13] and mixed incontinence may be associated with a lower cure rate after needle suspension procedures.

TECHNIQUES

There are five needle suspension procedures commonly used to correct GSI:

1. Pereyra procedure
2. Stamey procedure
3. Raz procedure
4. Gittes procedure
5. Muzsnai procedure

Each procedure is described in the following discussion, and pertinent aspects of the techniques are illustrated. A comparison of the various anchoring sutures used in all five procedures is provided in Figure 5-2.1. Table 5-2.1 notes the differences among the procedures.

Pereyra Procedure

The Pereyra procedure was first described in 1959.[1] In the original technique a special needle is passed through an abdominal stab incision and penetrates the unopened vaginal mucosa. Extension of a stylet results in a Y-shaped, double unilateral vaginal penetration. Subsequent placement of a suture and needle withdrawal results in vaginal wall elevation. The original suture material described was no. 30 steel wire, which ultimately penetrated the epithelium into the fibrous tissue of the vaginal wall. Thus the original technique was a no-incision needle suspension and is almost identical to a recently popularized procedure (the Gittes procedure),[10] which is discussed in more detail later.

Because the wire loops eventually cut through the vagina, resulting in recurrent anatomic defects, Pereyra and Lebherz, working independently, reported on their first modification in 1967. This report summarized their experience with a technique for suprapubic urethrovesical angulation and suspension in conjunction with vesical neck plication to create a suburethral shelf. The theory was that the plication sutures helped relieve some of the strain placed on the suspensory sutures.[14]

Because longer follow-up of the 1967 modification revealed recurrences due to cutting through and pulling out of catgut sutures from the periurethral tissue, Pereyra and Lebherz described their second modification in 1978. They believed that, to minimize the incidence of bladder injury, the retropubic space had to be exposed completely per vagina, so that each step of the operation could be performed under direct vision.

In this modification, Pereyra and Lebherz described entering the retropubic space through the vagina. The anterolateral attachments of the periurethral tissue to the inferior pubic ramus are released by means of blunt dissection from the level of the urethrovesical junction up to, but not including, the attachments of the urethral meatus (Figure 5-2.2). The endopelvic fascia is then brought down into the vaginal field (Figure 5-2.3), and a polypropylene suture is passed in a helical fashion several times through this detached fascia (endopelvic fascia). Traction on both suture ends results in ruffling and

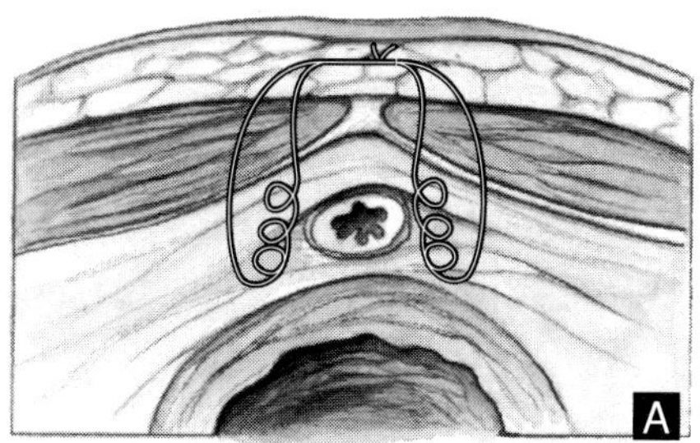

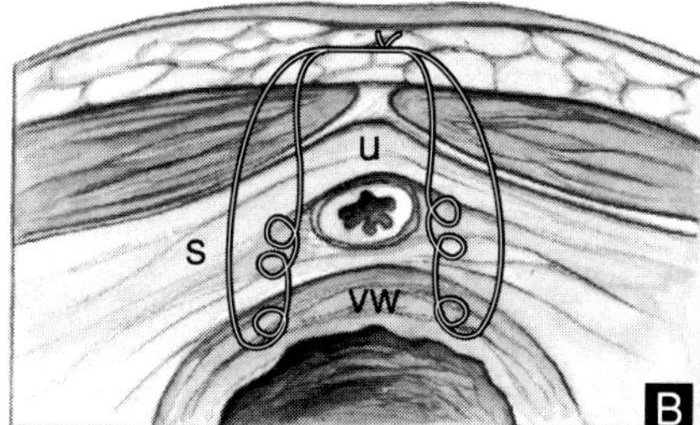

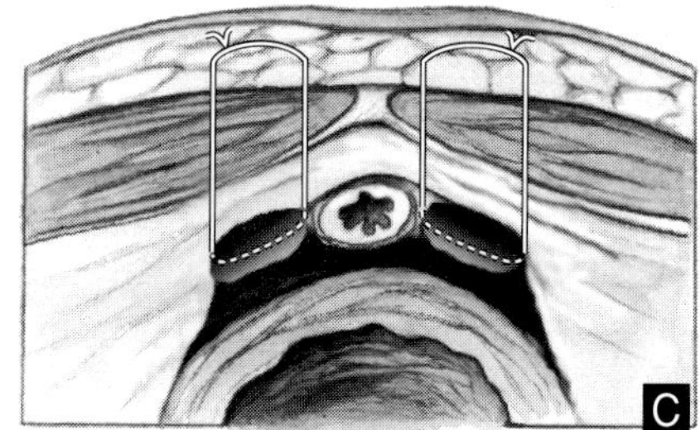

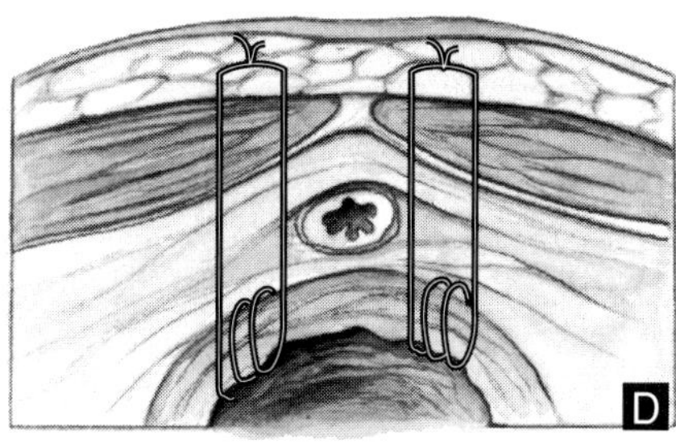

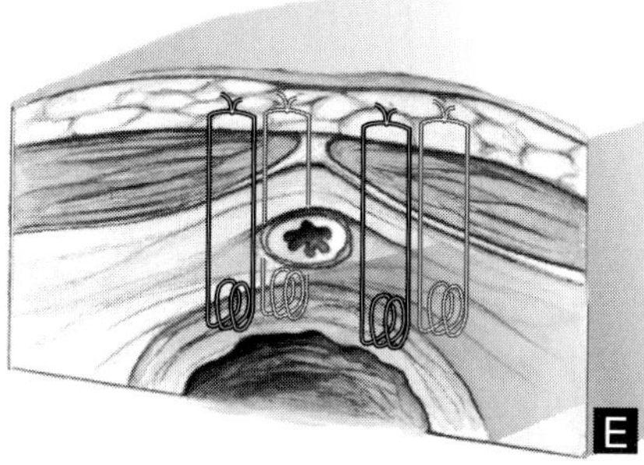

Figure 5-2.1 Cross-sectional view of various anchoring sutures used in commonly performed needle procedures. **A,** Modified Pereyra procedure—helical stitch through pubourethral ligament and detached endopelvic fascia. **B,** Raz procedure—helical stitch through detached endopelvic fascia and anchored in vaginal wall. **C,** Stamey procedure—buttresses placed in pubocervical fascia on each side of bladder neck. **D,** Gittes procedure—stitches through full thickness of vaginal wall. **E,** Muzsnai procedure—two stitches on each side through vaginal wall (excluding epithelium).

Table 5-2.1 Differences among Various Needle Suspension Procedures

Procedure	*Vaginal Incision*	*Needle Passage*	*Anchoring Tissue*	*Use of Cystoscopy*
Modified Pereyra	Midline	Under direct finger guidance	Pubourethral ligament and endopelvic fascia	To ensure no injury has occurred
Stamey	T-shaped	Blindly	Pubocervical fascia	To confirm proper needle and suture placement
Raz	Inverted U	Under direct finger guidance	Endopelvic fascia and vaginal wall	To ensure no injury has occurred
Gittes	None	Blindly	Full thickness of vaginal wall	To confirm proper needle and suture placement
Muzsnai	Midline	Under direct finger guidance	Vaginal wall (excluding epithelium)	To ensure no injury has occurred

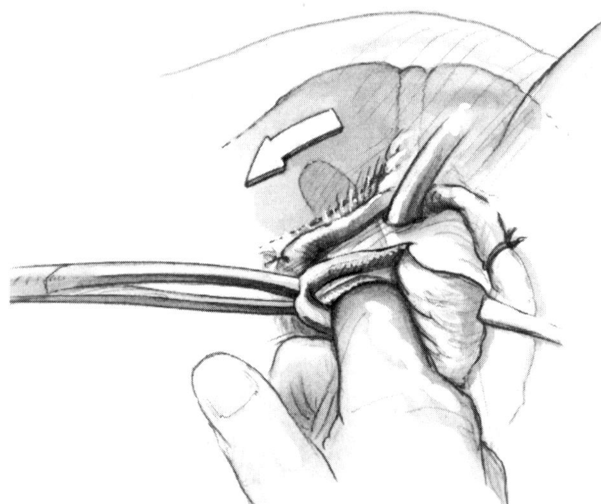

Figure 5-2.2 Technique of blunt dissection into retropubic space. With tip of index finger flexed anteriorly against posterior symphysis pubis, paraurethral attachment to pubic bone is perforated downward (in direction of *arrow*) toward ischial spine, completely detaching endopelvic fascia.

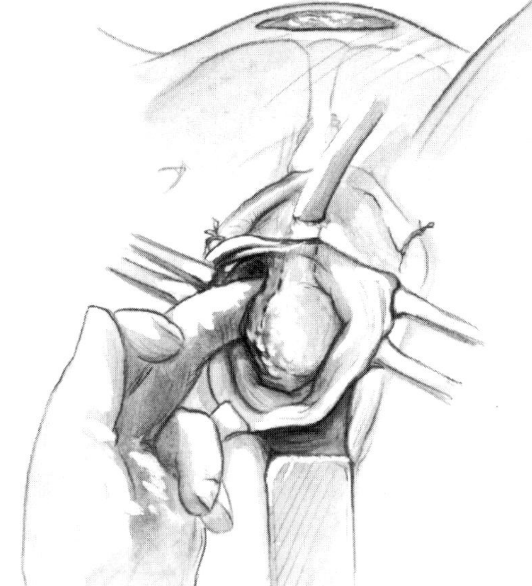

Figure 5-2.3 One finger is placed behind detached endopelvic fascia, mobilizing it into vaginal field to facilitate placement of helical suture.

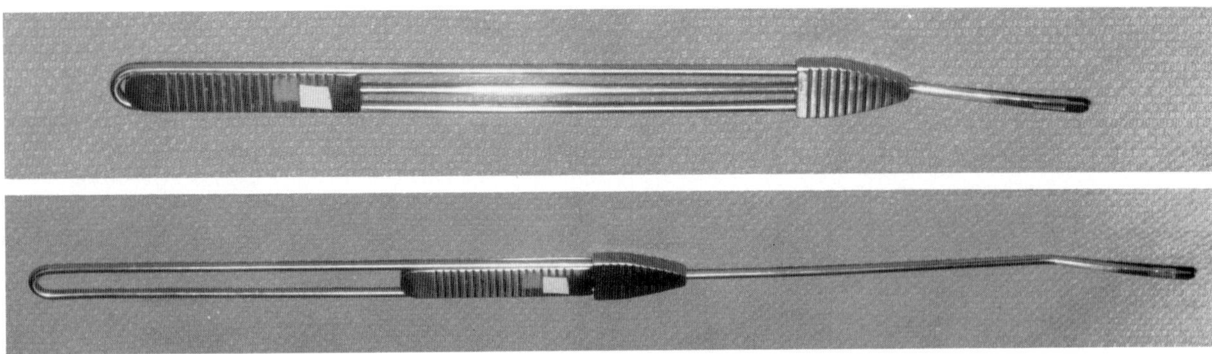

Figure 5-2.4 Pereyra ligature carrier. *Source:* Courtesy of El Ney Industries, Inc., Upland, CA.

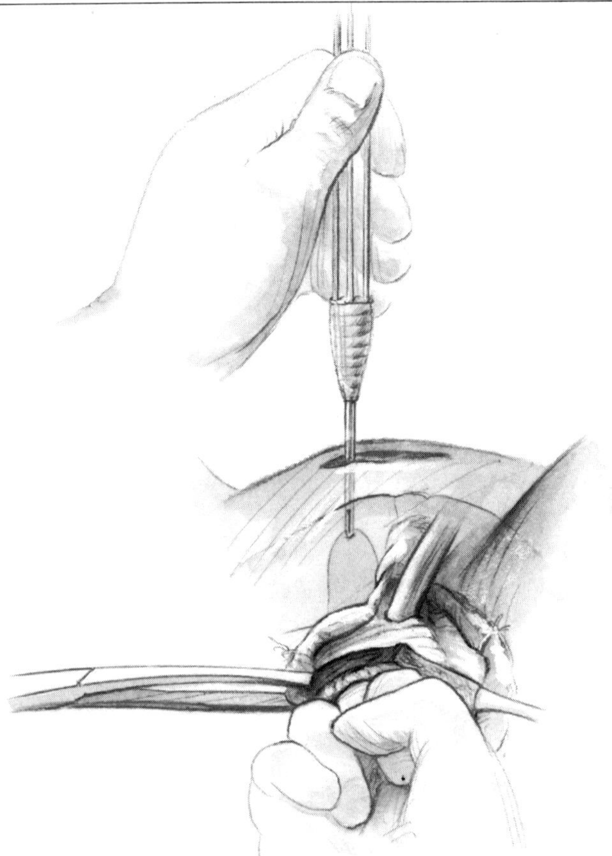

Figure 5-2.5 Passage of needle is under direct finger guidance. Finger in vagina is inserted to posterior aspect of rectus muscle.

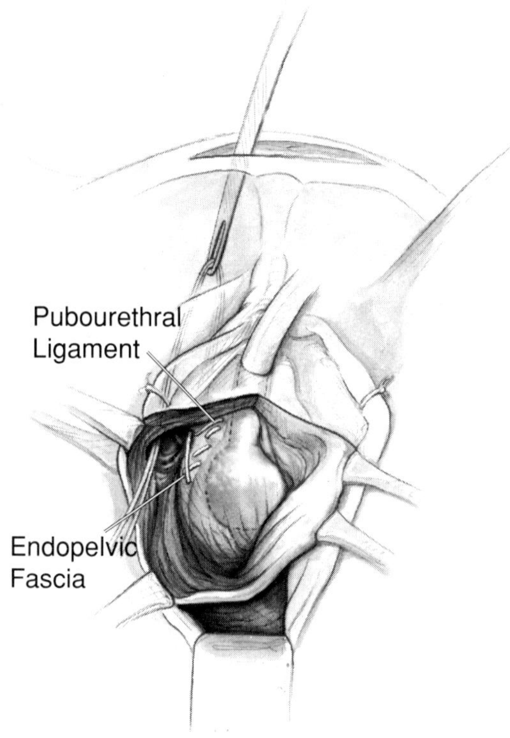

Figure 5-2.6 Modified Pereyra procedure. Permanent suture is anchored in pubourethral ligament. Numerous passes are then taken through detached endopelvic fascia.

thickening of the periurethral tissues, producing multiple pleats to impede the polypropylene sutures from pulling through. This revised procedure was safer because the surgeon's finger could be inserted vaginally to the rectus muscle to provide direct guidance of the Pereyra ligature carrier (Figure 5-2.4) through the retropubic space (Figure 5-2.5). With the use of an aneurysm needle, the suspensory sutures are anchored into the anterior rectus fascia.

Reports on the second modification included procedures performed on patients between 1974 and 1977.[14] In the latter portion of 1978, Pereyra believed that the revised procedure was incomplete because it did not include the posterior pubourethral ligaments in the suspensory sutures, even though the procedure laid open to view laterally the posterior pillars of the pubourethral ligaments.[15] He believed that including the posterior pubourethral pillars in the helical suture with the detached endopelvic fascia would provide maximal resistance to suspensory suture penetration. This final modification is what is known today as the modified Pereyra procedure[7] (Figure 5-2.6).

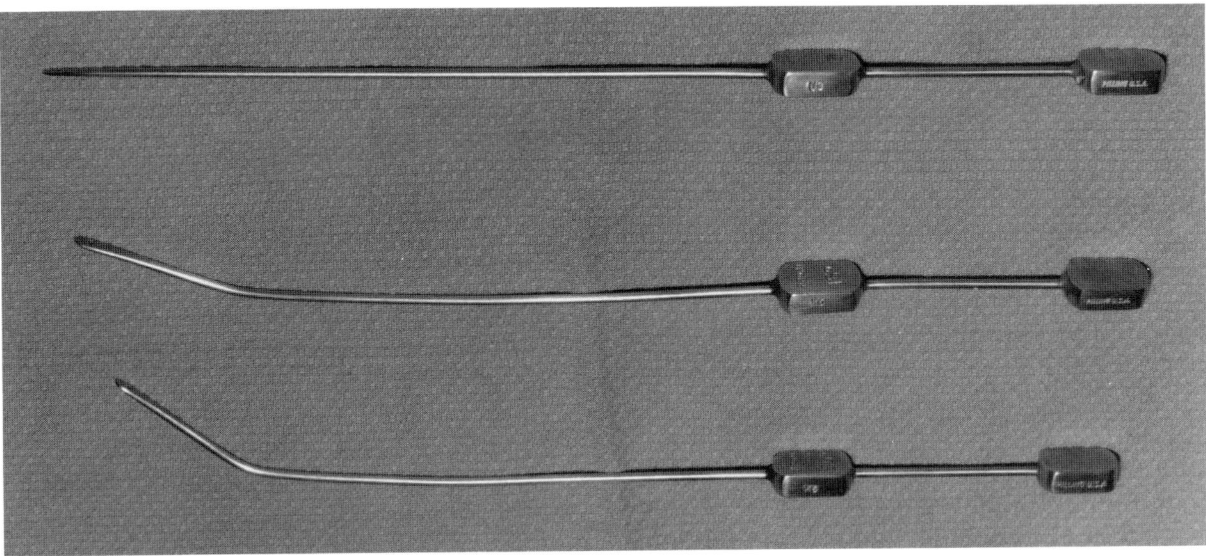

Figure 5-2.7 Series of Stamey needles: straight needle (*top*), 15-degree angled needle (*middle*), and 30-degree angled needle (*bottom*). *Source:* Courtesy of Pilling Company, Fort Washington, PA.

Stamey Procedure

Once Pereyra demonstrated the feasibility of suspending the pubocervical fascia to the abdominal wall by passing a suture through a special needle, many other investigators began to modify his techniques. Stamey believed that an appealing way to restore the posterior urethrovesical angle with great accuracy was to visualize the urethrovesical junction directly through the cystoscope while placing heavy monofilament suture on each side of the vesical neck. The idea was to raise a broad band of tissue on each side of the vesical neck, extending from the pubocervical fascia to the anterior rectus fascia.

In the Stamey procedure, 2 transverse suprapubic skin incisions are made on each side of the midline, 2 to 4 cm in length and about 2 to 3 fingerbreadths above the upper border of the symphysis pubis. A T-shaped vaginal incision is then made, and the vaginal wall is separated from the overlying urethra and trigone. One of three special long needles, angled at different degrees, is passed vertically alongside the vesical neck (Figure 5-2.7). A cystoscope is inserted to ensure that lateral motion of the needle produces an indentation on the bladder wall at the vesical neck. Once proper placement of the needle is assured, the tip is passed into the vagina and threaded with a no. 2 monofilament nylon suture and then withdrawn suprapubically. The needle is again passed through the same incision about 1 to 2 cm lateral to the original entry. It should exit in the vagina about 1 cm distal to the nylon suture. The vaginal end of the nylon suture is threaded through the eye of the needle and pulled out suprapubically. A broad band of tissue along one side of the vesical neck is within the nylon loop. If the integrity of the pubocervical tissue is poor and the tissue is unlikely to hold, the nylon suture can be passed through a 1 cm length of 5 mm surgical polyester fiber (Dacron) to buttress the vaginal loop (Figure 5-2.8).[16,17,18]

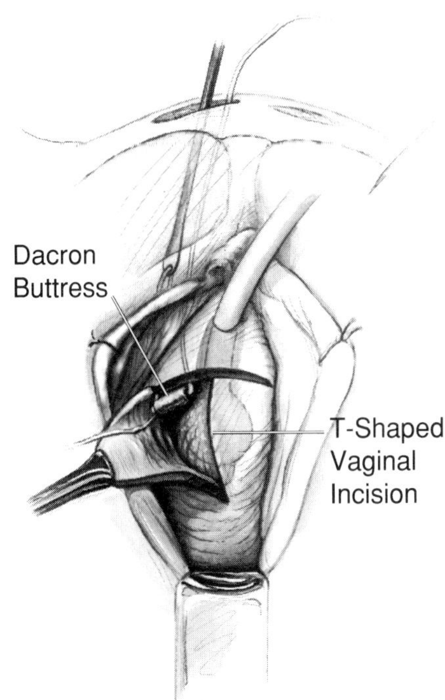

Figure 5-2.8 Stamey procedure. Surgical polyester fiber (Dacron) loops are placed in pubovesical–cervical fascia on each side of bladder neck. They are suspended to anterior rectus fascia with nylon sutures.

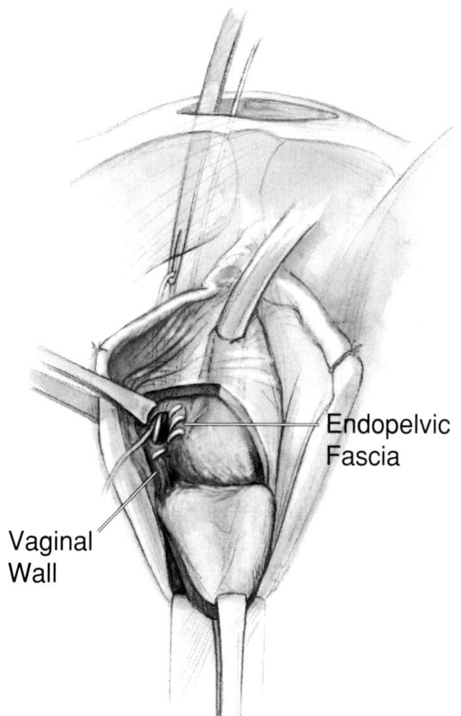

Figure 5-2.9 Raz procedure. Helical suture is taken through detached endopelvic fascia and anchored in full thickness of vaginal wall (excluding epithelium).

Raz Procedure

The Raz modification differs from the 1978 modification of the Pereyra procedure in that an inverted U incision is used on the anterior wall of the vagina to allow vaginal dissection lateral to the urethra and bladder neck. The suspension sutures are anchored not only in the endopelvic fascia but also through the full thickness of the vaginal wall, excluding the epithelium (Figure 5-2.9). Sutures are passed suprapubically under direct finger guidance. Cystoscopy is performed to inspect for any injury to the urethra, the bladder, or the ureters and to verify adequate bladder neck elevation. The claimed advantage over the modified Pereyra procedure is that anchoring the suspension sutures in the vaginal wall lateral to the urethra precludes the possibility of permanent urinary retention caused by overzealous traction on the sutures.[19]

Gittes Procedure

In 1987, Gittes and Loughlin described a no-incision pubovaginal suspension procedure for stress incontinence.[10] No vaginal incision is made in this procedure.

A small puncture is made in the suprapubic skin and subcutaneous tissue, 2 cm superior to the pubic bone and 5 cm lateral to the midline on each side. A long mattress-type needle, or Stamey needle, with a 30-degree deflection is passed through the subcutaneous tissue and rectus fascia. The tip is advanced carefully down the posterior aspect of the pubic bone. The surgeon's other hand elevates the anterior wall of the vagina lateral to the bladder neck, as palpated with the aid of a Foley catheter balloon. The tip is then popped through the vaginal wall.

A no. 2 nylon suture is threaded into the eye of the needle and withdrawn to the suprapubic area. A second pass of the needle is then made through a different site on the rectus fascia. The second perforation site on the vaginal wall is selected tactilely and visually to be 1.5 to 2 cm cephalad or caudad to the first puncture site. A free needle is used to anchor the suture into the anterior vaginal wall that stretches between the first and the second vaginal perforations. The mattress suture is threaded and passed forward (Figure 5-2.10). Cystourethroscopy is performed during passage of the sutures to detect any bladder damage or penetration by suture material. The sutures are tied tightly into the stab incision, resulting in elevation of the anterior wall of the vagina. The tied sutures are pulled upward and trimmed just above the knot, which then retracts below the skin. The tension on these tissues has been noted to relax slightly after 1 to 2 days.[10]

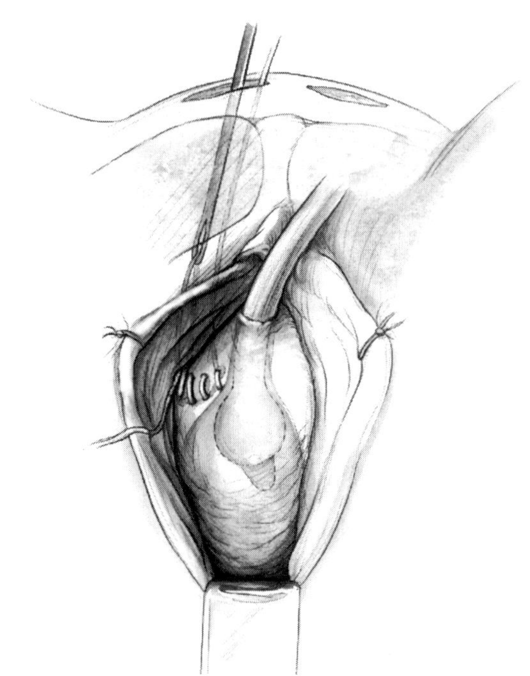

Figure 5-2.10 Gittes procedure. Stitches are taken through full thickness of vaginal wall and transferred suprapubically. No vaginal incision is made.

Muzsnai Procedure

In 1982, Muzsnai and co-workers reported results on a new needle suspension procedure that used the full thickness of the vaginal wall, excluding the epithelium, as anchoring tissue, thus performing a vaginal colposuspension.[11] A Foley catheter with a 30-cc balloon is used for easy identification of the bladder neck. The level of the bladder neck is marked on each side of the vagina before surgery is begun.

A midline anterior vaginal wall incision is used, extending to approximately 2 cm proximal to the external urethral meatus. The incision should be carried through the full thickness of the vaginal wall, including the loose connective tissue. Sharp dissection is used to separate the vaginal wall from the bladder anterior and lateral to the pubic rami. Thus two vaginal flaps are created, leaving the urethra and the vesical wall denuded.

At the level of the bladder neck, the anterolateral attachment of the periurethral tissue to the inferior ramus of the pubic bone is sharply (Figure 5-2.11) or bluntly (see Figure 5-2.2) separated, allowing access into the retropubic space. The endopelvic fascia is completely detached and freed from the pubic bone, thus mobilizing the bladder neck. Nonabsorbable suture is then placed through the inner surface of the vaginal wall. One helical suture is taken from the level of the midurethra to the bladder neck, and a second suture is placed from the bladder neck down to the level of the bladder base. A finger is placed on the outside of the vagina to ensure that the sutures do not penetrate the vaginal epithelium. These sutures are taken approximately 1.5 to 2 cm inside the edge of each vaginal flap (Figure 5-2.12). In patients with severe relaxation of the anterior vaginal wall, in which the surgeon anticipates trimming some vaginal wall, the sutures should be 2 cm inside the trimmed edge. In instances in which the vaginal wall is very thin, the sutures can be passed through the detached endopelvic fascia, either in conjunction with or separate from the vaginal wall. A Pereyra needle (Figure 5-2.4) is then used to transfer these sutures to the suprapubic area under direct finger guidance. If necessary, an anterior colporrhaphy is performed at this time. Cystourethroscopy is performed to ensure that no inadvertent bladder injury or stitch penetration has occurred. Five milliliters of indigo-carmine solution is given intravenously to help visualize and ensure patency of the ureters.

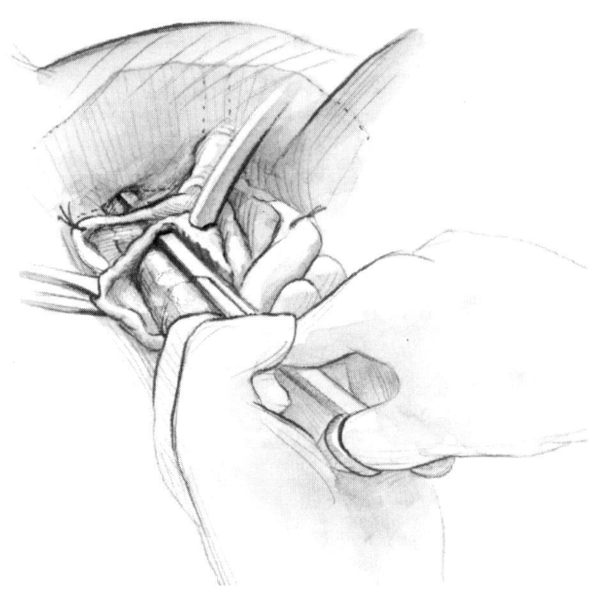

Figure 5-2.11 Technique of vaginal entrance into retropubic space with use of Metzenbaum scissors. Endopelvic fascia is perforated at inferior margin of pubic bone, as guided by surgeon's index finger. Blades of scissors are separated, and dissection is completed by inserting one finger into space created (as demonstrated in Figure 5-2.2).

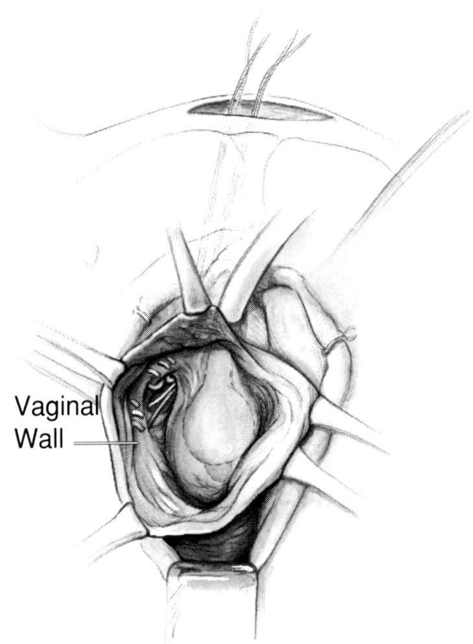

Figure 5-2.12 Muzsnai procedure. Permanent sutures are taken through full thickness of vaginal wall (excluding epithelium). Two stitches are placed on each side and transferred suprapubically under direct finger guidance.

The vagina is closed with interrupted 3-0 sutures. With a hand elevating the anterior vaginal wall, the suprapubic stitches are tied down, so that there is a small amount of dimpling in the lateral area of the vaginal fornix on each side, thus simulating the abdominal colposuspension (modified Burch procedure).

COMBINED NEEDLE SUSPENSION–SLING PROCEDURES

Some investigators have advocated a simplified sling procedure, with the use of a suburethral patch of tissue suspended by sutures to the anterior rectus fascia, for patients with stress incontinence related to a poorly functioning urethra (type III urethra).[20,21] The proposed advantages over more conventional sling procedures are that there is less extensive dissection, less postoperative voiding dysfunction, and it is also easier and quicker to perform.

A patch of autologous or synthetic tissue is fixed to the suburethra from a level just distal to the midurethra to approximately 1 cm beyond the bladder neck. One or two permanent sutures are passed through the long axis of the patch. These sutures are then passed to the suprapubic area with the use of a Pereyra needle and tied above the anterior rectus fascia (Figure 5-2.13).

Raz and co-workers published their experience with a vaginal wall sling. A full-thickness island of the anterior wall of the vagina with its squamous epithelium left in place is suspended with sutures to the anterior rectus fascia. A posterior flap of the vagina is then advanced to bury the suspended vagina.[22]

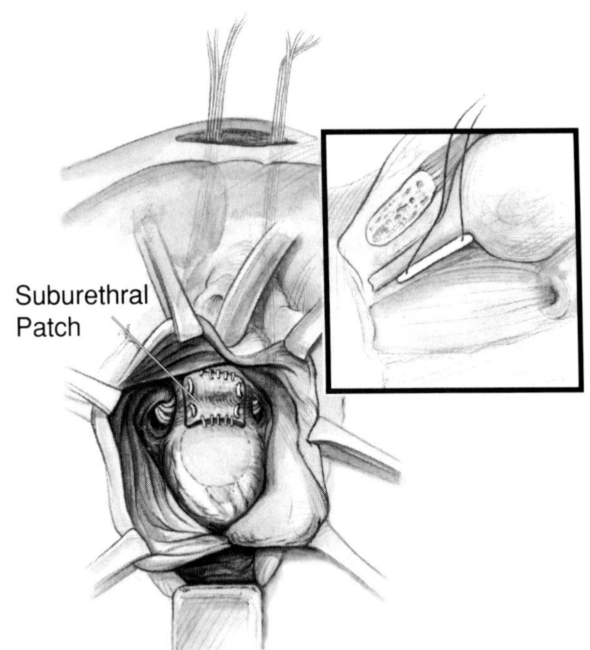

Figure 5-2.13 Combined needle suspension–sling procedure. Suburethral patch of tissue is suspended with permanent sutures to anterior rectus fascia.

RESULTS

The evaluation of any surgery for the correction of stress incontinence is hampered by several factors. First, the diagnostic criteria, including the need for urodynamic testing, are controversial. Second, variations in patient populations, including history of prior pelvic surgery, age, weight, childbearing history, associated medical conditions, and coexistent detrusor instability, influence the surgical success rates. Third, variations in surgical technique, including modifications of a so-called standard procedure, may be significant. Finally, and probably most importantly, the length and method of follow-up for these patients vary greatly. How long must a patient remain continent, and what constitutes a cure or failure?

Many investigators have reported clinical experiences with needle suspension procedures. Unfortunately, most of these studies are by modern standards methodologically flawed. The major problem with most studies is that objective parameters were not used preoperatively and postoperatively to establish diagnosis and outcome of surgery. In a review of published results of needle suspension procedures a cure rate of 85% for more than 1950 procedures was noted. However, most of these studies were based on subjective criteria for cure, and the follow-up periods were relatively short. Also, it was noted that in only three studies, with a total of 60 patients, were objective urodynamic criteria used preoperatively and postoperatively.[2]

Other investigators have reported objective results with much lower cure rates. Probably the best published data are two prospective randomized studies by Bergman and co-workers.[23,24] They compared the Burch urethropexy, to the modified Pereyra procedure, to an anterior colporrhaphy in patients with GSI with associated pelvic relaxation defects (289 patients)[24] as well as in patients with the isolated finding of GSI (107 patients).[23] The studies were randomized both for the procedure and for the surgeon. All patients underwent preoperative and postoperative urodynamic studies, and the minimum follow-up time was 1 year. The cure rate for the Burch procedure (88%) was significantly higher than that for the anterior colporrhaphy (67%) and the modified Pereyra procedure (68%). Weil and co-workers studied 86 patients clinically and urodynamically at least 6 months following a Burch urethropexy, modified Pereyra procedure, or anterior colporrhaphy and noted similar results[25] (see Table 5-2.2). Reports on the Stamey procedure have also noted objective cure rates in the 65% range at 3 to

Table 5-2.2 Published Studies on Needle Suspension Procedures in Which Preoperative and Postoperative Urodynamic Studies Were Performed

			Cure Rate (%) by Procedure				
Investigator(s)	*No. of Patients*	*Follow-up Period*	*Stamey*	*Pereyra*	*Burch*	*AR*	*Sling*
Bergman et al[24]	289	1 yr		70	87	69	
Bergman et al[23]	107	1 yr		65	89	67	
Weil et al[25]	86	6 mo		50	91	57	
Griffith-Jones and Abrams[29]	17	9 mo	76				
English and Fowler[26]	45	6 mo	58				
Peattie and Stanton[27]	44	3 mo	40				
Mundy[28]	51	1 yr	40		73		
Hilton[30]	21	6 mo	80				90
Karram et al[31]	103	1 yr		60			
Bhatia and Bergman[32]	64	1 yr		85	98		
Leach et al[33]	20	14 mo		90			

AR, Anterior repair

6 months' follow-up.[26] Peattie and Stanton noted only a 40% success rate after a Stamey procedure in women over the age of 65.[27] Mundy also noted an objective cure rate of only 40% in patients 12 months after a Stamey procedure.[28]

To date, there are no published objective data on the results of the no-incision urethropexy (Gittes procedure).[10] The only study on the Muzsnai procedure involved 98 patients.[11] All patients were monitored for a minimum of 6 months with a 95% cure rate (four failures) reported. Cure was defined as no subjective complaints of incontinence, and no visual loss of urine during coughing at the time of follow-up.

Table 5-2.2 lists all published studies on needle suspension procedures in which preoperative and postoperative urodynamic studies were performed.

COMPLICATIONS

Complications of needle suspension procedures can be classified broadly into those mutual to all needle suspension procedures and those associated with specific modifications of the procedures.

1. Infection

Infection can occur after any of the procedures but is probably more common in Stamey-type procedures in which Dacron or silicon buttresses are used. Because most surgeons use permanent suture when performing these procedures, stitch abscesses can occur and present vaginally or suprapubically. Abscesses rarely occur in the immediate postoperative period but can present months and even years postoperatively. Whether the routine use of prophylactic antibiotics is indicated has not been adequately addressed in the literature.

2. Hemorrhage

Hemorrhage is more common after modifications in which the retropubic space is entered. While doing this, a significant amount of venous bleeding, which is usually from perforating vessels at the medial edge of the periurethral attachment to the pubic bone, may occur. Surprisingly, bleeding from the retropubic space is almost always self-limited, even though it can appear to be severe at the time of surgery. A recent study reported on the results of 103 modified Pereyra procedures in which 7% of patients required blood transfusion and no patient required re-exploration to control active bleeding or evacuate a hematoma.[31] When excessive, uncontrollable bleeding occurs from the retropubic space, transvaginal tamponade can be achieved by inserting a Foley catheter with a 30 cc balloon into the bleeding space, as described by Katske and Raz.[34] Gauze packing is inserted around the catheter, and the catheter balloon is inflated until adequate tamponade is achieved.

3. Voiding Dysfunction

Voiding dysfunction is a potential complication of any anti-incontinence procedure. In this author's experience, needle suspension procedures have been more obstructive than retropubic procedures in the immediate postoperative period. In numerous studies, however, a low incidence of long-term voiding dysfunction has been noted.[35,36] Patients with severe anterior vaginal wall relaxation, those with preoperative high postvoid residual urine volumes, and those with underactive or areflexic detrusor muscles, as demonstrated with pressure-flow studies, are at high risk for prolonged voiding dysfunction[37] and should be taught intermittent self-catheterization preoperatively.

4. Detrusor Instability

Detrusor instability is a common cause of either persistence or recurrence of incontinence following surgery for GSI. Its presence should be aggressively sought out when anti-incontinence surgery is being contemplated as it has been shown to coexist in up to 30% of patients with GSI.[12,13] The postoperative course of detrusor instability is unpredictable as it may persist, worsen, improve, or develop de novo.[12,13] Its course has been studied more thoroughly after retropubic bladder neck suspensions than after needle suspension procedures.[38] All patients should be warned preoperatively that they may require anticholinergic medications postoperatively.

5. Lower Urinary Tract Injury

Cystotomy can occur during any of the steps of vaginal dissection and is probably more common during secondary procedures. In the modified Pereyra procedure, dissection directly on the medial aspect of the ischial pubic ramus, during mobilization of the bladder neck and entrance of the retropubic space, minimizes bladder injury. The modified Pereyra procedure permits finger-tip control of needle passage through the retropubic space to the vagina, thus minimizing the risk of injury to the bladder and the urethra. This advantage is not offered with the Stamey or Gittes modifications. With routine use of intraoperative cystoscopy, urinary tract injury should always be recognized. If a suture is inadvertently passed through the anterolateral part of the bladder, it should be removed and passed again under finger-tip guidance. Nonrecognition of a penetrating suture or intravesical migration of a permanent suture can lead to chronic infection and stone formation. Thus any patient with recurrent urinary tract infection or irritative symptoms who has undergone a previous suspension should have a radiographic and endoscopic evaluation to rule out this diagnosis.

Urethral injuries are rare but may occur. When urethral injury is recognized, immediate closure with long-term catheter drainage is recommended.[39]

6. Nerve Damage

Because the patient is in a dorsal lithotomy position during needle suspension procedures, neural injury can occur. This injury is most commonly related to direct compression of the nerve against various structures and may result in a first-degree injury (neuropraxia), which spontaneously resolves in 1 to 6 weeks. Rarely, a second-degree injury (axonotmesis) may occur, which takes 2 to 6 months to resolve. The most frequent nerve involved is the common peroneal nerve, but injury to the obturator, sciatic, tibial, femoral, or saphenous nerves can also occur (Table 5-2.3). After early recognition, appropriate neurologic and physical medicine consultations are recommended.[40]

Another category of nerve injury is a nerve entrapment of the ilioinguinal nerve which can occur when the sutures used in suspension of the bladder neck are tied above the anterior rectus fascia. Patients with this injury will complain of localized pain in the medial portion of the groin, labia, or inner thigh. The character of the pain varies from severe constant burning pain to sharp shooting pain. The pain is uniformly aggravated by straining and by attempts to lift the ipsilateral leg. This type of nerve injury has been reported in as many as 16% of patients undergoing transvaginal needle suspensions.[36,41] The nerve is most vulnerable to entrapment near its exit from the superficial inguinal ring, which lies almost directly above the pubic tubercle. Thus, to avert injury, sutures should always be passed medial to the pubic tubercle. When injury is suspected, the diagnosis is confirmed by means of a local nerve block in the inguinal canal, with 10 to 15 mL of 1% lidocaine hydrochloride (xylocaine). Initial management of this type of pain should include administration of analgesics and anti-inflammatory agents. The decision to untie and reposition the offending sutures depends on the severity and duration of pain.

Table 5-2.3 Nerves That Can Be Injured during Needle Suspension Procedures

Nerve	*Mechanism of Injury*	*Clinical Presentation*
Common Peroneal	Direct compression between fibular neck and leg brace	Footdrop
Sciatic	Pressure against sciatic notch or stretching of nerve during hip flexion	Weakness during knee flexion, or variable loss of common peroneal or tibial nerve function
Obturator	Compression of nerve at undersurface of pubic ramus	Weakness of ipsilateral thigh on adduction
Femoral	Hyperflexion of hips, compressing femoral nerve against inguinal ligament	Quadriceps weakness; gait impairment; decreased sensation over anterior thigh and medial calf
Saphenous	Hyperflexion of hips, creating undue stretch of nerve against medial aspect of knee	Burning or aching pain in medial calf
Ilioinguinal	Entrapment of nerve by suture when needle passed lateral to pubic tubercle	Pain in medial groin, labia, or inner thigh

7. Immediate Postoperative Urinary Incontinence

The immediate demonstration of urinary incontinence after surgery for stress incontinence is a very distressing finding to both patient and physician. The surgeon must differentiate among persistent stress incontinence, overflow incontinence, detrusor instability, lower urinary tract fistula, urinary tract infection, or a watery vaginal discharge simulating urinary incontinence.

Persistent stress incontinence is due most commonly to failure of the surgical procedure to stabilize and support the bladder neck (anatomic genuine stress incontinence). Rarely it is due to the development of a type III or poorly functioning urethra.

Overflow incontinence is a manifestation of iatrogenic retention, and can be managed with a combination of fluid restriction and self-catheterization.

As has been previously mentioned, detrusor instability can develop de novo after bladder neck suspension. This type of detrusor instability usually responds to anticholinergic therapy and is self-limited, undergoing spontaneous resolution within 3 months after surgery.[12,13]

CONCLUSION

On the basis of recently published objective studies, in the author's opinion, the procedure of choice for anatomic genuine stress incontinence is a retropubic urethropexy. Needle suspension procedures are reserved for elderly patients with medical disabilities, in whom anesthetic and operative times are best kept at a minimum; continent patients with marked relaxation of the anterior vaginal wall (potential stress incontinence); and patients with severe pelvic prolapse as a primary complaint who also have coexistent mild stress incontinence as a secondary complaint.

The author's needle procedure of choice is a vaginal colposuspension similar to that described by Muzsnai. The potential advantages of this modification are (1) use of a strong anchoring tissue (ie, full thickness of the vaginal wall); (2) complete mobilization of the bladder neck; (3) passage of the needle under direct finger guidance; and (4) facilitation of anterior vaginal wall support. These potential advantages await confirmation through controlled randomized trials.

These operations are still evolving as many procedural details remain controversial. Many of the currently held beliefs have been advocated empirically with very little supportive data. There is a definite advantage, in certain patients, to correct stress incontinence vaginally. It is hoped that continued experience with these procedures will lead to modifications, resulting in better long-term cure rates.

REFERENCES

1. Pereyra AJ. A simplified surgical procedure for the correction of stress incontinence in women. *West J Surg*. 1959;67:223–226.

2. Karram MM, Bhatia NN. Transvaginal needle bladder neck suspension procedures for stress urinary incontinence: a comprehensive review. *Obstet Gynecol*. 1989;73:906–914.

3. DeLancey JOL. Correlative study of paraurethral anatomy. *Obstet Gynecol*. 1986;68:91–97.

4. Richardson AC, Lyon JB, Williams NL. A new look at pelvic relaxation. *Am J Obstet Gynecol*. 1976;126:568–573.

5. DeLancey JOL. Structural aspects of the extrinsic continence mechanism. *Obstet Gynecol*. 1988;72:296–301.

6. Stamey TA. Endoscopic suspension of vesical neck for urinary incontinence. *Surg Gynecol Obstet*. 1973;136:547–554.

7. Pereyra AJ, Lebherz TB, Growdon WA, Powers JA. Pubourethral supports in perspective: modified Pereyra procedure for urinary incontinence. *Obstet Gynecol*. 1982;59:643–648.

8. Mostwin JL. Current concepts of female pelvic anatomy and physiology. *Urol Clin North Am*. 1991;18:175–197.

9. DeLancey JOL. Pubovesical ligament: a separate structure from the urethral supports ("pubo-urethral ligaments"). *Neurourol Urodyn*. 1989;8:53–61.

10. Gittes RF, Loughlin KR. No-incision pubovaginal suspension for stress incontinence. *J Urol*. 1987;138:568–570.

11. Muzsnai D, Carrillo E, Dubin C, Silverman I. Retropubic vaginopexy for correction of urinary stress incontinence. *Obstet Gynecol*. 1982;59:113–117.

12. Karram MM, Bhatia NN. Management of coexistent stress and urge urinary incontinence. *Obstet Gynecol*. 1989;73:4–7.

13. McGuire EJ, Savastano JA. Stress incontinence and detrusor instability/urge incontinence. *Neurourol Urodyn*. 1985;4:313–316.

14. Pereyra AJ, Lebherz TB. Combined urethral vesical suspension vaginal urethroplasty for correction of urinary stress incontinence. *Obstet Gynecol*. 1967;30:537–546.

15. Pereyra AJ, Lebherz TB. The revised Pereyra procedure. In: Buchsbaum H, Schmidt JD, eds. *Gynecologic and Obstetric Urology*. 1st ed. Philadelphia, Pa: WB Saunders Co; 1978:208–222.

16. Pereyra AJ. Revised Pereyra procedure using colligated pubourethral supports. In: Slate WG, ed. *Disorders of the Female Urethra and Urinary Incontinence*. Baltimore, Md: Williams & Wilkins Co; 1978:143–159.

17. Stamey TA, Schaffer AJ, Condy M. Clinical and roentgenographic evaluation of endoscopic suspension of the vesical neck for urinary incontinence. *Surg Gynecol Obstet*. 1975;140:355–360.

18. Stamey TA. Endoscopic suspension of the vesical neck for urinary incontinence in females. *Ann Surg*. 1980;192:465–471.

19. Raz S. Modified bladder neck suspension for female stress incontinence. *Urology*. 1981;17:82–84.

20. Karram MM, Bhatia NN. Patch procedure modified transvaginal fascia lata sling for recurrent or severe stress urinary incontinence. *Obstet Gynecol*. 1990;75:461–463.

21. Hadley RH, Zimmern PE, Staskin DR, Raz S. Transvaginal needle bladder neck suspension. *Urol Clin North Am*. 1985; 12:299–303.

22. Raz S, Siegel AL, Short JL. Vaginal wall sling. *J Urol*. 1989;141:43–46.

23. Bergman A, Ballard CA, Koonings PP. Comparison of three different surgical procedures for genuine stress incontinence: prospective randomized study. *Am J Obstet Gynecol*. 1989; 160:1102–1106.

24. Bergman A, Kooning PP, Ballard CA. Primary stress urinary incontinence and pelvic relaxation: prospective randomized comparison of three different operations. *Am J Obstet Gynecol*. 1989;161:91–101.

25. Weil A, Reyes H, Bischoff P, Rottenberg RD, Krauler F. Modification of the urethral rest and stress profile after different types of surgery for stress incontinence. *Br J Obstet Gynaecol*. 1984;91:46–55.

26. English PJ, Fowler JW. Videourodynamic assessment of the Stamey procedure for stress incontinence. *Br J Urol*. 1988; 62:550–552.

27. Peattie AB, Stanton SL. The Stamey operation for correction of genuine stress incontinence in the elderly woman. *Br J Obstet Gynaecol*. 1989;96:983–986.

28. Mundy AR. A trial comparing the Stamey bladder neck suspension procedure with colposuspension for the treatment of stress incontinence. *Br J Urol*. 1983;55:687–690.

29. Griffith-Jones MD, Abrams PH. The Stamey endoscopic bladder neck suspension in the elderly. *Br J Obstet Gynecol*. 1990;65:170–172.

30. Hilton P. A clinical and urodynamic study comparing the Stamey bladder neck suspension and suburethral sling procedures in the treatment of genuine stress incontinence. *Br J Obstet Gynecol*. 1989;96:213–220.

31. Karram MM, Angel O, Koonings P, Taber B, Bergman A, Bhatia NN. The modified Pereyra procedure. A clinical and urodynamic review. *Br J Obstet Gynecol*. 1991. In press.

32. Bhatia NN, Bergman A. Modified Burch versus Pereyra retropubic urethropexy for stress urinary incontinence. *Obstet Gynecol*. 1985;66:255–261.

33. Leach GE, Yip CM, Donovan BJ. Mechanism of continence after modified Pereyra bladder neck suspension. *Urology*. 1987; 29:328–331.

34. Katske FA, Raz S. Use of Foley catheter to obtain transvaginal tamponade. *Urol Urotech*. May 1987:8.

35. Ashken MH, Abrams PH, Lawrence WT. Stamey endoscopic bladder neck suspension for stress incontinence. *Br J Urol*. 1984; 56:629–634.

36. Kelly MJ, Knielsen K, Bruskewitz R, Roskamp D, Leach G. Symptom analysis of patients undergoing modified Pereyra bladder neck suspension for stress urinary incontinence. Pre and postoperative findings. *Urology*. 1991;37:213–219.

37. Bhatia NN, Bergman A. Use of preoperative uroflowmetry and simultaneous urethrocystometry for predicting risk of prolonged postoperative bladder drainage. *Urology*. 1986;28:440–444.

38. Cardozo LD, Stanton SL, Williams JE. Detrusor instability following surgery for genuine stress incontinence. *Br J Urol*. 1979;51:204–207.

39. Zimmern PE, Schmidbauer CP, Leach GE, Staskin DR, Hadley HR, Raz S. Vesicovaginal and urethrovaginal fistulae. *Semin Urol*. 1986:424.

40. Kelly MJ, Zimmern PE, Leach GE. Complications of bladder neck suspension procedures. *Urol Clin North Am*. 1991;18:342–346.

41. Diaz DL, Fox BM, Walzak MP, Nieh PT. Endoscopic vesicourethropexy. *Urology*. 1984;24:321–323.

5-3

Paravaginal Repair

A. Cullen Richardson

Most cystourethroceles are the result of a separation of the pubocervical fascia from its lateral attachment to the pelvic side wall. They may be a cause of stress urinary incontinence (SUI). The paravaginal repair is a procedure that is specific for the correction of cystourethroceles that are the result of a lateral detachment of the pubocervical fascia. When properly performed, it provides excellent anatomic and functional support to the anterior wall of the vagina. It will almost always correct SUI that is the result of such a cystourethrocele.

EVOLUTION OF THE PROCEDURE

It has been taught that cystoceles result from a generalized stretching or attenuation of the pubocervical fascia and that this attenuated or stretched fascia is found beneath the vaginal covering of the bulging mass of the cystocele. A chance observation in a single patient caused me to doubt this traditional explanation of the pathogenesis of a cystocele. When my patient strained and pushed out her cystourethrocele, I noticed that she also everted the right superior sulcus of her vagina. Subsequently, when I supported this area during straining, the bladder and the urethra no longer descended. It was clear to me that the supporting tissues had broken away from their lateral attachments to the pelvic side wall. If this was true, it was incompatible with what I had been taught—first, because there must be an isolated break in the anterior vaginal support system and, second, because it appeared that the break was at the pelvic side wall and not beneath the bulging mass that was protruding through the vaginal opening.

My partner and I went to the autopsy room and dissected freshly autopsied bodies and fixed cadavers with and without cystourethroceles. It became clear that my patient, who had an isolated break in the tissues supporting the right superior vaginal sulcus, was not an exception among our findings. Indeed, most of the patients we examined who had cystourethroceles were deemed to have isolated defects in their anterior vaginal support system, and the defect was most often at the pelvic side wall.

After a year of dissections, we operated on our first patient in whom we reattached the anterior vaginal fascia to the right pelvic side wall. We cured her cystourethrocele and relieved her SUI. After performing 65 similar procedures, we reported our concept that cystoceles or urethroceles (or both) are caused by isolated breaks in the anterior vaginal support system and that they are not the result of generalized stretching of the fascial attachments of the vagina.[1] Continuing observations documented the isolated nature of the defects but revealed that the break in the fascial attachment was not always at the pelvic side wall.

When we described the paravaginal repair in 1976, we made no claim as to its originality. In fact, the paravaginal defects were so obvious that, although we could find no description of their repair in the surgical literature, we felt that someone must have suggested the operation we were performing.

In 1982, David H. Nichols, MD, discovered a synopsis of a talk given by George R. White, MD, of Savannah, Georgia, in 1912 entitled, "An Anatomic Operation for the Cure of Cystocele."[2] In the published article, he described the vaginal approach to the paravaginal repair. It was subsequently discovered that White had also written an article in 1909 on "Cystocele, a Radical Cure by Suturing Lateral Sulci of Vagina to White Line of Pelvic Fascia."[3] Clearly, White was a man of vision and ahead of his time. His articles were based on careful thought and meticulous anatomic dissections. Unfortunately, his opinions differed so much with the teachings of his day that he was ignored.

At the time of his second report, White apparently had only performed his procedure vaginally on living patients but with uniformly successful results. He described doing the operation abdominally in the autopsy room and stated that some day the abdominal approach would likely be the "easiest and simplest way to accomplish [the attachment of the vagina to the pelvic side wall]."[2] He further stated, in his paper of 1912, "I doubt not that the transperitoneal suture of the vagina to the white line of the pelvic fascia will form a part of the ideal operation for procidentia."[2]

After studying the vaginal support system and performing paravaginal repairs for more than 20 years, I find nothing in White's report with which to differ, except that most but not all cystoceles are the result of lateral separation of the vaginal fascia from the pelvic side wall.

Dr. Nichols has also called my attention to an article in the Russian literature of 1948 in which K.M. Figurnov, MD,[4] described a vaginal operation for urinary incontinence very similar to Dr. White's original procedure. Although Figurnov's anatomic description and logic leave a lot to be desired, it is clear that he too was advocating a suspension of the anterior wall of the vagina to the fascial arcus. He reported that he had done the operation more than 200 times and that he had experienced only one failure.

In 1948, Goff[5] reported that in anatomic studies he had been unable to find any evidence of the attenuation of the pubocervical fascia in patients with cystoceles. He stated in his report that his next article would discuss the true cause of cystoceles, but unfortunately he died before he was able to publish further on his work.

Others have advocated the use of the white line or other points on the lateral aspect of the pelvic wall for vaginal suspensions. Inman[6] suggested suturing the fibromuscular wall of the vagina to the fascia of the pelvic side wall at the level of the vaginal apex when adequate cardinal and uterosacral ligaments could not be found. Durfee,[7] in his modification of the Burch procedure, recommended anchoring the fibromuscular wall of the vagina to the obturator fascia with a single suture on either side of the urethrovesical junction.

In 1976, I became aware that Wayne Baden, MD, and Tom Walker, MD, of Temple, Texas, had identified a subset of patients with SUI who had detachment of the lateral supports of the urethra from the pelvic side walls. They were performing in these patients a vaginal operation that was designed to reattach the tissues lateral to the urethra and the bladder neck to the pelvic side wall and correct their SUI. Baden helped me describe and classify the various paravaginal defects. It was he who suggested that we call our surgical procedure a paravaginal repair.

ANATOMY

The pelvic support system is described in Chapter 3. The mechanics of the support system, that is, the interplay between the active striated musculature and the passive connective tissue, are emphasized. To appreciate fully the role of the paravaginal repair in the cure of a cystourethrocele it is necessary to focus from a slightly different perspective on those tissues that support the vesical neck that, when damaged, may result in the development of a cystocele or a urethrocele (or both).

The peritoneal cavity extends from the diaphragm to the pelvic floor. It contains all the abdominal and pelvic viscera. In the erect position the most dependent portion of the peritoneal cavity is surrounded, in a cylindric fashion, by the bony pelvis. Attached to the bony pelvis are various contractile and noncontractile flexible supporting tissues, which close the space between the pelvic bones and maintain the viscera within the pelvic portion of the peritoneal cavity. Collectively, the soft tissues supporting the pelvic viscera may be referred to as the *pelvic floor*. It contains openings that allow for the passage of the urethra, the vagina, and the rectum.

The pelvic floor comprises three layers. They are from inside out (1) endopelvic fascia, (2) levator ani muscles, and (3) perineum. The endopelvic fascia (Figures 5-3.1–5-3.4) is a network of fibromuscular tissue that lies immediately beneath the peritoneum. It surrounds the viscera and fills the space between the peritoneum above and the levator ani muscles below. It extends from symphysis pubis to sacrum and ischial spine to ischial spine, providing a continuity of support from front to back and side to side. In places, portions of

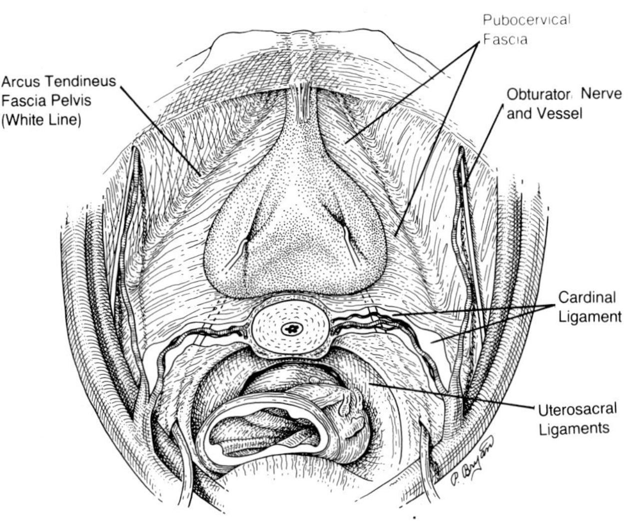

Figure 5-3.1 Endopelvic fascia viewed from above. *Source*: Reprinted with permission from *Contemporary Ob/Gyn* (1990;35[9]:100–109), Copyright © 1990, Medical Economics Company Inc.

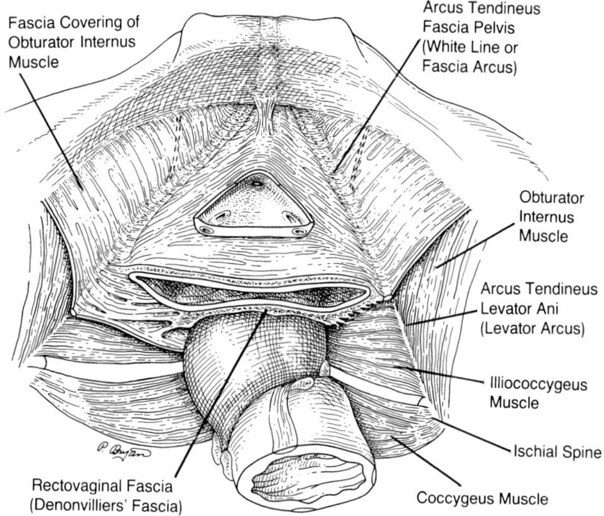

Figure 5-3.2 Relation of pubocervical fascia and edge of vagina to pelvic side wall. *Source*: Reprinted with permission from *Contemporary Ob/Gyn* (1990; 35[9]:100–109), Copyright © 1990, Medical Economics Company Inc.

the endopelvic fascia are referred to as *ligaments* (eg, uterosacral, cardinal), though the distinction is a weak one. In other areas it is simply called *fascia*. Histologically, the endopelvic fascia is a mixture of collagen and varying amounts of smooth muscle that is suspended in a matrix of ground substance. It contains some elastin fibers, which are most abundant in the perivascular areas.

The levator ani muscles are a bilaterally paired group of three striated muscles: pubococcygeus (to include the puborectalis), iliococcygeus, and coccygeus. The endopelvic fascia just described is densely connected to the fascial covering of the levator ani muscles. Contractions of these muscles can alter the contour and the position of the endopelvic fascia.

The perineum is the outermost layer of the pelvic floor and is composed of the urogenital diaphragm (urogenital membrane, deep transversus perinei muscle) and its attached striated perineal muscles (external genital muscles) and their fascial covering. The perineal structures give back-up support to the levator ani musculature (pelvic diaphragm) above.

The pelvic organs are always supported from inside out. They never fall out of the pelvic cavity; they are always pushed out as a result of increases in intra-abdominal pressure. The bladder, the uterus, the vagina, and the rectum are essentially extraperitoneal structures that rest on, or are contained in, the pelvic floor. When there is a defect in the integrity of the soft tissue supporting these organs, they can be pushed outward. The resultant protrusion into the vagina is named according

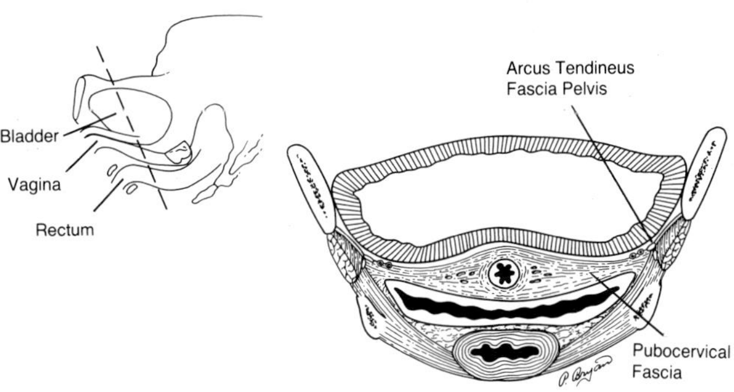

Figure 5-3.3 Diagrammatic cross-section at vesical neck. *Source*: Reprinted from *Hernia: Surgical Anatomy and Technique* (pp 244–250) by JE Skandalakis et al (eds) with permission of McGraw-Hill, © 1989.

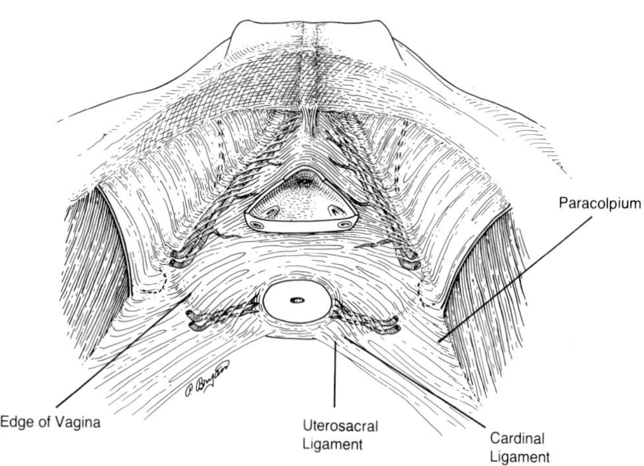

Figure 5-3.4 Pubocervical fascia with bladder removed. *Source*: Reprinted from *Hernia: Surgical Anatomy and Technique* (pp 244–250) by JE Skandalakis et al (eds) with permission of McGraw-Hill, © 1989.

to the displaced viscera (ie, urethrocele, cystocele, uterine prolapse, enterocele, and rectocele). This designation has led to much confusion because the problem is not with the visceral structure that is displaced but with the pelvic floor on which the structure rests or in which it is contained. For any of the pelvic organs to be pushed out, there must be a break in the continuity of support within the uppermost layer known as the *endopelvic fascia*.

The bladder (see Figure 5-3.1) rests on, and is attached to, that portion of the endopelvic fascia referred to as the *pubocervical fascia*. This layer of fibromuscular tissue attaches centrally to the pericervical tissue and extends ventrally to pass under the symphysis pubis and merge with the urogenital diaphragm. Bilaterally, it fuses into the fascial covering of the muscles of the pelvic side wall at the arcus tendineus fasciae pelvis (white line). The urethra traverses this layer tangentially, beginning above it at the vesical neck and terminating below it at the external meatus.

Many observers have tried to subdivide the urethral support system into pubourethral ligaments, and so on, but anatomic dissections reveal many variations. There are no consistent structures to which one can assign the term *ligament* because there is in fact a continuous hammock-like structure that blends laterally into the fascia over the muscles of the pelvic side wall (obturator internus and levator ani muscles) and centrally into those fibers referred to as *cardinal ligaments* and *bladder pillows*. The pericervical tissue maintains mechanical continuity through the uterosacral fibers all the way to the sacrum.

Anatomically, the fibromuscular tissue, referred to as the pubocervical fascia, is the principal supporting structure of the bladder, the vesical neck, and the urethra. As noted earlier, it constitutes a hammock-like diaphragm into which the trigone and the vesical neck are imbedded and on which the base of the bladder rests. The urethra traverses this layer and is supported by it throughout its entire length.

Mechanically, when a structure is subjected to stress, areas of stress concentration develop in the stressed structure. One of the first principles of mechanics is that there tends to be a concentration of the stress anywhere the lines of force change direction. Structures break or fail where the stress is concentrated. Because the pubocervical fascia is attached at its periphery to the pelvic side walls, when stressed, the lines of force would change direction at this peripheral attachment, and the expected break would be along the lines of this peripheral attachment. It is only with inherent other areas of weakness that other breaks would occur.

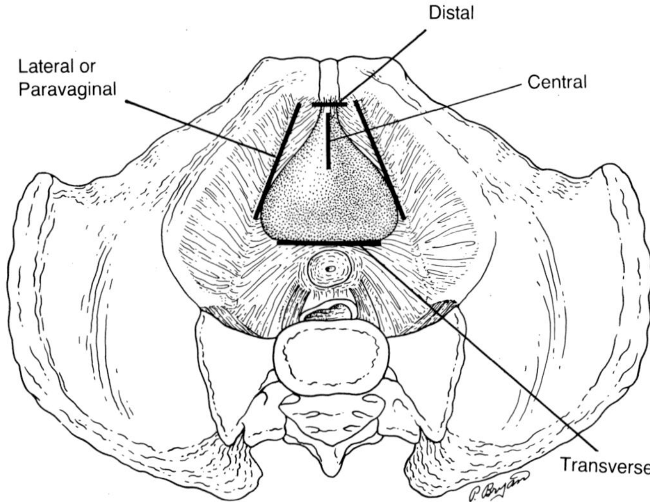

Figure 5-3.5 Four areas in which pubocervical fascia can break or separate—four defects. *Source*: Reprinted with permission from *Contemporary Ob/Gyn* (1990;35[9]:100–109), Copyright © 1990, Medical Economics Company Inc.

There are four areas in which breaks in the pubocervical fascia have been observed (Figure 5-3.5). In each there is some loss of support to the bladder. They are referred to as the four defects responsible for cystourethroceles. As one notes from the diagram, three of four defects are in the area of the peripheral attachment of the pubocervical fascia, and only one is located centrally.

DIAGNOSIS OF VAGINAL SUPPORT DEFECTS

A knowledge of normal anatomy and a careful physical examination will distinguish the various anatomic defects. It is important to recognize the various defects because the surgical correction of each requires a different operative procedure. The classification and the findings of each of the defects of the anterior vaginal support system are as follows.

1. Paravaginal Defect

In the paravaginal defect (Figures 5-3.6 and 5-3.7), the lateral attachment of the pubocervical fascia separates from its attachment to the fascia covering the obturator internus and levator ani muscles. This separation may be unilateral or bilateral. It usually results in a cystourethrocele. Because the vagina is attached to the pubocervical fascia, when there is a break in the fascia the lateral superior vaginal sulcus descends, the bladder neck becomes hypermobile, and often there is SUI.

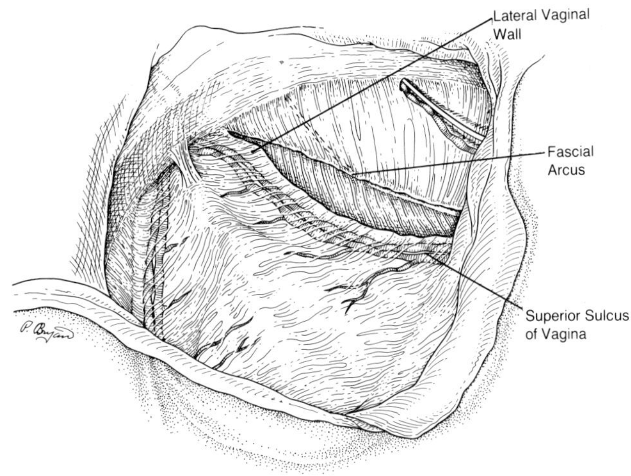

Figure 5-3.6 Paravaginal defect. *Source*: Reprinted with permission from *Contemporary Ob/Gyn* (1990;35[9]:100–109), Copyright © 1990, Medical Economics Company Inc.

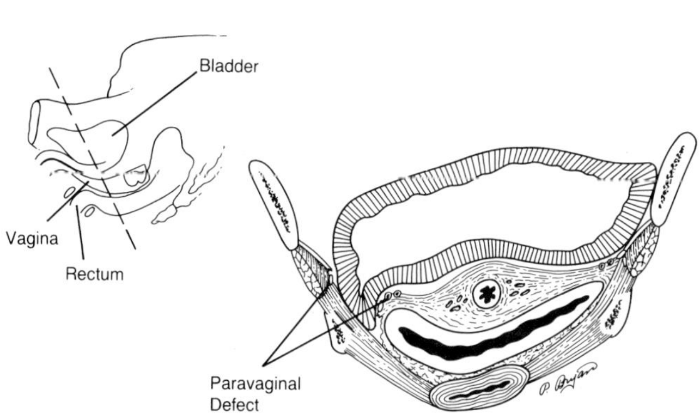

Figure 5-3.7 Diagrammatic cross-section of paravaginal defect. *Source*: Reprinted with permission from *Contemporary Ob/Gyn* (1990;35[9]: 100–109), Copyright © 1990, Medical Economics Company Inc.

When the superior sulcus is supported on each side, the cystourethrocele disappears. If the defect is unilateral (more often on the right), support of the sulcus on the side of the defect will correct the cystourethrocele. For this type of defect, and only this defect, is it appropriate to perform a paravaginal repair.

2. Transverse Defect

The transverse defect is the result of a separation of the pubocervical fascia from its attachment to the pericervical ring of fibromuscular tissue into which not only the pubocervical fascia but also the cardinal and uterosacral ligaments merge. This defect, when it occurs alone, produces a large cystocele, but the vesical neck remains well supported. The descent of the bladder obliterates the anterior vaginal fornix. Supporting the lateral vaginal sulci will have little effect on the descent of the bladder. The transverse separation of the pubocervical fascia away from the cervix will not cause SUI. Patients with this anatomic defect may have increased residual urine. The transverse defect is often seen in patients with total prolapse.

I prefer the vaginal surgical approach to correct transverse defects. The break in the fascia should be closed in an anteroposterior direction, not from side to side.

3. Distal Defect

The distal defect is the most rare of all defects of the anterior vaginal support system. When there is a distal defect, the distal portion of the urethra is avulsed or separated from its attachment by way of the urogenital diaphragm (urogenital membrane or deep transversus perinei muscle) to the overlying symphysis pubis. The physical findings are unusual in that the vesical neck does not descend, and no downward rotation of the urethra can be demonstrated with the applicator (Q-tip) test. Rather, there is direct outward projection of the external urethral meatus and the entire urethra. Usually there is a slight bulge in the mucosa just above the urethral meatus during Valsalva's maneuvers.

Patients with a distal defect often have distressing urinary incontinence that is difficult to cure. Currently, it is not clear just what is the best surgical approach. Suburethral sling procedures usually work, but my experience in managing these cases is limited.

4. Central Defect

Central defects are uncommon. They are diagnosed when there is any break in the central portion of the pubocervical fascial hammock. On casual inspection, patients with central defects have cystourethroceles that look very similar to those that accompany paravaginal defects. Support of the lateral superior vaginal sulcus on each side, however, will not correct the accompanying cystocele.

A central defect can occur after high suspension of the lateral portion of the vaginal fascia as the result of performing a Burch modification of the Marshall-Marchetti-Krantz procedure. It has also been observed rarely after paravaginal repairs. Central defects can be located immediately beneath the vesical neck. When this is the case and a sound is placed into the urethra, vaginal palpation of the tip of the sound at the vesical neck will reveal a thinning of the tissues to such an extent that it appears there is only vaginal and urethral mucosa between the examining finger and the sound.

The treatment of a central defect is a traditional anterior colporrhaphy. After reflection of the vaginal mucosa from the underlying fascia, one can distinguish the edges of the defect and repair it by reapproximation.

In my patient population, about 80% or more of patients with cystoceles have only paravaginal defects, about 5% have only a transverse defect, and 1% to 2% have central or distal defects. The remaining 10% to 15% have a combination of transverse and paravaginal defects. When two or more defects occur together, as in patients with complete prolapse who may have both a transverse defect in front of the cervix and a paravaginal defect laterally, the transverse defect and the paravaginal defect should be repaired individually.

Of the patients I see with cystourethroceles *and* SUI, more than 95% have paravaginal defects; therefore, in my experience, the paravaginal repair is the operation of choice in 95% of patients with SUI.

TECHNIQUE

In the paravaginal repair, a Pfannenstiel's incision is made through the skin, the subcutaneous tissue, and the fascia. The peritoneum is freed from the undersurface of the rectus muscles, and the recti are retracted. (Better exposure can be obtained by detachment of the rectus muscles from the superior pubic ramus, as in the Cherney incision. Once experience is gained, however, the Pfannenstiel's incision will be sufficient.) The retropubic space is entered by incising the transversalis fascia at its attachment to the superior pubic ramus. The transversalis fascia is then separated bluntly from the superior pubic ramus laterally until the obturator notch can be palpated or visualized. The bladder is drawn medially away from the side wall of the pelvis. The left hand of the operator is inserted into the vagina. While holding the bladder with a sponge stick (Figure 5-3.8), the lateral superior vaginal sulcus is elevated, and the prominent veins coursing down the lateral vaginal sulcus are exposed. The separation of the lateral sulcus (as indicated by the veins in the sulcus) from the pelvic side wall can be appreciated.

The object of the procedure is to reattach the lateral vaginal sulcus with its overlying pubocervical fascia to the pelvic side wall at the level to which it was originally attached. Remember, this is the level of the arcus tendineus fasciae pelvis (white line) that runs from the back of the lower edge of the symphysis pubis to the ischial spine. It is well, at this point, to palpate these two landmarks because this is the level to which the fascia is

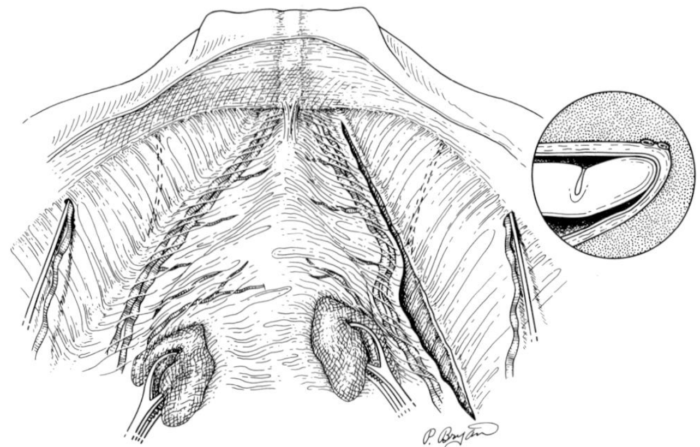

Figure 5-3.8 Elevation of lateral superior sulcus of vagina with hand in vagina. *Source*: Reprinted with permission from *Contemporary Ob/Gyn* (1990;35[9]:100–109), Copyright © 1990, Medical Economics Company Inc.

to be reattached. The first stitch placed on either side is the key suture because it is the placement of this stitch that determines where along the pelvic side wall the vagina is to be reattached.

The vesical neck can be palpated with the hand in the vagina. If the surgeon then draws an imaginary arc in a convex manner toward the symphysis pubis at the level of the vesical neck, the lateral extent of this arc will be the location along the lateral vaginal sulcus of this first stitch.

While elevating the lateral superior sulcus, a full-thickness stitch is placed through the lateral sulcus *beneath* the prominent veins (Figure 5-3.9). Before releasing the needle, traction is placed on the needleholder, moving its tip toward the ischial spine. While palpating with the hand in the vagina, this traction is carried toward the ischial spine until the external meatus of the urethra can be felt to be drawn immediately beneath the middle of the lower edge of the symphysis pubis (Figure 5-3.10). The needle is then passed through the lateral pelvic wall fascia. The suture is held and not tied.

After the placement of this first stitch, additional sutures are placed between the vaginal sulcus, with its overlying fascia, and the pelvic side wall. These are at about 1-cm intervals, both dorsally (toward the ischial spine) and ventrally (toward the pubic ramus). Dorsally, the last stitch should be approximately 1 cm in front of the ischial spine. Ventrally, the last stitch should be as close as possible to the pubic ramus. Once all sutures are placed, they are tied (Figure 5-3.11).

Permanent sutures should be used. I have used silicone-treated Dacron on a medium gastrointestinal needle (Davis & Geck; 3-0 Ticron on a T-5 needle). Because

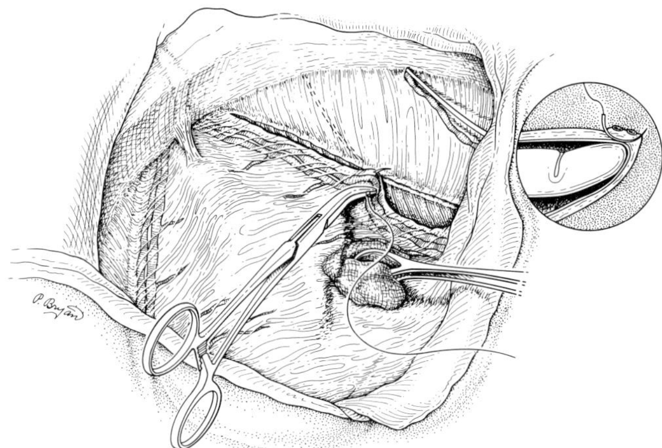

Figure 5-3.9 First medial bite in repair. *Source*: Reprinted with permission from *Contemporary Ob/Gyn* (1990;35[9]:100–109), Copyright © 1990, Medical Economics Company Inc.

this is a coated and very slick suture, at least six loops must be placed for knot security.

The procedure is repeated on the opposite side. Generally, I do the right side first because most patients have a defect only on the right side (reason unknown). Even if there is no defect on one side, the junction between the vagina and the pelvic side wall should be reinforced by placing sutures around the junction of the pubocervical fascia to the fascia over the obturator internus muscle, as described earlier.

Often, when sutures are placed, some bleeding will occur at the needle puncture sites. This usually stops when the sutures are tied. After the sutures are tied, the retropubic space is irrigated with warm lactated Ringer's injection. I rarely place drains in the retropubic space unless there is bleeding related to previous surgery and an extensive dissection.

The illustrations in Figures 5-3.6–5-3.10 show a defect that occurred by a separation immediately medial to the arcus. Although this may be the case, it is more common to find the entire arcus separated from the lateral aspect of the pelvic wall. Rarely, the separation will be down the middle of the arcus, and remnants can be identified on both the pelvic and the vaginal sides.

When the entire arcus is pulled away, it is necessary to locate the level at which it was originally attached. Remember, the arcus extends from a point 1 cm superior and 1 cm lateral to the midline of the lower edge of the symphysis pubis posteriorly to the ischial spine. For the dorsal two thirds of its length, the fascial arcus (white line) overlies the levator arcus (arcus tendineus levator ani), which is the semitendinous origin of the iliococcygeus muscle. Usually, when the fascial arcus is torn, careful palpation will locate the levator arcus. Nevertheless, establishing a mental image of a line between the two points of reference will help locate the line of reattachment of the vagina. When the fascial arcus is pulled completely away from the side wall, it is well to incorporate the levator arcus into the lateral tissue in the upper two thirds of the repair, because it is a structure with some strength and increased ability to hold a suture.

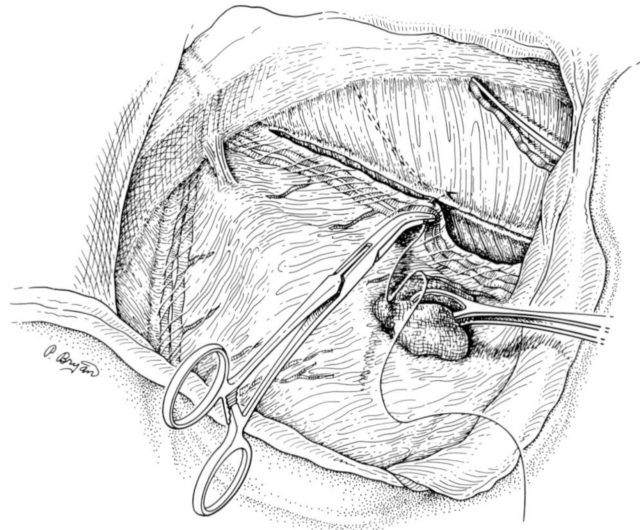

Figure 5-3.10 Completed first or key suture. *Source*: Reprinted with permission from *Contemporary Ob/Gyn* (1990;35[9]:100–109), Copyright © 1990, Medical Economics Company Inc.

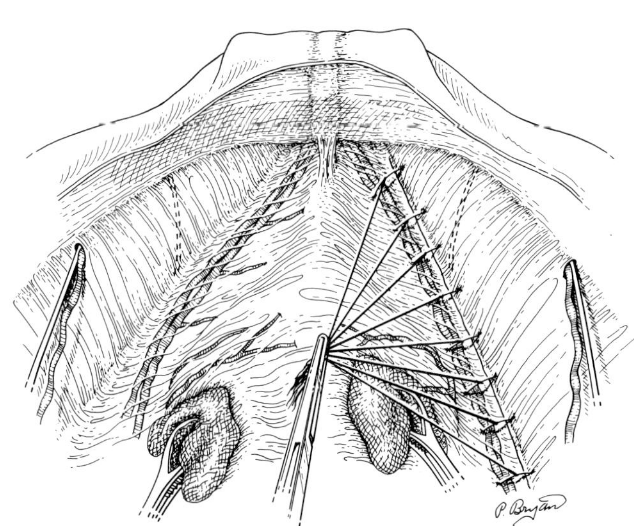

Figure 5-3.11 Completed paravaginal repair. *Source*: Reprinted with permission from *Contemporary Ob/Gyn* (1990;35[9]:100–109), Copyright © 1990, Medical Economics Company Inc.

Although I do not usually use an indwelling urethral catheter during or after a paravaginal repair, it may be helpful in locating the urethra and the bladder neck for those who are less experienced in performing the procedure.

CONCLUSION

The paravaginal repair is an attempt to restore normal anatomy when there have been isolated breaks in the anterolateral vaginal support system. Because I believe that normal anatomy has the best chance of restoring normal function, I prefer the paravaginal repair.

The paravaginal repair is not an operation for SUI. It is a procedure designed to correct a cystourethrocele that is the result of a paravaginal defect. The cystourethrocele may or may not be accompanied by the symptom of SUI.

Why SUI occurs frequently, but not uniformly, with paravaginal defects has yet to be determined. The mechanism of urinary incontinence in women is complex. Urodynamic studies show sphincteric activity along the entire length of the urethra. This sphincteric activity is the result of the combined interaction of the urethral mucosa, the periurethral vascular plexus, the connective tissues, the smooth and striated musculature, and the urethral and bladder neck support system.

When there is damage to the urethral and bladder neck support system, the paravaginal repair will reattach those supports lateral to the vesical neck and urethra to the fascia overlying the striated muscles of the pelvic side wall. It creates no rigidity, as is the result of attaching these structures to the pubic bone (as in the Marshall-Marchetti-Krantz procedure) or to the Cooper's ligament (as in the Burch procedure). The paravaginal repair preserves the delicate interrelation that should exist between the passive connective tissues and the contracting striated musculature.

My partner (James B. Lyon, MD) and I have performed the paravaginal repair more than 800 times, either as a primary operation for cystourethrocele with SUI or as a secondary operation in those who have had failed prior surgery for SUI or cystourethrocele (or both). We have obtained 95% satisfactory results in this group of patients.[8] By this we mean that we (1) correct the cystourethrocele, (2) provide satisfactory relief of SUI, (3) preserve normal voiding function, and (4) have no persistent postoperative bladder dysfunction. Similar results have been obtained by others who have used this approach.[9,10]

One of the most gratifying aspects of our procedure is that there have been no ongoing voiding difficulties, as commonly seen after the Marshall-Marchetti-Krantz procedure and its various modifications. All except one of the 800 patients have been able to void normally within 72 hours of their surgery. The one patient who was an exception voided on the fifth day. More than 80% of our patients void immediately after their surgical procedure. We use straight catheterization two or three times if necessary. If the patient is still unable to void, we will leave an indwelling Foley catheter in for 24 hours. Less than 5% of our patients have required a Foley catheter. In none of our patients did an unstable bladder develop as a result of their paravaginal repair.

Our functional failures have been due to a failure to correct fascial defects. As a result, the patients in follow-up have a residual urethrocele and vesical neck descent. Some of these failures have been due to our failure to recognize a coexisting central defect. In other cases, it is apparent that the sutures were improperly placed or simply did not hold.

The paravaginal repair is only for patients whose cystourethrocele is the result of the paravaginal defect (or defects) we have described. In the patient with genuine stress incontinence (according to the definition of the International Continence Society) in whom a paravaginal defect can be demonstrated, one can predict with 99% assurance that if the normal anatomy is restored, the patient will be cured of her SUI.

REFERENCES

1. Richardson AC, Lyon JB, Williams NL. A new look at pelvic relaxation. *Am J Obstet Gynecol*. 1976;126:568.

2. White GR. An anatomic operation for the cure of cystocele. *Am J Obstet Dis Women Children*. 1912;65:286.

3. White GR. Cystocele, a radical cure by suturing lateral sulci of vagina to white line of pelvic fascia. *J Am Med Assoc*. 1909; 53:1707–1711.

4. Figurnov KM. Surgical treatment of urinary incontinence in women. *Akush Ginekol*. 1948;5:6–11.

5. Goff BR. The surgical anatomy of cystocele and urethrocele with special reference to the pubocervical fascia. *Surg Gynecol Obstet*. 1948;87:725–751.

6. Inman WB. Suspension of the vaginal cuff and posterior repair following vaginal hysterectomy. *Am J Obstet Gynecol*. 1974; 120:977–981.

7. Durfee RB. Anterior vaginal suspension operation of stress incontinence. *Am J Obstet Gynecol*. 1965;92:615–619.

8. Richardson AC, Edmonds PB, Williams NL. Treatment of stress urinary incontinence due to paravaginal fascial defect. *Obstet Gynecol*. 1981;57:357–363.

9. Shull BL, Baden WF. A six-year experience with paravaginal defect repair for stress urinary incontinence. *Am J Obstet Gynecol*. 198;160:1432–1436.

10. Youngblood JP. Paravaginal repair. *Contemp Ob Gyn*. 1990;35:28–38.

5-4

Retropubic Urethropexy or Colposuspension

W. Glenn Hurt

Marshall, Marchetti, and Krantz made a significant contribution to the treatment of stress urinary incontinence (SUI) when they described their vesicourethral suspension procedure. They are responsible for shifting the emphasis in the surgical approach from vaginal to abdominal. Abdominal retropubic urethropexy or colposuspension procedures of the Marshall-Marchetti-Krantz or Burch type have become the gold standard for the treatment of primary and recurrent SUI.

This chapter discusses the indications for retropubic urethropexy or colposuspension; the evolution of the procedure currently used; and the physiologic alterations, complications, and therapeutic results associated with the procedure.

INDICATIONS

Retropubic urethropexy or colposuspension procedures are recommended for the treatment of SUI and are most successful in patients who have pure SUI. Patients who have mixed urinary incontinence as a result of a combination of SUI and detrusor instability (DI) incontinence can expect the component that is due to stress to be cured by a retropubic urethropexy or colposuspension. Its effect on incontinence caused by DI, however, is unpredictable.[1]

Because the effect of a retropubic urethropexy or colposuspension on DI is unpredictable and because transient or long-term DI may develop as a result of the procedure, I believe that all patients who have a mixed form of incontinence should have nonsurgical therapy before any surgical procedure.[2,3] The primary aim of the nonsurgical therapy should be optimum control of that component of the patient's urinary incontinence that is due to DI.

A retropubic continence procedure may improve or cure urinary incontinence that is due to DI.[1,4] This is most likely to occur when there is funneling of the proximal segment of the urethra. The presence of urine in the urethra can cause a reflex detrusor contraction, resulting in urinary leakage. If a retropubic continence procedure prevents urine from entering the urethra, the reflex detrusor contraction will be prevented and the urinary incontinence will be eliminated.

Retropubic urethropexy or colposuspension procedures are more likely to fail in patients who have low urethral closure pressures.[5–7] It has been recommended by several investigators that patients with urethral closure pressures of less than 20 centimeters of water (cm H_2O) should be treated routinely by using a sling urethropexy.[8] The issue has not been resolved as to whether a retropubic colposuspension (a type of sling procedure), which results in higher elevation of the urethrovesical junction and the proximal segment of the urethra being located closer to the retrosymphysis, can cure most patients with a urethral closure pressure of less than 20 cm H_2O.

Prophylactic retropubic urethropexy or colposuspension procedures have been recommended for patients who are predisposed to experience SUI as a result of a radical vulvectomy or abdominal colposacropexy. A vulvectomy may cause SUI by shortening the functional length of the urethra and injuring the urethral sphincteric mechanism. An abdominal colposacropexy may cause SUI by elevating the upper portion of the vagina, so that it nullifies the beneficial effect of the urethrovesical angle and prevents posterior rotational descent of the bladder base. Prophylactic retropubic procedures are being performed with increasing frequency in patients undergoing these procedures.

Two factors must be considered when recommending a retropubic colposuspension for the treatment of SUI: mobility and length of the anterior wall of the vagina. Retropubic colposuspensions of the urethrovesical junction elevate and shorten the anterior wall of the vagina. These procedures should not be recommended for patients who have a vagina that is scarred, immobile, and inadequate in caliber and depth.

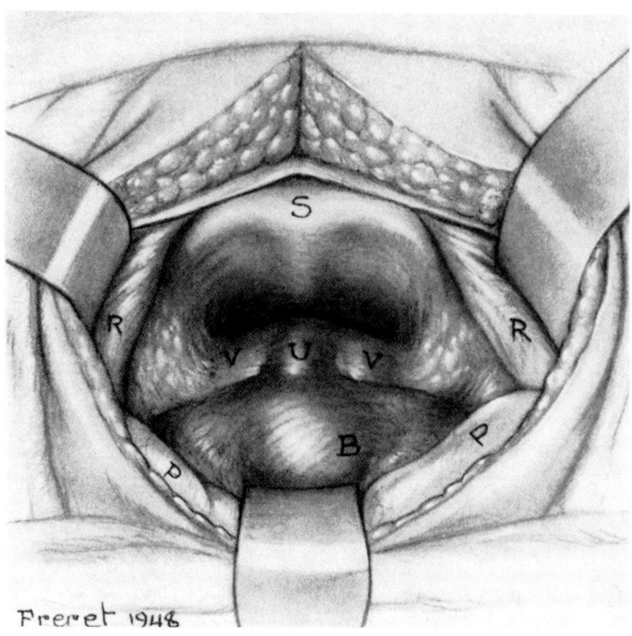

Figure 5-4.1 Marshall-Marchetti-Krantz procedure. Operative area exposed, and urethra (U) separated from symphysis pubis (S). R, Rectus muscles; B, bladder; P, peritoneum; V, upper surface of vagina. *Source:* Reprinted with permission from *Surgery, Gynecology and Obstetrics* (1949;88:510), Copyright © 1949, Surgery, Gynecology and Obstetrics.

EVOLUTION OF THE PROCEDURE

Marshall-Marchetti-Krantz Procedure

In 1949, Marshall, Marchetti, and Krantz[9] described their vesicourethral suspension procedure and recommended it as treatment for SUI in patients with "mobility and marked sagging of the vesical base and outlet." The case they cite as the one responsible for encouraging them to pursue the procedure, in fact, involved a man. (The initial series included 5 men and 45 women.) The male patient on whom the procedure was used had complete urinary retention after abdominoperineal removal of the rectum. Two subsequent transurethral resections were performed in an effort to relieve his urinary retention. Unfortunately, total urinary incontinence developed in the patient. The favorable result obtained by performing an abdominal retropubic vesicourethral suspension led the investigators to apply the principles of elevation and fixation of the bladder outlet to the problem of stress incontinence in women. In women, the operation was recommended for patients with urinary incontinence who responded favorably to their modification of the Bonney stress test and in whom previous continence surgery had failed.

In the original Marshall-Marchetti-Krantz (MMK) procedure,[9] the retropubic space (Retzius space) was widely dissected (Figure 5-4.1). In the midline, the dissection was carried down to within 1 cm of the external urethral meatus. To quote the authors

> An assistant's fingers in the vagina aided the palpation of the catheter and balloon which corresponded to the urethra and vesical neck, respectively. Three sutures of No. 1 chromic catgut were placed equidistant from each other on either side of the urethra [Figure 5-4.2]. The suturing needle was inserted deeply into the upper wall of the vagina adjacent to the urethra and through the lateral wall of the urethra, caution being exercised to avoid entering the urethral lumen. A double bite was taken to insure a secure hold and also to place eventually as large an amount of tissue as possible in apposition to the pubis. A similar suture was then placed on either side of the vesical outlet, in the angle between the balloon and the catheter after the balloon had been pulled down to mark the outlet. When upward traction was made on the long ends of these eight sutures, the urethra and vesical neck were lifted away from the introitus, which change was particularly noticeable by the assistant who had two fingers in the vagina. At this stage additional sutures were placed at points of advantage lateral to the urethra where the vaginal wall apparently sagged: that is, one additional suture on each side, but the number has varied according to circumstances in subsequent cases. With a curved,

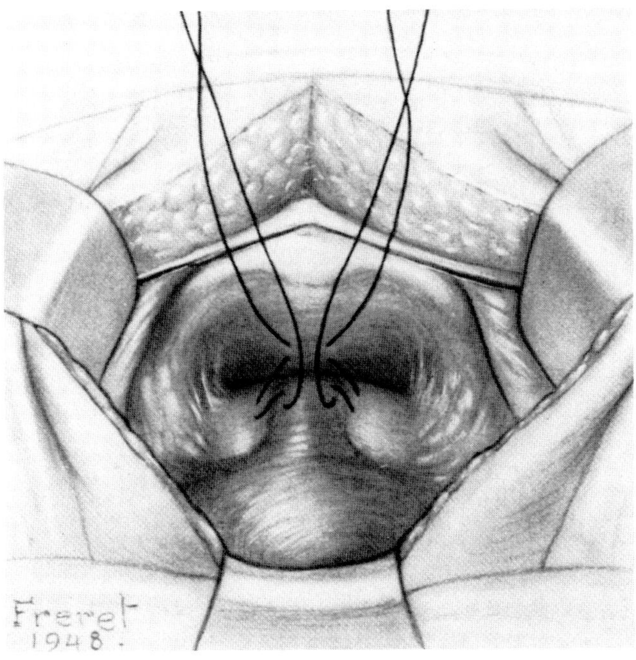

Figure 5-4.2 Marshall-Marchetti-Krantz procedure. Lowest suture on either side of urethra. *Source:* Reprinted with permission from *Surgery, Gynecology and Obstetrics* (1949;88:511), Copyright © 1949, Surgery, Gynecology and Obstetrics.

> round-edged needle the long ends of these sutures were placed securely through the periosteum of the pubis, especially into the cartilage of the symphysis whenever feasible [Figure 5-4.3]. The locations for these sutures in the pubis, or rectus muscles when indicated, were carefully selected in order that when the sutures were tied they would move the urinary passage upward and backward from the introitus. Upward displacement by the assistant's fingers in the vagina aided the selection of these sites and avoided undesirable tension until a sufficient number of the sutures had been tied. Thus, the space of Retzius was closed and a wide area of the superior surface of the urethra and vesical neck opposed to the symphysis and the posterior surfaces of the rectus muscles. Additional sutures were now placed into the musculature of the lower and lateral portions of the bladder with their long ends in the posterior parts of the rectus muscles and tied to further pull the bladder anteriorly into the space of Retzius [Figure 5-4.4].

In the original series (50 patients) with urinary incontinence treated by using the MMK procedure, the effectiveness of the procedure was reported as 82% excellent (does not wear protection, does not get damp during usual activities, and voids without difficulty), 7% improved, and 11% failures. The investigators' reasons for not obtaining cures were insecure suture placement related to inexperience of the surgeon; excessive scarring, which limited elevation; and wound infection. Complications reported were urethral injury, hematomas, wound infection, urinary urgency and frequency, ventral hernia, osteitis pubis, and failure to cure urinary incontinence.

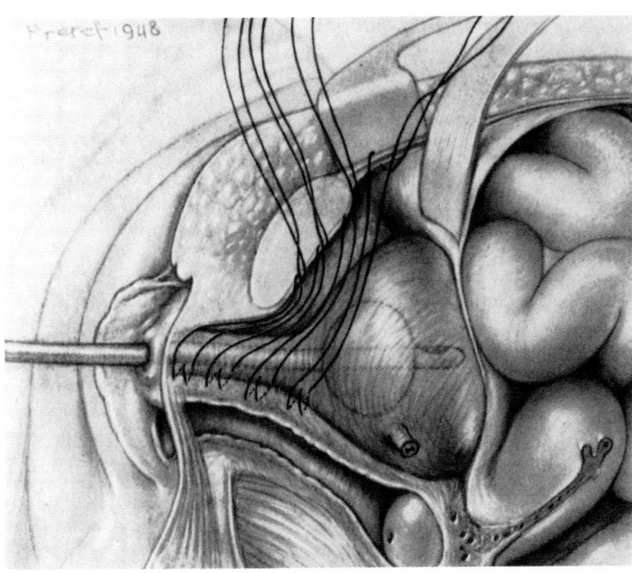

Figure 5-4.3 Marshall-Marchetti-Krantz procedure. Sagittal section showing location of four paraurethral sutures on left. *Source:* Reprinted with permission from *Surgery, Gynecology and Obstetrics* (1949;88:514), Copyright © 1949, Surgery, Gynecology and Obstetrics.

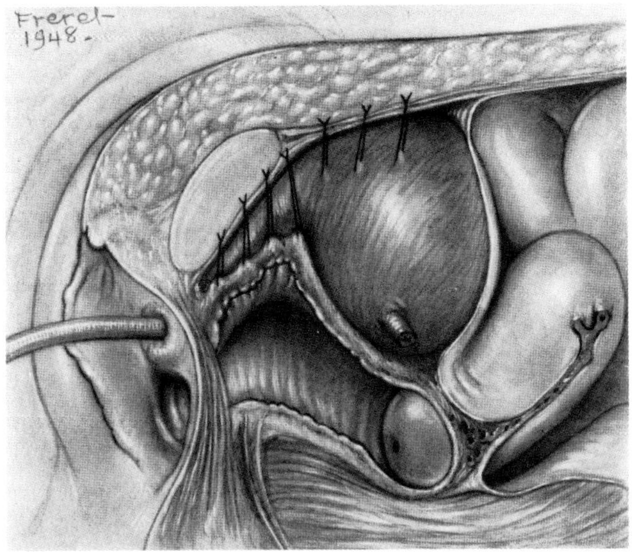

Figure 5-4.4 Marshall-Marchetti-Krantz procedure. Same as Figure 5-4.3 except sutures tied—diagrammatic, as actually less space remains between origin and insertion of sutures. *Source:* Reprinted with permission from *Surgery, Gynecology and Obstetrics* (1949;88:515), Copyright © 1949, Surgery, Gynecology and Obstetrics.

Burch Modification

In 1961, Burch[10] suggested a modification of the MMK procedure in an effort to find more secure points of urethrovaginal fixation than could be obtained by using the periosteum of the pubic bones. He had noticed at the time of the MMK procedure that, with fingers in the vagina, the anterior wall of the vagina could be elevated to the white line, which is the origin on the pelvic side walls of the paravaginal fascia and the underlying levator ani muscles. Suturing the anterior wall of the vagina to the white line restored anatomic relations about the bladder neck and often corrected any accompanying cystocele. After performing seven operations in this manner, he concluded that the white line, as the periosteum, was a weak point for fixation. Burch then selected Cooper's ligaments (Sir Astley Paston Cooper, English anatomist and surgeon, 1768–1841; the ligaments otherwise known as the iliopectineal ligaments), thick bands of fibrous tissue that run along the superior surfaces of the superior rami of the pubic bones, for the suspension of the anterior wall of the vagina (Figure 5-4.5).

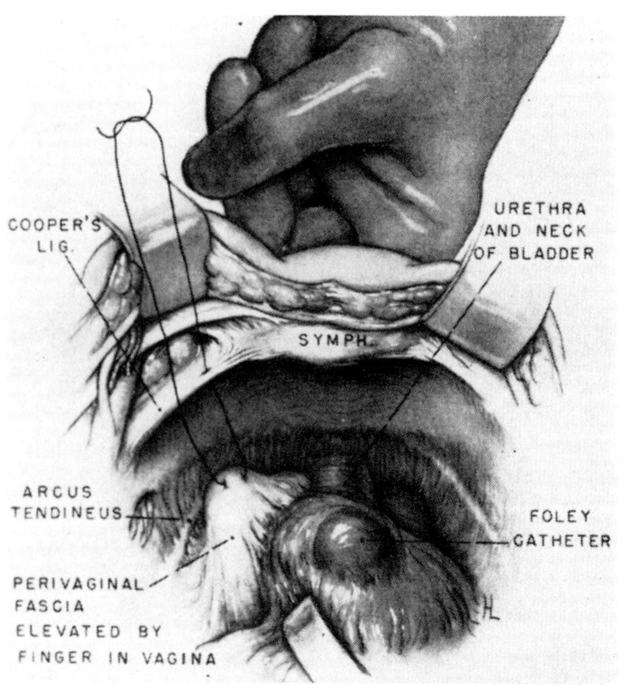

Figure 5-4.5 Burch modification. Suture has been passed through perivaginal fascia and wall of vagina, but not through mucous membrane. Sutured point is now matched to that point on Cooper's ligament to which it is most easily approximated, and suture is passed through this point and tied. *Source:* Reprinted with permission from *American Journal of Obstetrics and Gynecology* (1961;81:283), Copyright © 1961, Mosby-Year Book.

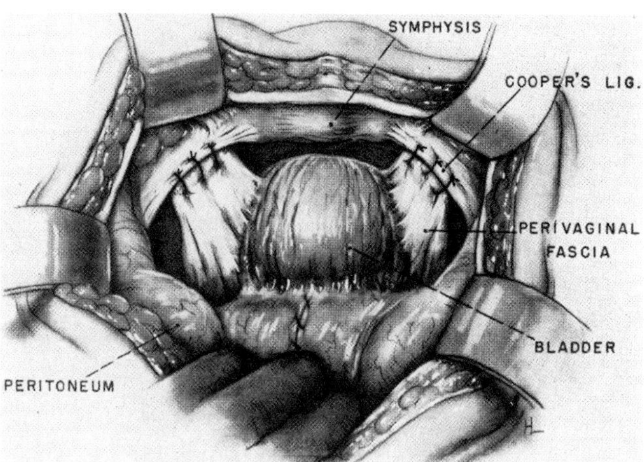

Figure 5-4.6 Burch modification. Lateral edges of vagina have been approximated to Cooper's ligament by using three interrupted sutures. *Source:* Reprinted with permission from *American Journal of Obstetrics and Gynecology* (1961;81:283), Copyright © 1961, Mosby-Year Book.

Burch placed three no. 2 chromic catgut sutures on either side of the urethrovesical junction into the paravaginal fascia and then suspended and fixed the anterior wall of the vagina on either side of the urethra directly above Cooper's ligaments (Figure 5-4.6). Although he used chromic catgut suture, he stated that a permanent substitute might be his eventual choice. The sutures were tied as the surgeon or the assistant elevated the anterior wall of the vagina with a finger placed in the vagina.

Burch noted that his modification of the MMK procedure, in addition to providing more secure points of fixation of the suspending sutures, often corrected an associated cystocele. He recognized, however, that, in the presence of uterine prolapse, the procedure could predispose to the development of an enterocele. Therefore he emphasized the role of hysterectomy, Moschcowitz's obliteration of the cul-de-sac, and high reperitonealization of the pelvis. If a posterior repair and perineorrhaphy are indicated, he recommended that they should be performed after the abdominal procedure.

Burch's reported complications were enteroceles, rectoceles, a ventral hernia, and a vesicovaginal fistula. The vesicovaginal fistula was believed to be a complication of a hysterectomy and not of the urethrovaginal suspension. In his initial series (53 patients), all patients were relieved of their SUI. On the basis of this success, he recommended that a retropubic suspension of the anterior wall of the vagina be considered as a primary procedure for patients with major degrees of SUI and that the procedure not be reserved only for those with recurrent incontinence.

Burch subsequently reported on nine years' experience with his procedure as performed in 143 patients.[11] With the use of lateral straining urethrocystograms, he defined the anatomic results of a successful procedure: (1) recession of the external urethral meatus, (2) elevation of the bladder neck, (3) development of an acute angle between the bladder and the urethra, (4) change in the angle of inclination of the urethra, and (5) possibly some lengthening of the urethra. With all patients monitored for at least 10 months, and some for 5 years, he reported a cure rate of 93% with rare recurrences after 20 months of follow-up. His most challenging complication was the development of an enterocele (7.6%). To prevent this complication, the need for obliteration of the cul-de-sac was reemphasized.

Symmonds (Mayo) Modification

In 1972, Symmonds[12] (and with Lee in 1975[13]) recommended the removal of periurethral and perivesical fatty tissue during dissection of the retropubic space to improve visualization of anatomic landmarks and approximation of tissues. He recommended routine opening of the dome of the bladder to look for and correct the characteristic atonicity and funneling of the bladder neck and, in patients who had previously had surgery, to aid in dissecting the bladder and the urethra from the rectus muscle and retropubis (Figure 5-4.7). The surgeon's index and middle fingers were inserted into the vagina to determine the placement of the paraurethral sutures. Two, and occasionally three, pairs of 3-0 permanent (Tevdek) sutures were placed in the fibromuscular layer of the anterior wall of the vagina next to and on either side of the urethra. The most distal pair of sutures was placed at the level of the midurethra, and the proximal and most crucial pair of sutures were placed on either side of the urethrovesical junction, as determined visually by looking through the cystotomy site.

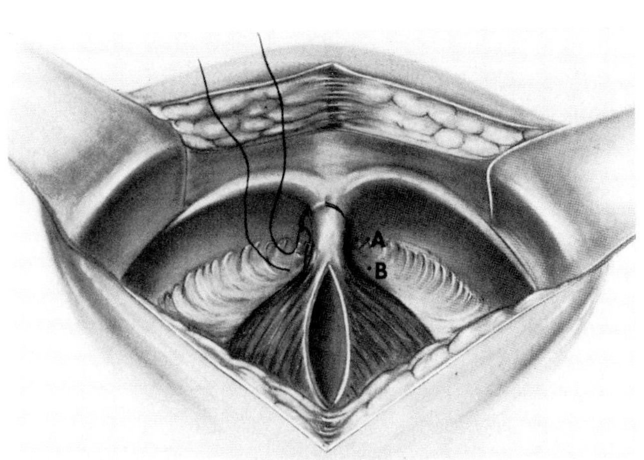

Figure 5-4.7 Symmonds (Mayo) modification. Retropubic dissection with perivesical fat removed and bladder open for inspection of neck and proximal aspect of urethra. Two (occasionally three) suspending sutures will be inserted at points *A* and *B* on each side of urethra and bladder neck. *Source:* Reprinted with permission from *Clinical Obstetrics and Gynecology* (1972;15:1114), Copyright © 1972, JB Lippincott Company.

Each suture was suspended toward the midline by a secure stitch into the fibrous tissue of the symphysis pubis (Figure 5-4.8). If there was a widely gaping urethrovesical junction, the anterior cystotomy was extended down the anterior upper half of the urethra and the upper portion of the urethra was tightly plicated about a Foley (16F) catheter with the use of interrupted 2-0 absorbable (chromic catgut) sutures placed in the muscular wall, but not through the epithelium of the urethra (Figure 5-4.9). When urethral plication was completed, the catheter's balloon was punctured, and the catheter was removed. The suspending pairs of sutures were tied to elevate and approximate the vaginal wall to the symphysis pubis. The cystotomy was closed about a suprapubic bladder drainage catheter with the use of two rows of continuous 2-0 absorbable (chromic catgut) suture. The suprapubic catheter was brought out of the lower portion of the abdominal wall through a separate stab incision.

Tanagho Modification

In 1976, Tanagho[14] recommended that the suspending sutures in the anterior wall of the vagina be placed as far lateral from the urethra as possible and that they pass through the full thickness of the vaginal wall, sparing the mucosa. He did this in an effort (1) to lift and support the urethrovesical junction forward and upward within the retropubic space, (2) to reduce the chance of compression or obstruction of the proximal portion of the urethra, and (3) to prevent surgical damage to the urethra and its sphincteric mechanism. Tanagho also recommended the removal of retropubic fat. He used two no. 1 delayed-absorbable (ie, polyglycolic acid) sutures placed through the anterior wall of the vagina on each side of the urethra, one opposite the midurethra and one (the more important one) far lateral to the urethrovesical junction, to suspend the proximal portion of the urethra (Figure 5-4.10A). He recommended the use of delayed-absorbable suture in the belief that permanent fixation would be the result of postoperative fibrosis.

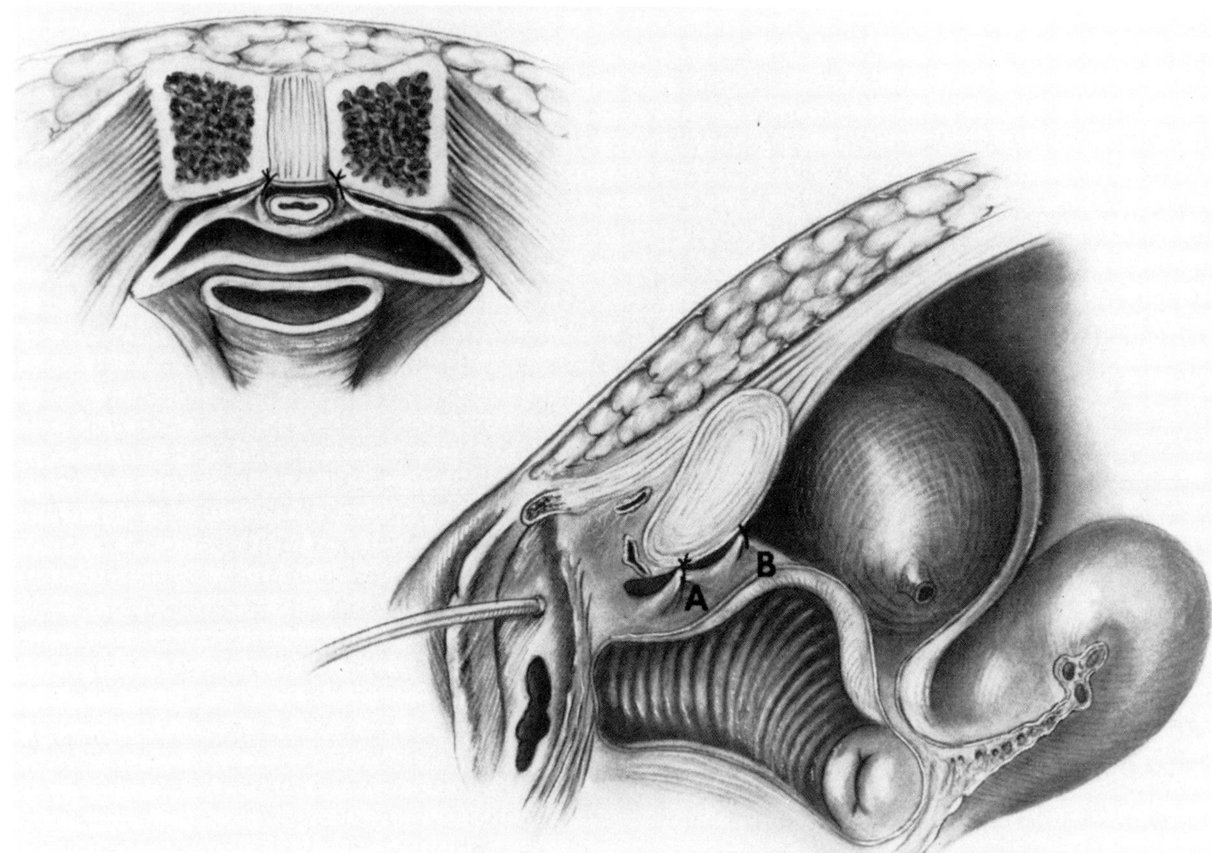

Figure 5-4.8 Symmonds (Mayo) modification. *Top*, Cross-section of symphysis pubis, urethra, and vagina at level of point *B* in lower figure. Suspending suture placed slightly medial into fibrocartilage of symphysis pubis, not in tenuous pubic periosteum. *Bottom,* When suspending sutures are tied, they provide smooth, nonobstructing *hammock* for entire length of urethra and bladder neck. *Source:* Reprinted with permission from *Clinical Obstetrics and Gynecology* (1972;15:1115), Copyright © 1972, JB Lippincott Company.

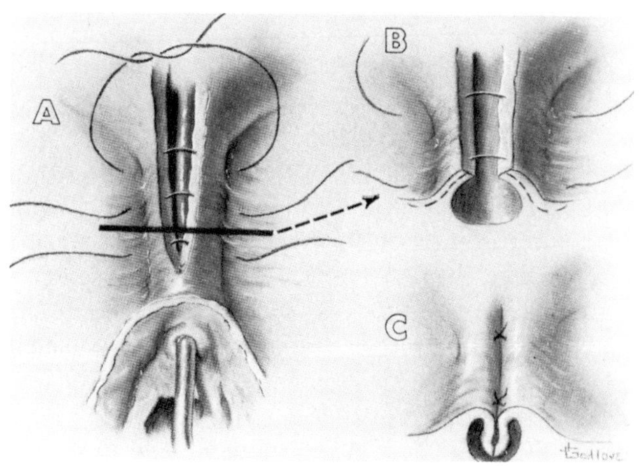

Figure 5-4.9 Symmonds (Mayo) modification. **A**, Cystostomy incision has been extended down through bladder neck and upper two thirds of urethra. Transverse line shows location of cross-section shown in **B** and **C.** (Symphysis pubis removed for clarity.) **B** and **C,** Cross-section of urethra showing method of inserting sutures in urethral smooth muscle (**B**) and diminished caliber of atonic funnel urethra (**C**). *Source:* Reprinted with permission from *Clinical Obstetrics and Gynecology* (1972;15:1118), Copyright © 1972, JB Lippincott Company.

The suspending sutures were attached to Cooper's ligaments, not toward the midline, but straight above their location within the vaginal wall. The tied sutures lifted the anterior wall of the vagina upward and forward within the retropubic space. Free suture material between Cooper's ligaments and the anterior wall of the vagina was not seen as a disadvantage (Figure 5-4.10B). Tanagho warned that the anterior wall of the vagina and Cooper's ligaments should not be brought into apposition if doing so might compress or obstruct the proximal portion of the urethra.

Recommended Technique

A retropubic colposuspension may be performed with the use of general or regional anesthesia. The patient is positioned supine on the operating table with her gluteal folds at the break between the middle and the lower

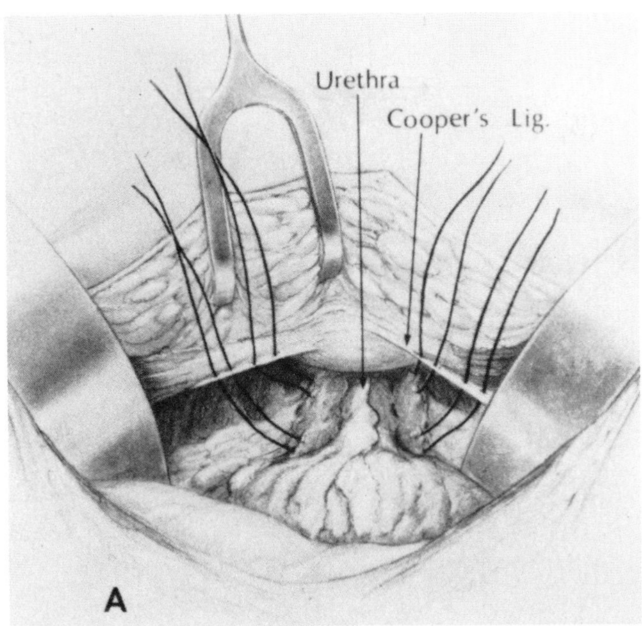

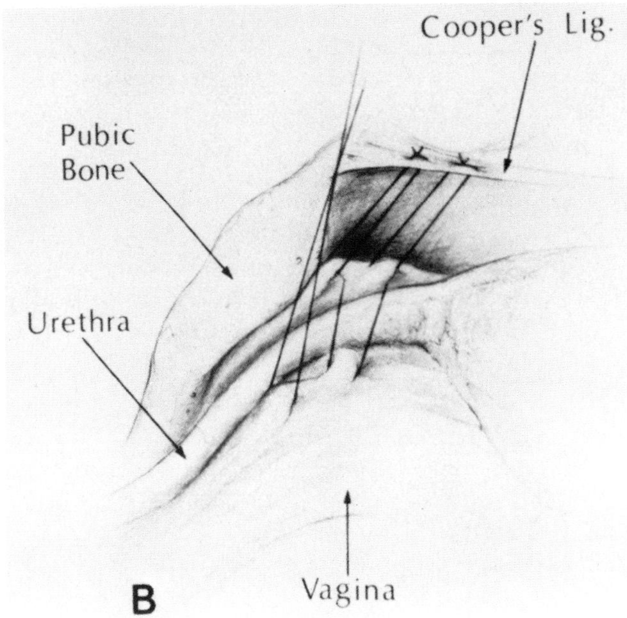

Figure 5-4.10 Tanagho modification. **A,** Diagrammatic illustration of retropubic space after mobilization of anterior wall of vagina and placement of sutures, two on either side and far lateral from midline. Distal sutures are opposite midurethra, whereas proximal sutures are at end of vesicourethral junction. Sutures are attached to Cooper's ligament. **B,** Side view of suture placement with one side tied. Anterior wall of vagina is acting as broad sling supporting and lifting vesicourethral segment. Yet, urethra is free in spacious retropubic space. *Source:* Reprinted with permission from EA Tanagho, "Colpocystourethropexy: The Way We Do It," *Journal of Urology* (1976;116:752), Copyright © 1976, Williams & Wilkins Company.

sections of the table. When the anesthesia reaches a satisfactory level, the patient's ankles and feet are placed in Allen Universal stirrups (Edgewater Medical Systems, Cleveland, OH), and she is positioned so that her legs are slightly flexed, abducted, and supported at a level just above that of the table top. The lower portion of the table is lowered (Figure 5-4.11). The abdomen, upper aspect of the thighs, vulva, vagina, perineum, and perianal areas are prepared and draped to allow the surgeon access to the abdomen and vagina. A sterile Foley (16F or 18F) catheter is placed transurethrally into the bladder. The catheter balloon is inflated, and its drainage port is connected to straight drainage.

The operation may be performed through a transverse (Pfannenstiel, Cherney, Maylard) or midline low abdominal incision. The incision is carried through the skin, the subcutaneous tissues, and the abdominal aponeurosis. The peritoneum is entered. If a hysterectomy or salpingo-oophorectomy (or both procedures) is to be a part of the procedure, it is performed, and the vaginal cuff is closed.[15]

To reduce the incidence of postoperative enterocele, the cul-de-sac (pouch of Douglas) is obliterated by using 2-0 permanent suture to perform either a Moschcowitz or Halban procedure. A Moschcowitz procedure[16] consists of placing two or three concentric sutures about the circumference of the cul-de-sac. The first suture is placed 1 to 2 cm above the deepest point within the cul-de-sac. A second, and perhaps a third, pursestring suture is placed in a similar fashion at 1 cm levels above the preceding suture. Suture placement must incorporate the channels on either side of the sigmoid colon and leave no spaces for entry and possible strangulation of the bowel. The plane of each pursestring suture should pass through the peritoneum and tinea of the colon at a higher level than its points of fixation to the peritoneum overlying the posterior wall of the vagina. The sutures must be placed so that they will not kink either ureter when they are tied. A Halban procedure[17] consists of placing a series of sutures within the cul-de-sac in sagittal planes so as to obliterate the cul-de-sac. Sutures placed in this manner are less likely to kink the ureters than are those placed in the Moschcowitz procedure. Again, it is important that no channels be left inside either uterosacral ligament that may permit entry and possible strangulation of the bowel.

After obliteration of the cul-de-sac and completion of any ancillary intra-abdominal procedures, the anterior parietal peritoneum is closed with a running 2-0 or 3-0 delayed-absorbable suture.

The patient is placed in a slightly reversed Trendelenburg's position. The medial edges of the rectus muscles

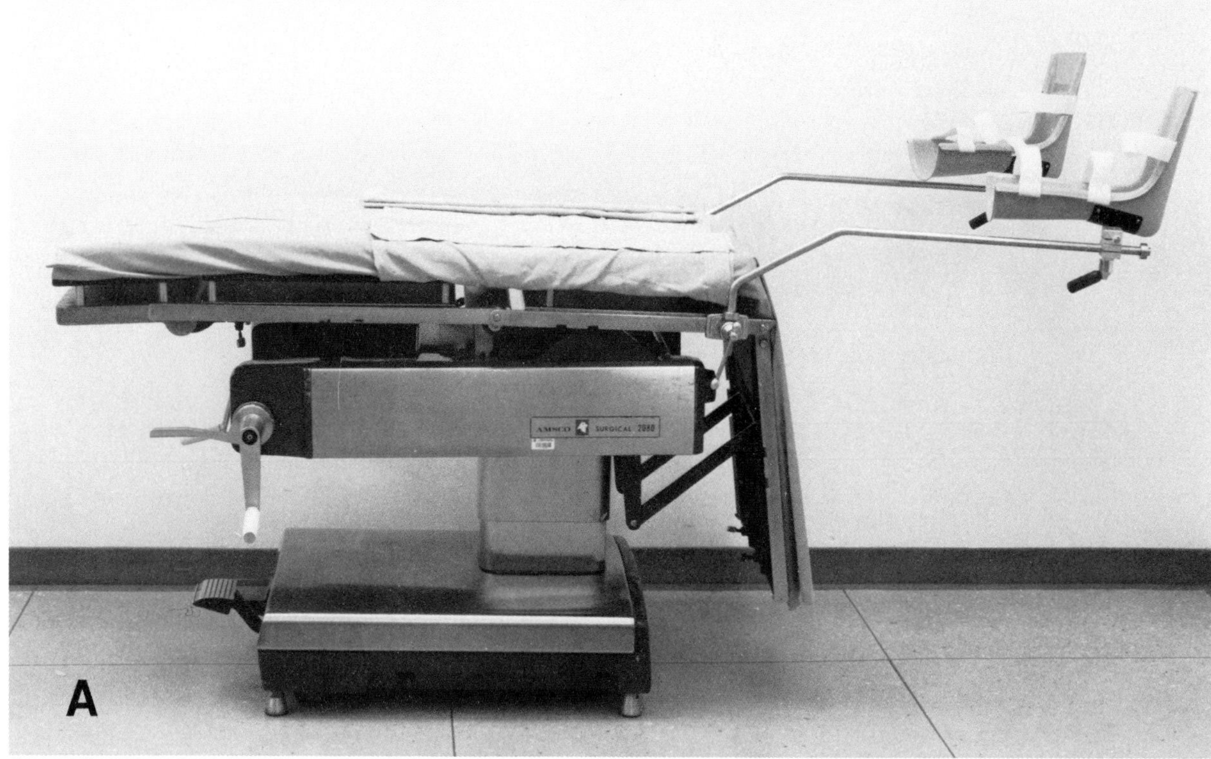

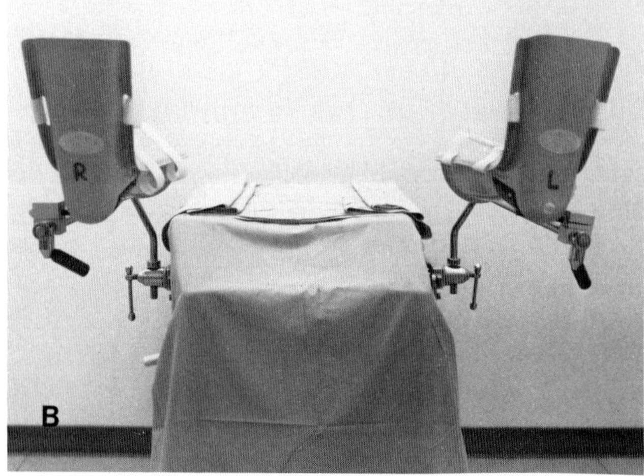

Figure 5-4.11 **A** and **B**, Allen Universal stirrups (Edgewater Medical Systems, Cleveland, OH) are used to position patient so that her legs are slightly flexed, abducted, and supported at level just above that of table top. *Source:* Courtesy of Edgewater Medical Systems, Cleveland, OH.

are retracted with the blades of a Balfour self-retaining retractor, placed so that its crossbar lies across the belly of each rectus muscle (Figure 5-4.12). As an alternative, especially in an obese patient, a Maylard muscle-cutting incision may be made and a Bookwalter retractor placed to increase lateral exposure. The transversalis fascia and parietal peritoneum are separated from beneath the lower ends of the rectus muscles. When there has been no previous surgery within the retropubic space, a moistened abdominal pack may be gently placed between the anterior wall of the bladder and the pubic bones and symphysis pubis to dissect the anterior wall of the bladder and peritoneum from the posterior surface of the pubis. The depths and lateral margins of the retropubic space may be better dissected with a moistened sponge on a sponge stick. Dissection of the retropubic space in patients who have had prior retropubic procedures is accomplished with greater ease and safety by performing an extraperitoneal vertical cystotomy in the dome of the bladder and by using a scalpel and Metzenbaum scissors under direct vision to dissect sharply the anterior wall of the bladder and the urethra from the pubic bones.

As a protective measure, approximately 5 mL of sterile infant's formula or indigo-carmine sterile solution should be instilled into the bladder by means of the drainage tube of the transurethral catheter. The tube is clamped shut to prevent the solution's escape. The escape of formula or blue solution into the operative field is evidence of bladder penetration or laceration and requires investigation.

It is advisable to prepare for the placement of the colposuspension sutures by ensuring the availability of three articles: (1) a malleable retractor, covered with a moistened and closely wrapped abdominal pack and bent

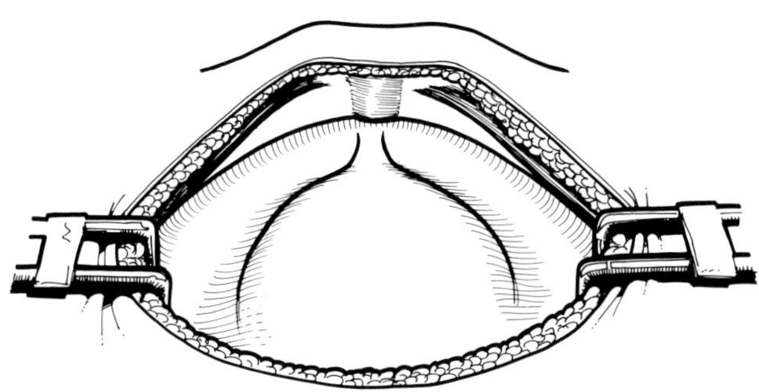

Figure 5-4.12 Abdominal wall is retracted, and retropubic space is exposed.

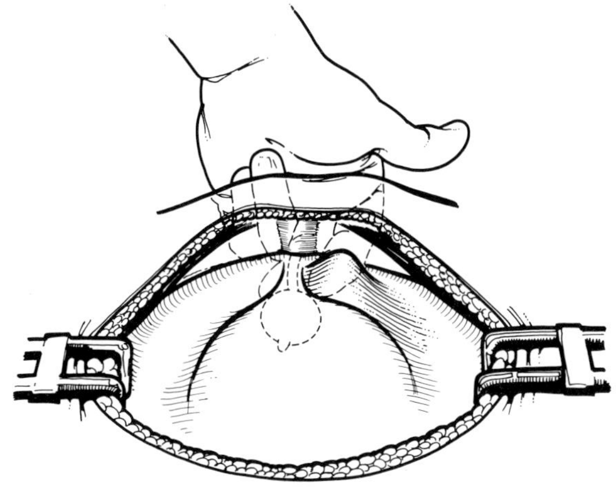

Figure 5-4.13 One finger within vagina elevates vaginal wall next to urethrovesical junction, and overlying tissues are displaced medially.

at the middle at an angle of approximately 20 degrees; (2) a gauze dissector (or peanut) on the end of a Kelly forceps; and (3) a Mayo (no. 5) taper needle threaded twice through its eye with 18 in of permanent suture material.

At this point, the surgeon should place a sterile sleeve and glove over the gown and glove on his or her non-dominant hand. The first and second fingers of the hand should be inserted into the patient's vagina. By flexing first one finger and then the other within the vagina, the anterior wall of the vagina on either side of the proximal portion of the urethra is elevated while the depths of the retropubic space are systematically dissected and de-fatted to a level that will allow visualization of the urethrovesical junction and the bladder neck. The glistening white fibromuscular layer of the anterior wall of the vagina on either side of the urethra should be exposed to the lateral vaginal fornices.

Normally, the distance between the middle crease of the index finger and the tip of that finger is about 4.5 to 5 cm. This is the average length of the female urethra. The surgeon should hold the drainage tube of the Foley catheter within the palmar surface of the hand that is within the vagina. The tips of the fingers are at the junction of the Foley catheter balloon and drainage tube, and the tip of the thumb of the same hand compresses the drainage tube as it exits the external meatus against the crevice between the first and second fingers at the level of the middle crease of the fingers. This establishes a method for determining the approximate level of suture placement on either side of the urethrovesical junction 4 to 5 cm from the external urethral meatus.

The surgeon should place the fingers of his or her dominant hand into one lateral wing of the retropubic space and with medial and upward traction move the anterolateral wall of the bladder and the more lateral posterior wall of the retropubic space to expose its depths. The assistant then places the malleable retractor between the dorsal aspect of the surgeon's fingers and the retrosymphysis and maintains exposure after removal of the surgeon's hand. The surgeon elevates one of the lateral vaginal fornices by flexing one of the fingers within the vagina (Figure 5-4.13). If necessary, a gauze (or peanut) dissector on a Kelly forceps is used to displace the proximal aspect of the urethra and bladder neck medially.

A long Allis forceps is used to grasp the entire thickness of the anterior wall of the vagina overlying the tip of one of the fingers in the vagina 2 cm lateral to the urethrovesical junction. Although the glove overlying the finger may be pinched by grasping the anterior wall of the vagina with the Allis clamp, the risk of puncturing the glove and penetrating the finger, in this era of concern about human immunodeficiency virus infection, is overcome by this maneuver. A permanent 0 suture is placed by two passes through the entire thickness of the anterior wall of the vagina, which has been grasped with the Allis forceps. The forceps are then removed, and the long ends of the suture are equalized and tagged. With placement of the malleable retractor in the opposite wing of the retropubic space, the entire thickness of the anterior wall of the vagina is grasped with a long Allis forceps in an identical location on the opposite side of the urethrovesical junction, and a 0 permanent suture is similarly placed and tagged with an identical type of small forceps. A second suture is placed on either side of the bladder neck with the use of the malleable retractor for exposure and long Allis forceps to grasp the anterior wall of the vagina 1.5 to 2 cm lateral and superior with respect to the first pair of sutures and to place and tag in a similar manner a second pair of 0 permanent sutures. It is helpful to tag each pair of sutures with dissimilar small forceps to distinguish their lateral location. If the patient has a significant cystocele, a third suture may be placed on either side of the bladder neck in a similar fashion lateral and cephalad to the second suture, with care being taken not to incorporate or otherwise compromise the ipsilateral ureter. All sutures are placed on both sides of the urethrovesical junction and bladder neck before any sutures are tied.

Upward traction on the tagging forceps determines the security of suture placement within the anterior wall of the vagina and the maximum degree of elevation of the proximal portion of the urethra. In a sequential fashion, the arms of each suspending suture are individually threaded onto a Mayo (no. 5) taper needle and passed through Cooper's ligaments directly above their location within the anterior wall of the vagina. The needle is removed, and the ends of the suture are tagged again. The ends of all sutures are placed through Cooper's ligaments before any sutures are tied (Figure 5-4.14). While the surgeon uses the tips of his or her fingers within the vagina to determine the desired amount of elevation of the urethrovesical junction, the assistant ties the suspending sutures to maintain the location of the urethrovesical junction and the bladder neck (Figure 5-4.15). Care is taken not to compress the urethra against the symphysis pubis or to obstruct the urethra by excessive elevation and kinking of the urethrovesical junction. When permanent suture material is used for the suspension, it is not necessary to have the anterior wall of the vagina in direct apposition with Cooper's ligaments, especially if doing so will unduly stretch the urethra and obstruct the bladder neck. Loops of permanent suture material should not compromise the overall result. Excessive tension on the suspending sutures may cause necrosis at their points of attachment to the anterior wall of the vagina and may contribute to suture release and surgical failure.

When there is excessive bleeding in the retropubic space, the use of disposable suction drains (Jackson-Pratt) is recommended. The drains should be placed under direct vision, and the drainage tubing should be brought out the anterior abdominal wall through separate stab incisions. The tubing should be secured to the skin by using 2-0 permanent suture.

The medial edges of the rectus muscles should be approximated across the midline with interrupted delayed-absorbable sutures to prevent ventral herniation of the dome of the bladder or the abdominal viscera (or both structures). The cut edges of the abdominal aponeurosis and the skin should be approximated in a routine fashion. The abdominal incision and all stab incisions should have an appropriate dressing.

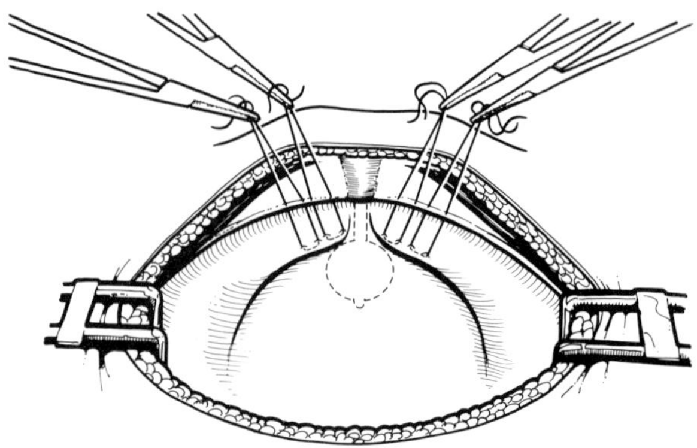

Figure 5-4.14 Figure-of-eight sutures are placed bilaterally through entire thickness of anterior wall of vagina lateral to urethrovesical junction and then directly through Cooper's ligaments (iliopectineal lines).

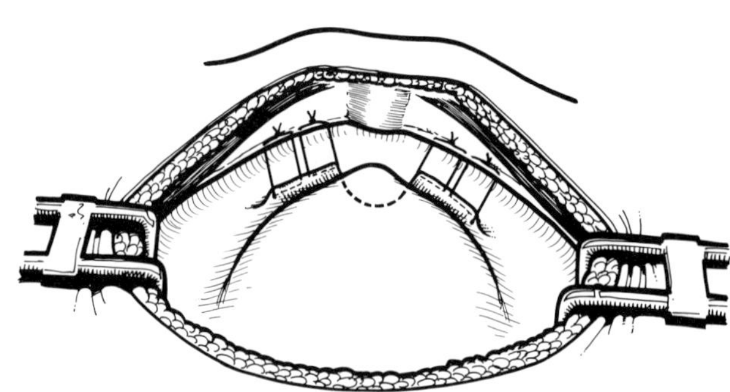

Figure 5-4.15 Colposuspension is performed by tieing suspending sutures. It should elevate, but not obstruct, urethrovesical junction.

When a cystotomy is performed, ureteric function and patency can be documented after urethrovesical suspension by administering intravenous indigo-carmine (5 mL) solution and observing the subsequent excretion of blue urine from the ureteral orifices. If a cystotomy is not performed, it is possible to document ureteral excretion of the blue urine by filling the bladder with a sterile liquid (eg, water, normal saline, or 10% glucose), placing a delayed-absorbable pursestring suture about a small area in the extraperitoneal portion of the anterior wall of the bladder, and inserting the telescope (teloscopy) of either a hysteroscope or cystoscope through a puncture incision in the portion of the bladder wall encompassed by the pursestring suture. Once it is determined that there are no suspending sutures within the bladder and that bilateral ureteral excretion is occurring, the bladder may be drained and a suprapubic catheter (Foley or Malecot) placed into the bladder through the cystotomy site. The bladder wall can then be closed about the catheter by tying the pursestring suture, and the suprapubic catheter can be brought out through a separate stab incision in the lower area of the abdominal wall. Transurethral cystoscopy is an alternative method of documenting that no sutures traverse the bladder mucosa and that there is bilateral ureteral function.

Postoperative bladder drainage is recommended. If there was no cystotomy and no significant bleeding within the bladder during the procedure, a disposable suprapubic catheter may be inserted, fixed to the skin, and attached to a closed straight drainage system. If a cystotomy was performed, or if there was significant bleeding within the bladder, a Foley or Malecot catheter should be inserted through a cystotomy site in the extraperitoneal portion of the dome of the bladder. All drainage tubes should be brought out of the abdominal wall through separate puncture sites.

I have the patient begin voiding trials on the third or the fourth postoperative day. I have noticed that bladder function usually does not return until bowel function returns. Therefore voiding trials may be postponed until the patient begins passing flatus or having bowel movements. In a voiding trial, the patient clamps the suprapubic tube to allow the bladder to fill with urine; attempts to void when there is the urge to do so; and measures the amount of urine voided and, by emptying the bladder by way of the suprapubic catheter, the postvoid residual. I usually do not remove the suprapubic catheter until the patient has a postvoid residual consistently less than 90 to 100 mL. When voiding trials are begun, the patient is instructed to unclamp the suprapubic catheter and drain the bladder if she experiences pain related to bladder distention or inability to void. The patient should never be allowed to collect more than 500 mL of urine in her bladder. One episode of overdistention of the bladder will delay the return of normal voiding for an indeterminate period. It may also cause anoxia of the urothelium and promote the development of a urinary tract infection.

PHYSIOLOGIC ALTERATIONS

Anatomically, a retropubic colposuspension elevates the proximal portion of the urethra and maintains the urethrovesical junction within the abdominal zone of pressure during sudden increases in intra-abdominal pressure. Repositioning the proximal portion of the urethra may well lengthen the urethra and reduce the caliber of its proximal segment. Suspending the suture on either side of the bladder neck will reduce an anterior cystocele.

I believe that the goals of retropubic surgery in the treatment of SUI are (1) to restore the urethrovesical junction to within the abdominal zone of pressure, (2) to allow posterior rotational descent of the bladder base as the result of the downward thrust of the more posterosuperior viscera, (3) to preserve the integrity of the urethral sphincteric mechanism, and (4) to preserve the compressibility of the urethra.[18,19]

Restoration and stabilization of the urethrovesical junction to a high retropubic position places the bladder outlet and proximal portion of the urethra within the abdominal zone of pressure in which increases in intra-abdominal pressure will be equally distributed to both organs and the pressure differential favoring continence will be preserved.[19,20] As long as the pressure within the urethra remains greater than the pressure within the bladder, no urinary leakage should occur.

When the bladder base and the more posterosuperior viscera retain their downward mobility, sudden increases in intra-abdominal pressure will result in their descent, which closes the urethrovesical junction and compresses the well-supported proximal portion of the urethra.[19] This mechanism is inherent to many continence procedures and is effective in preventing the involuntary escape of urine. Both lifting the bladder base in an effort to correct a cystocele and straightening the anterior wall of the vagina as a result of too much tension on the suspending strap of an abdominal colposacropexy or cystopexy sutures (such as those used in the original version of the MMK procedure) are believed to be counterproductive with respect to the cure of SUI.

The urethra of most patients with primary SUI is anatomically and neurologically normal. The bladder sphincter, however, is at an anatomic disadvantage as a result of damage to its supporting mechanism. Sudden increases in intra-abdominal pressure displace it from within the abdominal zone of pressure and result in unequal distributions of pressure to the bladder outlet and proximal segment of the urethra. When bladder pressure exceeds urethral pressure, urinary leakage may occur. Chronic downward displacement of the urethrovesical junction can further compromise urethral function by dilating the proximal segment of the urethra. Such proximal funneling of the urethra shortens its functional length. If urine enters the proximal portion of the urethra, it may in itself be responsible for urethral relaxation and involuntary leakage of urine. The urethral sphincteric mechanism has three components, each of which contributes to approximately one third of the urethral closure pressure: (1) smooth muscle; (2) skeletal muscle; and (3) mucosa, connective tissue, and vascular plexus. It is important to preserve the integrity of the urethral sphincteric mechanism when continence procedures are performed. Because the urethra and the urethral sphincteric mechanism are rarely involved pathologically in cases of SUI, there is no reason for a direct surgical attack on the urethra itself. In fact, surgery on the urethra can damage it indirectly through devascularization or denervation injuries or directly through disruption of the various components of its delicate wall.

Preserving the compressibility of the urethra is important in the restoration of urinary continence.[19] The functionless, ''drain-pipe'' urethra has no sphincteric action and is only a urinary conduit. If the compressible urethra is so aligned with the retrosymphysis that it can be closed at the bladder neck and its proximal segment compressed, it will not permit the involuntary escape of urine during sudden increases in intra-abdominal pressure.

Urodynamically, a successful retropubic colposuspension has little or no effect on the passive (resting) urethral pressure profile. It does, however, enhance the stress urethral pressure profile by increasing the total profile length, functional urethral length, and maximum urethral closure pressure. It also improves pressure transmission ratios. Uroflowmetry often reveals a slightly reduced flow rate, reduction in the peak flow rate, and increase in maximum voiding pressure. Failed retropubic colposuspensions do not show significant changes in these parameters.

Table 5-4.1 Complications of Retropubic Urethropexy or Colposuspension Procedures

Bleeding
Extraperitoneal hematoma
Infections and Inflammation
Retropubic abscess
Urinary tract infection
Osteitis pubis
Osteomyelitis
Thrombophlebitis
Urinary Tract Injury
Ureter
Bladder
Genitourinary fistula
Urinary Tract Dysfunction or Incontinence
Urinary retention
Detrusor instability
Stress incontinence
Pelvic Organ Prolapse
Enterocele
Rectocele
Cystocele
Sexual Dysfunction
Dyspareunia
Vaginal shortening

COMPLICATIONS

A list of the more common complications associated with retropubic urethropexy and colposuspension procedures is given in Table 5-4.1.

The retropubic space is a potential space bounded anteriorly by the pubic bones and symphysis pubis and posteriorly by the anterior wall of the bladder, the urethra, and the vagina. It contains a loose network of areolar tissue, a variable amount of fat, and many blood vessels, including the inferior vesical artery and large veins of the perivesical plexus. When fully exposed by the abdominal approach, the retropubic space is triangular and has no dependent drainage. Initial dissections of the retropubic space can usually be performed with ease and with minimal blood loss. Repeat dissections complicated by fibrosis and fixation of the anterior wall of the bladder, the urethra, and the vagina to the retropubis are more likely to be accompanied by blood vessel or organ injury.

There is a longitudinal venous plexus that courses along the undersurface of each anterior lateral fornix of the vagina. More often than not, it is located in the area of placement of the suspending sutures for retropubic colposuspension. If this is the case, it is best to incorporate these vessels by placing the suspending sutures about, rather than through, this longitudinal venous plexus. Inevitably, in the course of some dissections and suture placements, some of these veins will be lacerated and bleeding will occur. It may be possible to encompass the venous plexus and control the venous bleeding by tying the suspending sutures. If this cannot be done, vascular clips should be applied or suture ligation used. If a large collection of blood within the retropubic space is likely to occur, or if there has been injury to the urethra, the bladder, or the ureter(s) that might result in the collection of urine within the retropubic space, pliable suction drains (eg, Jackson-Pratt drains) should be placed into the depths of the space and brought out separate stab incisions anteriorly in the lower aspect of the abdominal wall. These drains should be kept activated and not removed as long as there are clinically significant accumulations of blood or urine.

The development of an abscess is rare when the retropubic space is approached abdominally.[21] Dissection of the retropubic space and placement of the suspending suture through-and-through the anterior wall of the vagina inevitably contaminate the retropubic space with vaginal organisms. Unless there is a collection of blood or serum, however, an abscess usually does not develop. Therefore it is important to prevent the collection of blood and serum within the retropubic space. A short course of prophylactic antibiotics (eg, cefazolin sodium, 1 g; given intravenously, before, during, and 6 to

8 hours after surgery) has been shown to reduce the postoperative febrile morbidity of patients undergoing retropubic surgery for SUI.[22]

Significant bacteriuria is common after continence surgery and usually is due to contamination by bladder catheter drainage. Patients who have suprapubic bladder catheters have much fewer symptomatic urinary tract infections than do patients with transurethral catheters. Intermittent urethral self-catheterization is less likely to cause a urinary tract infection than is an indwelling catheter. To prevent urinary tract infections it is important not to operate on patients who have bacteriuria, to avoid direct bladder injury as a result of the surgical procedure or indirect injury related to overdistention or denervation of the bladder, to use a closed-catheter drainage system with an antireflux valve, and to limit the use of indwelling catheters. It is difficult to render free of infection the urine of patients who have an indwelling catheter; however, it is important to do so when catheterization is no longer required.

Osteitis pubis occurs in about 2% to 3% of patients who have their suspending sutures placed into the periosteum of the symphysis pubis.[21] Its cause is unknown. It does not appear to be related to the type of suture material used in the suspension procedure. Osteitis pubis usually becomes symptomatic within 2 months of the procedure and is characterized by the abrupt onset of pubic pain that may radiate down the inner aspect of the thighs. It is aggravated by physical exertion. There is tenderness over the symphysis pubis. The diagnosis is confirmed radiologically by the rarefaction and loss of cortical bone. Sclerosis is evidence of healing. The condition tends to be self-limiting. Treatment is symptomatic and consists of bed rest and the administration of analgesics and cortisone acetate (300 mg on day 1, 200 mg on day 2, and 100 mg per day for 8 days). Therapy usually results in the relief of pain and adductor spasm. Noninfectious osteitis pubis should be differentiated from infectious osteitis pubis, which is more commonly referred to as osteomyelitis and is a rare complication of retropubic urethropexy and colposuspension procedures. If there are signs of an overt bacterial infection, intravenous antibiotic therapy is indicated.

Pelvic surgery predisposes patients to the development of deep thrombophlebitis and to pulmonary embolization. Patients who are at risk for thrombophlebitis may be candidates for mini-dose heparin prophylaxis, intermittent pneumatic compression stockings, and early ambulation.

Continence operations predispose the lower urinary tract to injury. The incidence in retropubic urethropexy and colposuspension procedures should be less than 5%.[21] Bladder and ureteral injuries are more common when prior pelvic surgery has resulted in fibrosis and fixation of the ureter(s), the bladder base, and the proximal segment of the urethra. In difficult cases, an extraperitoneal cystotomy will allow the surgeon to dissect the anterior portion of the bladder and urethra from the retropubis under direct visualization and reduce the incidence of inadvertent injury to these organs. It will also enable the surgeon to see that no sutures traverse the bladder and, by the intravenous injection of indigo-carmine (5 mL) solution, to test bilateral ureteral function. Unrecognized injuries should be almost eliminated if the integrity of the lower urinary tract is tested during surgery. Genitourinary fistulas rarely occur after retropubic urethropexy and colposuspension procedures. When they do occur, they are often the result of concomitant procedures.

Some degree of urinary retention occurs in 15% to 20% of patients who undergo MMK or Burch procedures.[23] These operations can compress the proximal segment of the urethra and unduly kink the urethrovesical junction.[1,24] Bladder outlet obstruction is a more important cause of urinary retention than is bladder denervation. Preoperative uroflowmetry and studies of the voiding mechanism can help predict patients who will have postoperative voiding difficulty. Patients who depend on a Valsalva's mechanism for voiding are more likely to have postoperative voiding difficulty than are those in whom a detrusor contraction initiates micturition. Overdistention of the bladder predisposes to urinary tract infection and delays the return of spontaneous and efficient voiding. Bladder catheterization should be used to prevent urinary retention. Because postoperative urinary retention is usually transient and is overcome by the "tincture of time," it is reasonable to use catheter drainage until the postvoid urinary residual is repeatedly less than 90 to 100 mL. Diazepam (2 to 10 mg, one to three times per day), as a striated muscle relaxant and anxietolytic, has proved to be more effective than bethanechol chloride in treating postoperative urinary retention.

In rare cases, prolonged postoperative retention after urethropexy and colposuspension procedures has required release of the suspending sutures or revision of the surgical repair.[24] Detrusor function should be evaluated before surgical release of the suspension because some patients might prefer intermittent self-catheterization to taking a chance that they may experience recurrent urinary incontinence.

Preoperative DI may or may not be cured by a retropubic continence procedure, and, unfortunately, DI is a recognized complication in 10% to 15% of patients who have undergone a retropubic continence procedure.[1,25]

The patient who has postoperative urinary incontinence related to DI will consider her surgical procedure a failure. It is important to diagnose DI preoperatively and to inform patients that it can develop as a consequence of continence surgery.[3] Once the patient has discontinued catheter use and had her urine rendered free of infection, she should have aggressive drug therapy, bladder training, and behavioral modification in an effort to control this cause of postoperative urinary incontinence.

Retropubic urethropexy and colposuspension procedures fail to cure approximately 15% of patients with SUI.[21] Many reasons can be given for the failure, including imprecise preoperative diagnosis, failure to accomplish the technical objectives of the procedure, and failure of suspending materials or tissues.

Ventral fixation of the pelvic organs exposes the cul-de-sac (of Douglas) to increases in intra-abdominal pressure and the development of an enterocele. This has been reported in 7% to 14% of patients in whom prophylactic obliteration of the cul-de-sac was not performed.[15] For this reason a Moschcowitz or a Halban procedure should be considered when performing a retropubic urethropexy and colposuspension procedure.

The development of cystoceles or rectoceles after surgery usually is due to a failure to recognize and correct such conditions at the time of surgery. Both may become more pronounced as a result of a procedure to suspend the anterior aspect of the vagina. Progressive descent of a cystocele or a rectocele may in itself become symptomatic and require surgery.

Sexual dysfunction can be the result of the development of a tender vaginal constriction at the level of the urethrovesical junction. It may take 3 months or more for the tenderness and the obstructive nature of this band to resolve. Elevating the urethrovesical junction can foreshorten an already shortened vagina. If, preoperatively, the patient has a scarred and foreshortened vagina, some other continence procedure may be considered. When colposuspensions are followed by vaginal constrictions and shortening of the vagina, vaginal dilators may be beneficial in overcoming vaginal inadequacy and dyspareunia.

THERAPEUTIC RESULTS

Review of the surgical literature reveals that retropubic urethropexy or colposuspension procedures of the type described can be expected (on the basis of objective testing) to cure 80% of patients with urodynamically proved SUI.[21,26] An additional, but unpredictable, number of patients will be improved to the extent that they will be satisfied with the results of surgery. The operation will fail to restore urinary continence in about 15% of patients. Failure to restore urinary continence may be due to a failure to accomplish the technical objectives of the procedure, release of the suspending sutures or tissues, preoperative DI not corrected by the procedure, or DI that developed as a consequence of the procedure. In many cases, DI can be managed with medical therapy, bladder retraining drills, and behavior modification.

As with all continence procedures, a retropubic urethropexy or colposuspension procedure is more likely to cure patients with SUI who have not had prior surgery for the problem than those who have had one or more failed continence procedures. The failure rate of all continence procedures tends to increase in proportion to the number of procedures performed for its cure. Although most surgical failures occur within the first 2 years of continence surgery, there is a gradual increase in the failure rate, which can be attributed to aging, systemic disease, and physical stresses of daily living.

REFERENCES

1. Langer R, Ron-El R, Neuman M, Herman A, Caspi E. Detrusor instability following colposuspension for urinary stress incontinence. *Br J Obstet Gynaecol*. 1988;95:607–610.

2. Korda A, Ferry J, Hunter P. Colposuspension for the treatment of female urinary incontinence. *Aust N Z J Obstet Gynaecol*. 1989;29:146–149.

3. Sand PK, Bowen LW, Ostergard DR, Brubaker L, Panganiban R. The effect of retropubic urethropexy on detrusor stability. *Obstet Gynecol*. 1988;71:818–822.

4. Jorgensen L, Lose G, Mortensen SO, Molsted-Pedersen L, Kristensen JK. The Burch colposuspension for urinary incontinence in patients with stable and unstable detrusor function. *Neurourol Urodynam*. 1988;7:435–441.

5. Bowen LW, Sand PK, Ostergard DR, Franti CE. Unsuccessful Burch retropubic urethropexy: a case-controlled urodynamic study. *Am J Obstet Gynecol*. 1989;160:452–458.

6. Koonings PP, Bergman A, Ballard CA. Low urethral pressure and stress urinary incontinence in women: risk facts for failed retropubic surgical procedure. *Urology*. 1990;36:245–248.

7. McGuire EJ. Urodynamic findings in patients after failure of stress incontinence operations. *Prog Clin Biol Res*. 1981;78:351–360.

8. Sand PK, Bowen LW, Panganiban R, Ostergard DR. The low pressure urethra as a factor in failed retropubic urethropexy. *Obstet Gynecol*. 1987;69:399–402.

9. Marshall VF, Marchetti AA, Krantz KE. The correction of stress incontinence by simple vesicourethral suspension. *Surg Gynecol Obstet*. 1949;88:509–518.

10. Burch JC. Urethrovaginal fixation to Cooper's ligament for correction of stress incontinence, cystocele, and prolapse. *Am J Obstet Gynecol.* 1961;81:281–290.

11. Burch JC. Cooper's ligament urethrovesical suspension for stress incontinence. *Am J Obstet Gynecol.* 1968;100:764–774.

12. Symmonds RE. The suprapubic approach to anterior vaginal relaxation and urinary stress incontinence. *Clin Obstet Gynecol.* 1972;15:1107–1121.

13. Lee RA, Symmonds RE. Repeat Marshall-Marchetti procedures for recurrent stress urinary incontinence. *Am J Obstet Gynecol.* 1975;122:219–229.

14. Tanagho EA. Colpocystourethropexy: the way we do it. *J Urol.* 1976;116:751–753.

15. Langer R, Ron-El R, Neuman M, Herman A, Bukovsky I, Caspi E. The value of simultaneous hysterectomy during Burch colposuspension for urinary stress incontinence. *Obstet Gynecol.* 1988;72:866–869.

16. Moschcowitz AV. The pathogenesis, anatomy, and cure of prolapse of the rectum. *Surg Gynecol Obstet.* 1912;15:7–21.

17. Halban J. *Gynäkologische Operationslehre.* Berlin and Vienna: Urban & Schwarzenberg; 1932.

18. Hertogs K, Stanton SL. Lateral bead-chain urethrocystography after successful and unsuccessful colposuspension. *Br J Obstet Gynaecol.* 1985;92:1179–1183.

19. Hertogs K, Stanton SL. Mechanism of urinary continence after colposuspension: barrier studies. *Br J Obstet Gynaecol.* 1985; 92:1184–1188.

20. Penttinen J, Lindholm EL, Kaar K, Kauppila A. Successful colposuspension in stress urinary incontinence reduces bladder neck mobility and increases pressure transmission to the urethra. *Acta Gynecol Obstet.* 1989;244:233–238.

21. Mainprize TC, Drutz HP. The Marshall-Marchetti-Krantz procedure: a critical review. *Obstet Gynecol Surv.* 1988;43:724–729.

22. Bhatia NN, Karram MM, Bergman A. Role of antibiotic prophylaxis in retropubic surgery for stress urinary incontinence. *Obstet Gynecol.* 1989;74:637–639.

23. Lose G, Jorgensen L, Mortensen SO, Molsted-Pedersen L, Kristensen JK. Voiding difficulties after colposuspension. *Obstet Gynecol.* 1987;69:33–38.

24. Galloway NTM, Davies N, Stephenson TP. The complications of colposuspension. *Br J Urol.* 1987;60:122–124.

25. Cardozo LD, Stanton SL, Williams JE. Detrusor instability following surgery for genuine stress incontinence. *Br J Urol.* 1979;51:204–207.

26. Van Geelen JM, Theeuwes AGM, Eskes TKAB, Martin CB. The clinical and urodynamic effects of anterior vaginal repair and Burch colposuspension. *Am J Obstet Gynecol.* 1988;159:137–144.

5-5

Pubovaginal Slings

Edward J. McGuire and Julian Wan

BACKGROUND

The use of fascia or other materials to partly encircle the urethra and to cure incontinence is not new. In 1917, Stoeckel[1] reported on the use of pyramidalis muscle as a sling. Millin[2] described the use of two strips of rectus fascia, and other workers[3,4] reported on the use of lyophilized dural strips or other, alloplastic, synthetic materials as slings.

In general, sling procedures have been used to correct incontinence that has failed to respond to a less severe method of therapy, rather than as a primary procedure to correct incontinence. In all these procedures, the initial success rate in the cure of stress incontinence was high.[5] The early and late complications, however, were multiple and serious and included erosion of the bladder or the urethra, particularly by the alloplastic material; sinus formation; abscess formation; obstructive uropathy; and, occasionally, permanent urinary retention. Although the primary indication for sling operations is failure of a prior procedure, some investigators have reported their use in patients with bladder and urethral dysfunction resulting from myelodysplasia and peripheral neuropathy.[6,7]

In spite of the fact that in some medical centers slings are used often, they have never gained widespread acceptance. This may be related in part to a perception that the procedure is technically difficult or that the potential complications are so severe that the operation is best left to experts in the area.

Unfortunately, a clear exposition of the indications for sling procedures, as opposed to a less complicated operation, is not apparent in the literature. It seems likely that this is the major reason why slings are not often used by urologists and gynecologists. If, for example, it were clearly established that a certain type of incontinence would respond reliably only to a sling procedure and that other procedures would fail to correct the problem, a true risk:benefit relation could be established. After 19 years and some 1340 sling procedures, we know that the situation described actually exists, but we appreciate that those who use slings have not been very adept at describing to others what seems obvious to them.

PATIENT SELECTION

Most articles on slings simply state that the procedure is reserved for patients in whom one or more prior operative procedures have failed. That these patients are cured by a sling does not establish the sling as superior unless more is known about the urodynamic findings in the patients treated with a sling. Failure of a prior operation to cure stress incontinence is not rare, and, by using a familiar procedure, a good surgeon can in many instances cure the incontinence with a standard retropubic or transvaginal needle suspension. Thus the mere fact that a prior operation has failed is not in itself sufficient reason to use a sling for the patient's next repair, given that the degree of difficulty with the procedure for both patient and surgeon is likely to be greater than with a standard repair.

Most patients with stress urinary incontinence show urinary leakage in association with a change in urethral position.[8] The increase in intra-abdominal pressure causes posterior rotational descent of the urethra, and urinary leakage occurs in association with that movement.[8,9] Most patients with incontinence related purely to hypermobility have a normal sphincteric mechanism at rest. In particular, the internal sphincter is closed, as confirmed both by radiographic observation and by direct pressure measurements.[10] Furthermore, urethral pressures are not changed by a successful operative repair of the stress incontinence. In other words, *cure* of the condition does not depend on compression of the urethra or on the engineering of a better closure mechanism. Rather, it depends on suspension of the urethra, so that it no longer moves with an increase in intra-abdominal pressure. These findings indicate that correction of urethral hypermobility alone, without any other measurable change, is sufficient to cure the incontinence in women in whom video urodynamic studies show that urethral hypermobility was present in association with stress.[11]

There is a much smaller group of women with stress incontinence who do not show urethral hypermobility with changes in intra-abdominal pressure but who, nonetheless, leak urine across the urethral sphincter with coughing and sneezing, just as do women with urethral hypermobility. On video urodynamic studies these women show a poorly closed or totally open internal sphincteric mechanism. In the first descriptions of these findings, most of the patients had already experienced two failed operative procedures, usually an anterior repair and a retropubic urethropexy.[9,11] Urinary loss occurred at lower intra-abdominal pressures in this group, as compared to the pressures in women with a hypermobile urethra, and the incontinence was more severe.

Although these findings indicated that there was a subgroup of women with stress incontinence that resulted from a pathophysiologic mechanism different from that encountered in most patients, this observation did not lead to a change in the usual diagnostic methods for women with stress incontinence. The standard evaluation continued to be clinical assessment supplemented by the use of provocative cystometry, urethral pressure profilometry, and other tests designed to characterize the degree of urethral hypermobility. Although there are reasons to do a cystometrogram in patients with stress incontinence, it is not as important as the identification of a poorly functioning internal sphincter. The latter problem is the underlying cause of failure of a prior operation to cure incontinence in most patients. Unfortunately, the urethral pressure profile, which concentrates on peak urethral closing pressure, does not identify these patients, and a dynamic pressure profile misses some 25% to 30% of an unselected population with stress incontinence, as demonstrated with the use of video urodynamic studies.

It is possible to obtain information on the strength of the closing mechanism of the internal sphincter by simply noting the intra-abdominal pressure (measured in the bladder) required to cause leakage while the patient performs a Valsalva's maneuver. A hypermobile urethra leaks at pressures greater than 70 centimeters of water (cm H_2O), and a poorly functioning urethra leaks at pressures less than 50 cm H_2O. There is a mixed incontinence area in the midrange, but at either end of the spectrum there are two clearly defined types of stress incontinence: one associated with a fixed immobile dysfunctional urethra (Figure 5-5.1) and one associated with urethral hypermobility (Figure 5-5.2). Although there are no true random, double-blind studies that have proved the superiority of one operative procedure over another for either of these types of incontinence, it does not take much vision to see the relative futility of a resuspension procedure in a patient whose urethra is already well supported as a result of a prior operation but who, nonetheless, leaks urine whenever she assumes the upright position as a result of a poorly functioning internal sphincteric mechanism. That some 85% to 90% of patients in that category can be made dry with a pubovaginal sling does not prove that the operation is superior to others for this condition, but it strongly supports that argument.

Patients with myelodysplasia, in whom function of the internal sphincter is absent but that of the external sphincter is preserved, are, as a group, more troubled by incontinence than any other patient population with bladder or urethral dysfunction. Despite using the same drug and intermittent catheterization regimen, it is easier to achieve continence in patients with spinal cord injuries or multiple sclerosis than in patients with myelomeningocele. The reason is clearly because of the absent function of the internal sphincter in the latter group. Continence can be achieved in men or women with myelodysplasia by using a sling or by injecting collagen into the area of the internal sphincter. The latter technique only increases the coaptation of the urethral walls,

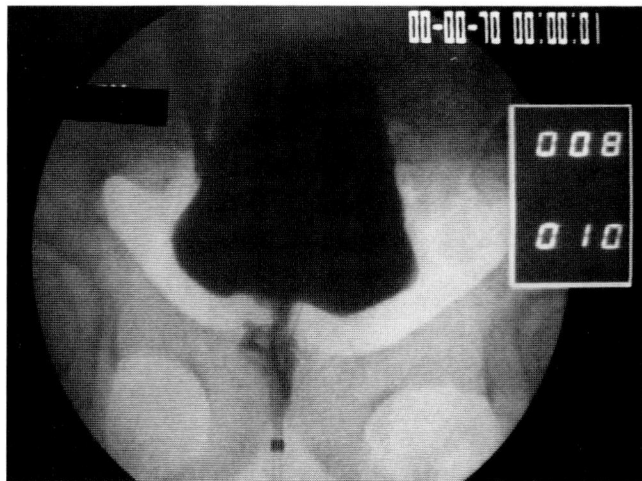

Figure 5-5.1 A videourodynamic snapshot of a patient with an open bladder neck and a dysfunctional proximal urethra.

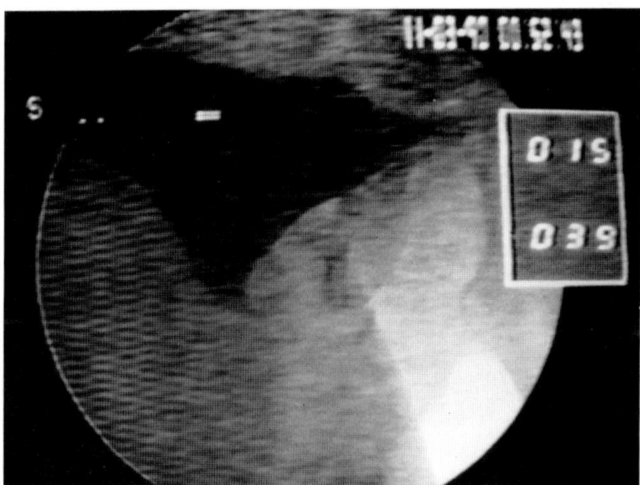

Figure 5-5.2 This patient has SUI associated with urethral hypermobility. Note the marked drop of the posterior urethra in this lateral view.

yet continence is achievable in 95% of patients with absent internal sphincter function. Also of interest, urethral pressure profile values are not influenced with the technique. Valsalva leak point pressures, however, are markedly improved, just as they are after sling procedures, which increase the closing pressure in the urethra just beneath the sling only by 5 to 6 cm H_2O. Given that most patients who are successfully treated with a sling procedure, or a collagen injection, have (before that treatment) maximal urethral closing pressures substantially higher than those produced either by the sling or the collagen injection, it seems obvious that urethral resistance to intra-abdominal pressure excursions is not related to pressure alone but to where that pressure is exerted. A small amount of pressure exerted in the proximal segment of the urethra is sufficient to induce continence if the internal sphincter is poorly functioning or nonfunctioning. In contrast, collagen treatment does not work well for stress incontinence related to hypermobility in which the function of the internal sphincter is normal. Slings, on the other hand, work well for both types of incontinence, even though they are not often necessary in patients with pure hypermobility stress incontinence.

In practice, sling procedures should be used for patients with an open, nonfunctional bladder outlet, as observed with fluoroscopy.[12] Because the bladder outlet is normally open only when the bladder is contracting, the examiner should ensure that the bladder is not contracting while the open urethra is being observed. This requires either placing a pressure monitor in the bladder or observing that the bladder outlet was open from the very beginning of filling and not suddenly during that process. The study should be done with the patient in the upright position for better filling of the proximal segment of the urethra. Without fluoroscopy, one can assess the Valsalva leak point pressure to determine whether the intra-abdominal pressure necessary to cause leakage is quite low (<50 cm H_2O). Endoscopy, as described by Robertson,[13] can also be used. The data obtained with the latter method, however, are subjective. The patient is in the lithotomy position, which makes identification of more subtle grades of internal sphincter dysfunction difficult, and using the endoscope requires practice. Better results are obtained if, while gaining experience, the examiner can correlate the endoscopic results with fluoroscopic findings. Also, endoscopic visualization, which was described as a method to identify a fixed, rigid nonfunctioning urethra, is not the equivalent of a fluoroscopically guided urodynamic study.

Other less firm indications for slings include failure of a prior needle or retropubic suspension, unless failure occurred immediately. (For example, the patient states that, as soon as the catheter was removed, she was "wetter than ever.") Such an occurrence almost always indicates severe incontinence associated with an open vesical outlet. Other indications include severe pulmonary disease, athleticism, as for example gymnastics etc., obesity, and finally the elderly presenting with new onset stress incontinence, since most such patients have poor urethral closing function. Recently we have treated most elderly, new onset stress incontinent patients with collagen injection, rather than a sling procedure with comparable results and less morbidity.

PREOPERATIVE PREPARATION

All patients are required to learn intermittent self-catheterization and are told that urinary retention may result from the sling procedure. Patients are instructed on the technique and receive assistance and assurance regarding the concept and the need for self-catheterization.

All patients are given antibiotics prophylactically, so that desired blood levels are achieved before the start of the procedure. No special bowel preparation is used unless a coexistent rectocele or enterocele needs to be repaired. Heparin prophylaxis is no longer used. Patients are admitted the day of surgery and are up and about the next day. The average length of stay is 4.3 days (range 2 to 7 days).

If the patient has a history of motor urge incontinence, or if an unstable detrusor contraction is noted on video urodynamic studies, she is counseled regarding the predicted outcome with these additional problems. In 85% of patients in whom we have performed sling operations the effect on these conditions has been good, although the exact outcome in an individual case is difficult to determine. Patients are told that the sling may cause pain in the suprapubic area and that the monofilament sutures used to hold the sling may cause pain, become infected, and, occasionally, need to be removed. Patients are also told that the sling may fail to resolve the problem of incontinence completely.

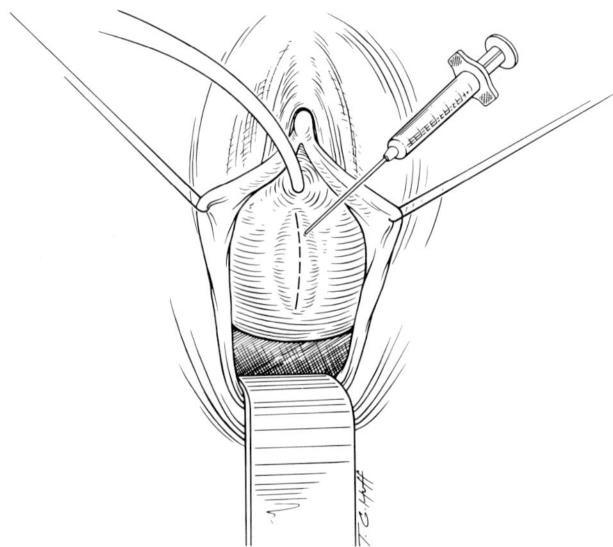

Figure 5-5.3 This vaginal epithelium is infiltrated with normal saline to facilitate the incision.

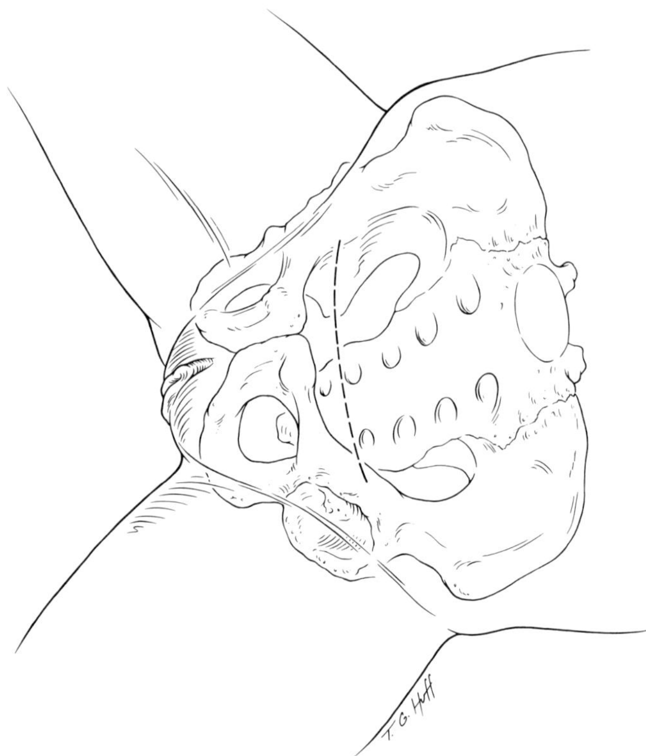

Figure 5-5.4 The location of the abdominal incision relative to the symphysis pubis.

OPERATIVE TECHNIQUE

The patient is placed in a modified lithotomy position with the legs elevated on Allen Universal stirrups (Edgewater Medical Systems, Cleveland, OH), which places all the patient's weight on the plantar surface of both feet. The legs are flexed at the hip only very gently so as to allow free access to the suprapubic area. A Foley (18F) catheter is placed in the bladder through the urethra, and a self-retaining vaginal speculum is used to provide access to the urethra and the bladder base.

Normal saline is injected beneath the vaginal epithelium, and a vertical incision is made in the vagina over the proximal segment of the urethra and the bladder base. The incision is about 3 to 4 cm in length (Figure 5-5.3). The vaginal epithelium is carefully dissected off the underlying periurethral fascia, which is white and glistening. In patients who have had previous vaginal surgery in this area, especially a Kelly-type plication, access is a little more difficult to achieve. Access to the retropubic space is gained on both sides by penetrating the dense attachments of the endopelvic fascia to the surface of the ischium sharply, and the area is then developed well lateral to the urethra by using blunt finger dissection.

At this point the vaginal wound is packed, and a transverse incision is made just above the symphysis pubis and carried down to the rectus fascia (Figure 5-5.4). The fascia is opened, and the upper and

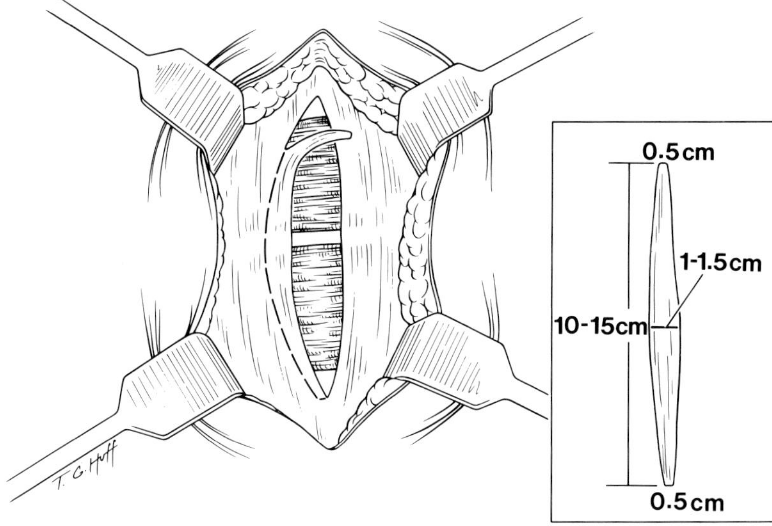

Figure 5-5.5 The sling is harvested from the lower leaf of the fascial incision. The fascial incision runs to the lateral border of the recti muscles.

lower leaves are developed and mobilized. The incision in the fascia should measure about 10 to 15 cm. The sling is cut from the lower leaf of rectus fascia. (Although the upper leaf can be used, fascial closure is easier if the sling is cut from the lower fascia.) The sling should be about 10 to 15 cm in length and about 1 cm in width, except at the very center where the fascia will bear on the urethra; here it should be slightly wider (Figure 5-5.5). The sling is oversewn at both ends with monofilament nonabsorbable suture material in such a way as to fix all the longitudinal fibers in the suture and the knots.

With the use of gentle finger dissection the lateral border of the rectus muscle is located on both sides. Just lateral to the insertion of the muscle into the pubic bone is a triangular opening in the abdominal musculature through which the retroperitoneal fat is visible (Figure 5-5.6). The fascia in this area is opened bluntly or sharply just at its junction with the pubic bone, and thereby access to the very lateral retropubic space is gained. Even in cases in which extensive retropubic dissection has already been done, this area is almost always unsullied, and easy finger dissection of the bladder and its surrounding fat from the back of the pubis is possible toward the vaginal operator and the entry from that area into the retropubic space. The dissection can be complicated by prior traumatic injuries associated with pelvic fractures and diastasis of the symphysis pubis, as well as by the residual effects of an extensive pelvic hematoma. When the landmarks described are used, however, bladder injury is extremely rare. Patients who have undergone prior surgical procedures involving the pelvis or the abdomen, particularly those associated with vertical incisions, may have no true retroperitoneal space anterior and lateral to the bladder. The peritoneal cavity simply extends inferiorly to the pubic bone and encompasses the dome and anterior wall of the bladder to the urethra (Figure 5-5.7). It is best to avoid this area entirely, and the method of approach outlined here permits that.

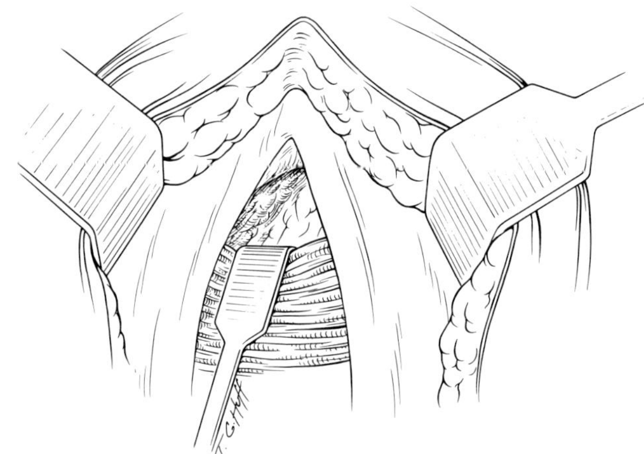

Figure 5-5.6 Close-up of the triangle formed by the lateral border of the rectus muscle (retracted), the back of pubis and the peritoneum.

The tunnel for the sling, which is made on both sides, is a product of sharp dissection from the vaginal wound into the retropubic space by means of a retropubic approach. To enter the retropubic space from below it is important that the dissection of the vaginal epithelium off the underlying urethra starts and stays in the correct plane, superficial to the periurethral fascia, because that fascia guards both the urethra and the bladder from inadvertent injury. By following the periurethral fascia laterally with the use of sharp scissor dissection, the junction of the fascial envelope around the urethra with

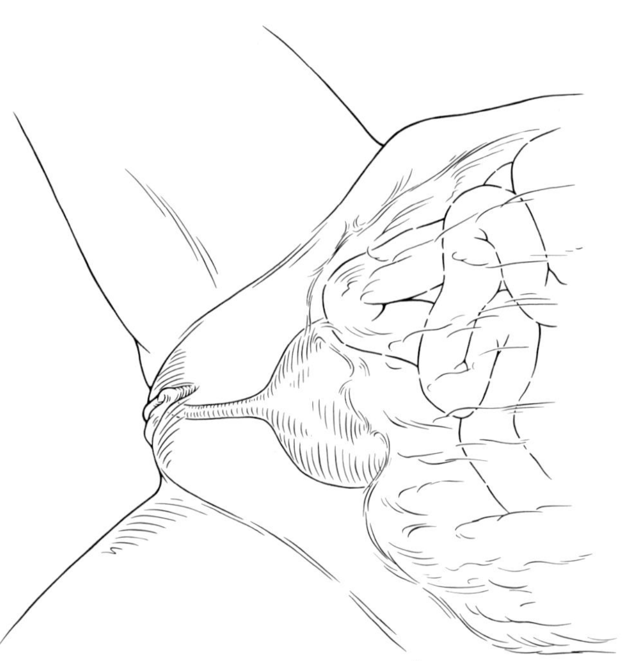

Figure 5-5.7 The peritoneum in patients with prior surgery can drape down over the bladder.

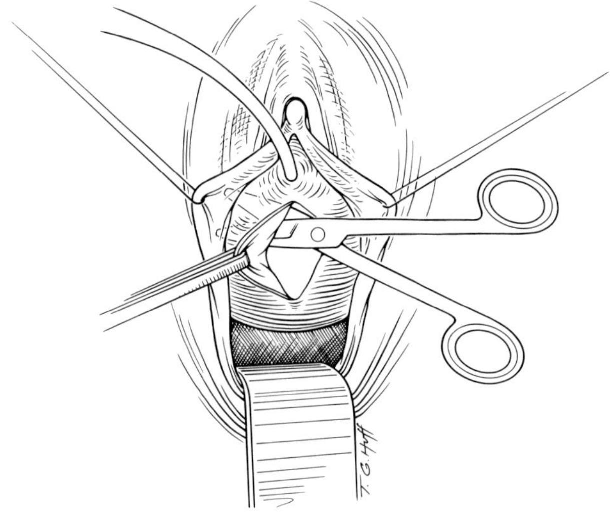

Figure 5-5.8 Entering the retropubic space from below. Keep the scissors flat parallel with the perineum.

its attachment to the endopelvic fascia, which inserts into the pelvic bone, is located. That insertion is opened with the scissors, pointed in a lateral direction toward the anterior superior iliac spine. The instrument is held almost parallel to the plane of the perineum, so that the points are directed away from the urethra and the bladder laterally into the free area of the retropubic space opened from above earlier (Figure 5-5.8).

At this point, the sling sutures on either side, which are kept at full length, are clamped in long slender clamps and advanced under bimanual control from below upward, or vice versa, depending on which technique is easier (Figures 5-5.9 and 5-5.10). In very obese women the above-toward-below direction is often the only possible route. Although longer instruments can be used, they are also larger and thus the opportunity for damage is greater. In the event that bladder injury occurs during the passage of the instruments (this is usually obvious by the sudden appearance of clear fluid in the wound, the Foley catheter having been clamped at the beginning of the procedure), the instrument is simply withdrawn and a new, more lateral, route is chosen.

At the end of the procedure, but before closure of the wounds, endoscopic inspection of the bladder should be performed to ensure that the sling is not in the bladder. Endoscopy (with the use of a 30-degree lens) is also useful to check the position of the sling behind the proximal segment of the urethra (Figure 5-5.11). At this point the sling is sutured to the periurethral fascia by using two absorbable sutures to spread the sling out along the urethra and increase its bearing area. Also, this maneuver holds the sling in place, so that when tension is applied the sling does not become dislodged from its selected position with the central widest portion of the sling in contact with the urethra. Both ends of the sling must be physically located within the retropubic space and not left below the endopelvic fascia, at the passageway, because that leads to an unequal distribution of tension on the sling and a poor result. The sling sutures are passed through the rectus fascia away from the midline on either side by using a small clamp to make the opening. Each suture is then passed through a small pledget by means of two towel clip point holes. The rectus fascia is closed, and no drains are used.

Once both the vaginal wound and the rectus fascia are closed, tension can be applied to the sling. The amount of tension applied varies, depending on whether the preoperative evaluation showed poor function of the proximal segment of the urethra or hypermobility. If the problem is hypermobility, enough tension is placed on the sling to prevent urethral motion when the Foley catheter is pulled downward, as a nonsupporting, examining finger is placed intravaginally just behind the urethra. With the sling just in place, the urethra will move readily into the vagina when downward traction is placed on the catheter. The sling sutures are tied down

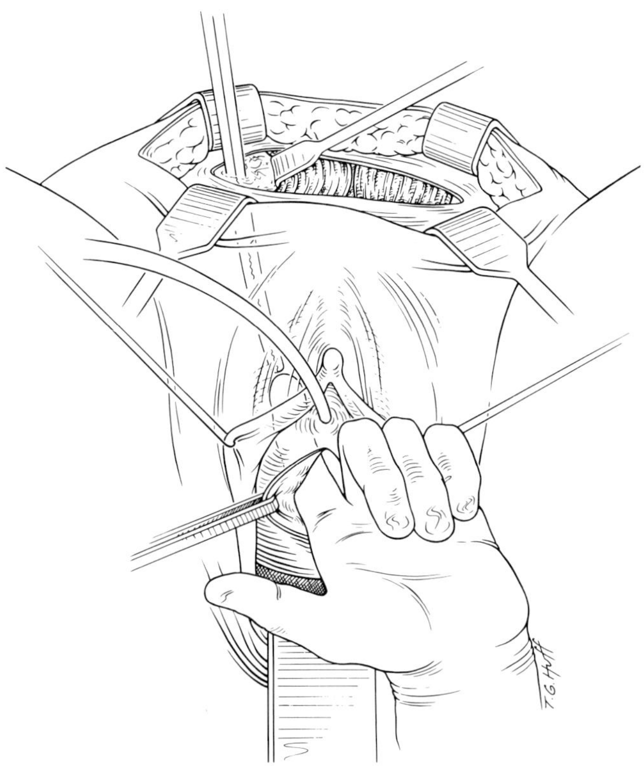

Figure 5-5.9 Passing the clamp down the tunnel.

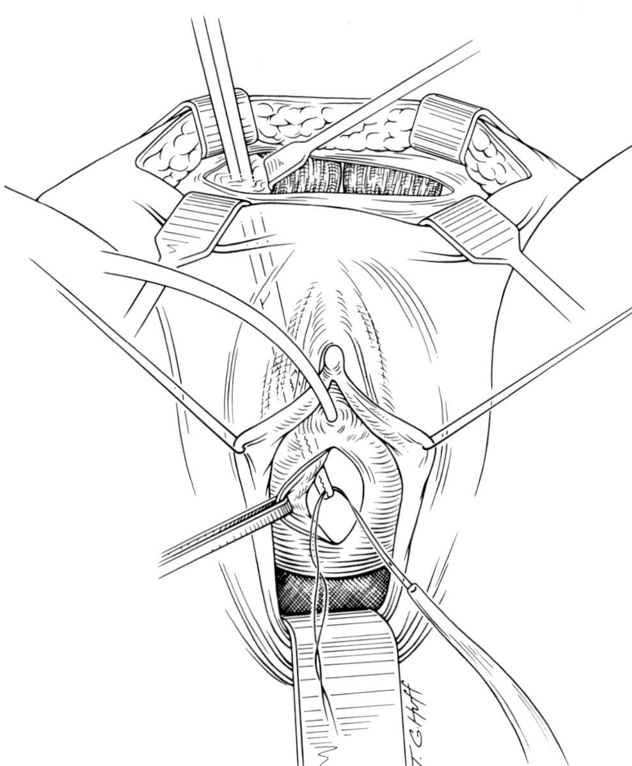

Figure 5-5.10 Grasping the sling sutures prior to passing them up into the abdomen.

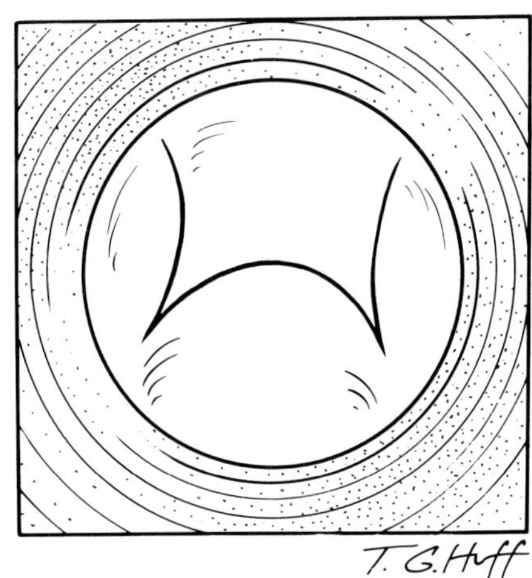

Figure 5-5.11 A drawing illustrating the endoscopic appearance of the bladder neck and proximal urethra when buttressed by the sling.

tightly enough to just stop motion (Figure 5-5.12). If the problem is a poorly functioning or nonfunctioning urethra, the tension must be slightly more than that used for support. How much is unfortunately a matter of practice, but those who embark on slings do not seem to have any more trouble than we do when it comes to selecting the proper amount of tension.

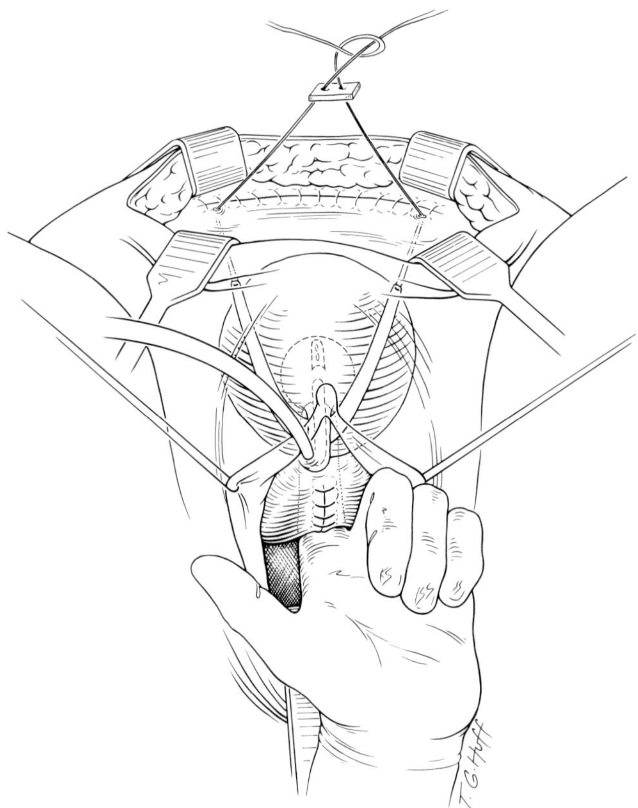

Figure 5-5.12 Checking the tension of the sling. The sling sutures are passed through the lower fascial leaf and tied over a pledget. The fascial incision should be closed prior to tying the knot.

POSTOPERATIVE CARE AND COMPLICATIONS

The Foley catheter is left in place until the patient is up and about, which usually is in 1 or 2 days. Once the catheter is removed, the nursing staff begins intermittent catheterization, to be performed every 4 hours or as needed. (An order for catheterization every 4 hours means just that and often that is not enough; hence, the as needed designation.) As mentioned earlier, all patients are taught intermittent self-catheterization. This facilitates independent care, and, thus, the inability to urinate does not prevent timely discharge from the hospital.

Some patients experience extreme urgency and bladder spasms associated with retention at this stage. In these cases we prescribe anticholinergic agents to prevent this, even though these agents delay the onset of normal micturition. Sudden nonpainful urgency and urge incontinence are common, and most women who undergo sling operations do not have a normal bladder capacity owing to defunctionalization related to long periods of severe incontinence. Therefore sudden urgency is usually very transient. In most cases if one explains to the patient (1) that the problem is temporary and (2) that, although anticholingeric agents will stop the urgency, they will also impair recovery of normal voiding, most patients elect not to take the drugs.

Complications of the procedure are the same as those encountered in any combined transvaginal and retropubic procedure in which a foreign body (the sutures) is left in place. They include bleeding, infection, pain, and erosion of the suture material through the bladder or the urethra. Prolonged or permanent urinary retention can also occur as a consequence of the sling, as it can with any suspension procedure. If prolonged retention occurs, it is important to document the presence of a bladder contraction, which is a prerequisite to resumption of voiding. If that can be demonstrated, the sling can be loosened by making a vertical vaginal incision and dissecting sharply along the pathway of the sling as it tracks up into the retropubic space, much as one would do to begin the sling procedure. The loss of tension on the sling can be measured by the downward traction maneuver on the Foley catheter. One can proceed with the dissection until some mobility is restored to the urethra and then stop. In practice, the temptation to undo the entire sling is easy to resist because both the patient and the surgeon know that the price paid will be incontinence. If one must undo a sling, it is better to wait 8 to 10 weeks before doing so, because in the interim many if not most patients begin voiding without difficulty, and early operative intervention is more likely to lead to recurrent incontinence.

Detrusor instability as a persistent problem plagues about 5% to 6% of patients who undergo sling procedures. A problem with urge incontinence antedated the sling procedure in 50% of patients, but in an equal percentage of patients it appears to be a problem brought on by the sling. The latter is difficult to prove, other than as a temporal relation, because some degree of urge incontinence could certainly be missed or underestimated in patients as incontinent as are most women who undergo sling operations. We initially believed that incontinence related to detrusor contractility without its owner's permission was more common after sling procedures than after other operative procedures for stress incontinence. In examining the data on anterior repairs, Burch suspensions, sling procedures, and needle suspensions performed by us, surprisingly, the only differences were observed between anterior repairs and the other procedures at 3 years and those were for recurrent stress incontinence.

Pain with exercise or movement in the area in which the sling sutures are tied together is common for the first 2 to 3 weeks after the procedure. Persistent pain in the area is an occasional problem. The pain is almost invariably on one side. Despite the fact that the pain is usually unilateral, percutaneous blockage with a local anesthetic of the central area of the sutures and pledget often provides significant pain relief. In some cases the relief lasts up to 3 to 4 weeks. If the block does not provide satisfactory relief, and at least 10 weeks have passed since the surgery, we will remove the sutures and the pledget under local anesthesia in the office. Incontinence has not recurred with this procedure thus far. It is impossible to state with any certainty whether over time slings will maintain tension without their suspending sutures.

REFERENCES

1. Stoeckel W. Über die Verwendung der Musculi Pyramidales bei der operativen Behandlung der Incontinentia Urinae. *Zentralbl Gynakol.* 1917;41:11–19.

2. Millin T. Some observations on the surgical treatment of urinary incontinence. *Proc R Soc Med.* 1939;32:777–778.

3. Morgan JE. A sling operation using Marlex polypropylene mesh for treatment of recurrent stress incontinence. *Am J Obstet Gynecol.* 1970;106:369–377.

4. Aldridge AH. Transplantation of fascia for the relief of urinary stress incontinence. *Am J Obstet Gynecol.* 1942;44:398–411.

5. McLaren HC. Late results from sling operations. *J Obstet Gynecol.* 1968;75:10–13.

6. McGuire EJ, Wang CC, Usitalo H, Savastano JA. Modified pubovaginal sling in girls with myelodysplasia. *J Urol.* 1986; 135:94–96.

7. McGuire EJ, Bennett CJ, Konnak JA, Sonda LP, Savastano JA. Experience with pubovaginal slings for urinary incontinence at the University of Michigan. *J Urol.* 1987;138:525–526.

8. Shapiro RA, Raz S. Clinical applications of the radiologic evaluation of female incontinence. In: Raz S, ed. *Female Urology.* Philadelphia, Pa: WB Saunders Co; 1983:123–136.

9. McGuire EJ, Lytton B, Pepe V, Kohorn EI. Stress urinary incontinence. *Obstet Gynecol.* 1976;47:255–264.

10. McGuire EJ, Lytton B. Pubovaginal sling procedure for stress incontinence. *J Urol.* 1978;119:82–84.

11. McGuire EJ. Urodynamic findings in patients after failure of stress incontinence operations. In: Raz S, Sterling DM, eds. *Female Incontinence.* New York, NY: Alan R Liss; 1981:351–360.

12. Woodside JR, Borden TA. Pubovaginal sling procedure for the management of urinary incontinence in a myelodysplastic girl. *J Urol.* 1982;127:744–746.

13. Robertson J. Dynamic urethroscopy. In: Ostergard DR, Bent AE, eds. *Gynecologic Urology and Urodynamics.* 3rd ed. Baltimore, MD: Williams & Wilkins Co; 1991.

6

Detrusor Instability Incontinence

Jerry G. Blaivas and Michael B. Chancellor

Detrusor instability (DI) is an enigmatic condition. With careful scrutiny of the cystometric examination it is demonstrated in as many as 10% of women with otherwise normal urogynecologic findings.[1] In women with bladder symptoms, the incidence of DI ranges from 9% to 50%.[2–4] Thirty percent of women with genuine stress incontinence (GSI) have DI, and, in women with recurrent incontinence after failed GSI surgery, the incidence of DI is as high as 76%.[5–8] Some women have DI, as confirmed with cystometric examination findings, but are virtually asymptomatic. Others have no cystometric evidence of instability and are plagued by the telltale symptoms of urinary urgency and frequency and urge incontinence.

In some patients, the DI is easily managed with small doses of an anticholinergic medication. Some patients, however, cannot tolerate the untoward side effects of the medication, and, in others, the DI is refractory altogether. During the past few decades, this unpredictable outcome has led to a number of alternative therapies. Although no single treatment has proved to be effective, most patients are treated adequately by using nonsurgical modalities. Only those who have experienced failure with all reasonable attempts at conservative management should be considered for surgical treatment. This chapter presents a brief overview of the definition, causes, diagnosis, and nonsurgical treatment of DI, as well as a critical analysis of surgical procedures to correct DI.

DEFINITION

According to the International Continence Society (ICS), "the unstable detrusor is one that is shown objectively to contract, spontaneously or on provocation, during the filling phase while the patient is attempting to inhibit micturition."[11] We believe that this definition is too restrictive. Approximately 50% of patients are able to abort unstable detrusor contractions voluntarily when asked to do so.[12] If, during cystometry, the patient is instructed to try to inhibit micturition, as per the recommendations of the ICS, 50% of patients with DI will remain undetected. For this reason, we recommend that the patient be instructed to neither try to void nor inhibit micturition but, simply, to report her sensations to the examiner. If the bladder contracts during bladder filling in this setting, we consider this to be DI.

In the ICS classification, the generic term for involuntary detrusor contractions is *detrusor overactivity*. When detrusor overactivity is due to a neurologic condition, the condition is called *detrusor hyperreflexia*; when it is idiopathic or associated with urethral obstruction, the proper term is *detrusor instability*. When there is insufficient clinical information to make this distinction, such as in the frail elderly woman, we prefer to use the generic term detrusor overactivity.

CAUSES

The cause of DI (ie, detrusor overactivity per the ICS) has been attributed to several conditions (Table 6-1). In some, such as certain neurologic disorders, the cause and effect relation is obvious and well documented; in others, such as inflammation and infection, the relation is mere conjecture. Nonneurologic causes that have been proposed include urethral and bladder infection or trauma, outflow obstruction, aging, and anxiety neurosis.[9–14]

The bladder is never really at rest. Spontaneous contractions of individual smooth muscle cells occur with a rhythmic quality, which some investigators have attributed to the presence of pacemaker cells within the bladder wall.[15,16] Coalescence of these contractions culminates in detrusor contractions, which can be measured by using a cystometer. Small, unmeasurable contractions, however, may be responsible for symptoms of urinary frequency and urgency.[15–17] Also, in all likelihood, a number of neurologic and nonneurologic factors mediate and regulate the timing and appearance of these contractions. For example, imbalances of the neurotransmitters that modulate the micturition reflex may be responsible for some cases of idiopathic DI. Vasoactive intestinal peptide, which inhibits detrusor contractions, has been found in reduced concentrations in the detrusor of patients with DI.[18] The spinal and supraspinal enkephalinergic system has also been implicated because of its inhibitory effect on the detrusor.[19]

Table 6-1 Causes of Detrusor Overactivity

Neurologic Causes
Detrusor Hyperreflexia (Neurologic Disorders)
Multiple sclerosis
Cerebrovascular accident
Spinal cord injury
Myelodysplasia
Parkinson's disease
Nonneurologic Causes
Detrusor Instability
Idiopathic
Primary vesical neck obstruction
Obstruction of distal segment of urethra
Postoperative urethral obstruction
Inflammation and Infection*
Pelvic Floor Prolapse*
Genuine Stress Incontinence (GSI)*

*Cause and effect relation is not definitively documented.

Neurologic Disorders

Several neurologic conditions may cause involuntary detrusor contractions (detrusor hyperreflexia). These include cerebrovascular accident, brain tumor, closed head injury, multiple sclerosis, Parkinson's disease, spinal cord injury, and myelodysplasia.[4,20–22]

From a urodynamic viewpoint, the cystometrogram cannot distinguish neurologic from nonneurologic causes of detrusor overactivity. This distinction often can be made, however, with the use of multichannel urodynamic studies, particularly when sphincter electromyography is performed.[21,23] When involuntary detrusor contractions are accompanied by involuntary contractions of the striated sphincter, the proper term is *detrusor–external sphincter dyssynergia*.[24] This condition always is due to a neurologic lesion of the spinal cord.[24,25] Its presence in a woman with otherwise normal urogynecologic findings should indicate such a lesion, until proved otherwise, and prompt neurologic assessment is essential. Involuntary detrusor contractions that are accompanied by sphincter relaxation are consistent with a neurologic diagnosis, but, unless there are other suggestive signs and symptoms, further neurologic assessment is generally unwarranted.

Outflow Obstruction

Detrusor instability is found in more than two thirds of men with prostatic obstruction. It has been postulated that urethral obstruction in women also causes an unstable bladder.[2,26] In the absence of prior urethral surgery, however, urethral obstruction is so rare in women that it is seldom considered in the differential diagnosis.[2,27] Nevertheless, because symptomatic DI usually subsides after relief of obstruction in men, it is worth excluding obstruction by performing screening uroflowmetry.

DIAGNOSIS

The diagnosis of DI is confirmed by using the urodynamic examination. The urodynamic technique may vary from "eyeball urodynamics"* to multichannel synchronous video, pressure, and flow electromyographic studies.[23] The specific examination to perform depends on several factors, including the patient's history, the outcome of prior diagnostic tests, the experience of the examiner, and the availability of urodynamic testing facilities.

The simultaneous measurement of intravesical, intra-abdominal, and intraurethral pressure with uroflowmetry and radiographic visualization of the lower urinary tract offers the most artifact-free, precise way of defining the cause of urinary incontinence.[23] Because of the cost, both in equipment and in work hours, however, it is not readily available in many locations. In many patients the diagnosis can be confirmed and effective treatment can be undertaken without more sophisticated studies. Multichannel studies are recommended routinely in certain patients; that is, in women (1) who complain of incontinence, but in whom it cannot be demonstrated clinically; (2) who have previously undergone corrective surgery for incontinence; (3) who have previously undergone radical pelvic surgery, such as abdominal-perineal resection of the rectum or radical hysterectomy; (4) who have known or suspected neurologic disorders that might interfere with bladder and sphincteric function, such as myelodysplasia, spinal cord injury, multiple sclerosis, and Parkinson's disease; and (5) with increased postvoid residual urine or an impaired urine flow.

Detrusor instability may be difficult to demonstrate during urodynamic studies. In the course of a day, when a woman is distracted by her activities, she may have sudden involuntary detrusor contractions that she cannot stop and, consequently, urge incontinence develops. During a urodynamic study with a catheter in place, however, the patient's attention is focused and her pelvic floor is tightened. In these circumstances, she may be able to prevent the onset of the involuntary detrusor contraction. Some study findings have shown that continuous ambulatory bladder monitoring is more sensitive than conventional urodynamics in detecting DI.[28–30]

We have previously demonstrated that some women perceive the involuntary detrusor contraction as a sudden urge to void and are able voluntarily to contract their sphincter, interrupt the urinary stream, and abort the detrusor contraction. In these patients, DI usually causes urinary frequency and urgency, but not urge incontinence. Other women perceive the involuntary detrusor contraction as a sudden urge to void but are unable to abort it. They usually complain of frequency and urgency as well as urge incontinence. Still others have no perception of the involuntary detrusor contraction and just find themselves wet.[25]

Sensory Urgency

Clinically, DI should be distinguished from sensory urgency. *Sensory urgency* is a syndrome characterized by urinary frequency and urgency, often accompanied by suprapubic pain and discomfort or a feeling of the constant urge to void, which occurs without any overt urodynamic abnormalities. Cystometry shows a flat curve, and the patient's symptoms are usually reproduced by bladder filling at low volumes. With sedational anesthesia, bladder capacity is usually normal.

The terms *urethral syndrome, trigonitis,* and *interstitial cystitis* are ample testimony to the lack of understanding of sensory urgency. Patients with this disorder void frequently, not because of involuntary detrusor contraction or infection but, simply, because it hurts so much if they do not void. Accordingly, neither anticholinergics nor antibiotics have any effect on their symptoms. Empiric treatment is often unsuccessful in these patients, and it is not surprising that many experience secondary psychologic manifestations. In some patients, a primary psychiatric disorder is believed to be responsible for their symptoms. Current diagnostic methods do not provide a clear-cut distinction between those patients with primary psychopathologic characteristics and those in whom secondary psychiatric symptoms have developed because of their incurable bladder condition. Regardless of the underlying cause, we have found structured behavior modification to be the most practical approach for these patients. Less than 2% of our

---

**Eyeball urodynamics* is performed with the patient in the lithotomy position after she has urinated. A catheter is inserted and postvoid residual urine is measured. A 60-mL catheter tip syringe is connected to the Foley catheter and its barrel removed. Water or saline is then poured in through the open end of the syringe and allowed to drip into the bladder by gravity. As the water level in the syringe falls, its meniscus represents the intravesical pressure, which can be estimated in centimeters of water above the symphysis pubis. When the water level in the syringe falls to the level of the catheter tip, it is refilled.

Any change in intravesical pressure will be manifest as a slowing down in the rate of fall or a rise in the level of the meniscus. As soon as a change in pressure is noted, the examiner should question the patient to determine if she is aware of any symptom, such as the urge to void. Visual inspection will usually belie abdominal straining, but in doubtful cases formal cystometry with rectal pressure monitoring is necessary.

patients with sensory urgency ultimately undergo a surgical treatment.

Urethral Obstruction

Urethral obstruction in women is exceedingly rare, appearing in less than 1% of patients evaluated for persistent urinary bladder symptoms.[2,27] In examining women with bladder outlet obstruction, almost all have previously undergone urethral surgery, such as urethropexy, pubovaginal sling, excision of urethral diverticula, and multiple urethral dilations. Rarely, a primary vesical neck obstruction is encountered.[27,31]

In our experience, the initial symptoms experienced by the patient are most often urgency and frequency of micturition. Poor urine flow rate alone is not diagnostic of urethral obstruction; the diagnosis must be made by using multichannel detrusor pressure and uroflowmetry studies.[32] Less commonly, the woman complains of classic obstructive symptoms, including hesitancy, weak stream, difficulty initiating micturition, and postvoid dribbling. Ironically, and unlike the situation in men, almost all women who complain of acute urinary retention have either impaired detrusor contractility or a psychogenic cause for the retention, not bladder outlet obstruction.

Empiric treatment of primary vesical neck obstruction may be attempted with alpha-adrenergic blocking agents, such as prazosin hydrochloride or terazosin hydrochloride. We believe urethral dilation is uniformly unsuccessful. Surgical treatment is rarely indicated, but both transurethral vesical neck incision[27] and Y-V plasty of the vesical neck have been effective.[31]

Mixed Incontinence

Genuine stress incontinence and an unstable bladder often occur in the same patient. Blaivas and Olsson,[5] and McGuire and Savastano,[33] have stated that 24% to 30% of patients with GSI also have DI. Only about half of patients with cystometrically demonstrable DI have symptoms; conversely, only half of women who complain of frequency, urgency, and urge incontinence have DI on cystometric examination.[23]

Does DI reduce the chances for surgical cure of GSI? Some investigators believe that DI is a relative contraindication to corrective surgery.[34–36] Others have concluded that its presence before surgery has no effect on the surgical outcome.[23,33]

In most of the reported series, DI was not a significant risk factor mitigating against successful surgery, provided that GSI was objectively demonstrated. The implication of this statement is that, if a patient complains of both GSI and urge incontinence, a successful outcome may be expected if the GSI is repaired. This, however, should not be construed to suggest that one may indiscriminately treat urinary frequency and urgency and urge incontinence with a surgical repair for GSI. Rather, the following guidelines should be observed. If a patient complains predominantly of urinary frequency and urgency and urge incontinence and examination findings show GSI, she should be treated for involuntary detrusor contractions, and surgical repair should be considered only if the GSI becomes a significant complaint. If a patient complains of GSI, which is clinically reproduced, and also has asymptomatic DI, she should undergo surgery for the correction of the GSI. If a patient complains of GSI and urge incontinence, and the former is a significant component of her symptoms, there is a greater than 85% chance that both conditions will be cured after corrective surgery.[5,8,37] In a series with 46 patients, Bent[38] found that 85% of those with both GSI and DI improved with a combination therapy of anticholinergics and surgery.

NONSURGICAL TREATMENT OF DETRUSOR INSTABILITY

Historically, the mainstay of therapy for DI has been pharmacologic treatment. During the past decade, however, a number of other therapies have been advocated, including behavior modification, biofeedback, electrical stimulation, and intermittent self-catheterization.

Pharmacologic Treatment

Pharmacologic treatment consists primarily of anticholinergic agents and the tricyclic antidepressants. Anticholinergic agents are competitive inhibitors of acetylcholine, and they block its muscarinic effects. All the active drugs must be given in a dose sufficient to ensure a physiologic effect. In practice, the dose may be increased every 3 to 5 days until the patient is improved clinically or until untoward side effects occur. These consist of dry mouth, blurred vision, or supraventricular tachycardia. Anticholinergic agents are contraindicated in patients with closed-angle glaucoma. In some patients, the drugs are so effective that the patient is unable to void at all. Intermittent self-catheterization is indicated in this situation. Propantheline bromide and oxybutynin chloride are the two most widely used anticholinergics. Subjective improvement is reported in 50% to 80% of patients with DI. Objective improvement, as demonstrated with urodynamic findings, however, occurs in only 40%.[39,40]

The exact mode of action of the tricyclic antidepressants has not been clearly demonstrated, but they exert anticholinergic and sympathomimetic actions and have a central effect as well. Imipramine hydrochloride is the prototype tricyclic antidepressant. Unlike with the anticholinergics, the blood level of imipramine builds up over several weeks. Its effect may not be apparent for at least that length of time. In our experience, the effects of imipramine on the bladder and the urethra are often additive to those of anticholinergic agents. Consequently, a combination of imipramine and oxybutynin is sometimes especially useful.

Several other pharmacologic agents have been tried with variable success. These include dicyclomine hydrochloride,[41] terodiline hydrochloride,[42] flavoxate hydrochloride,[43–46] indomethacin, scopolamine, baclofen, and bromocriptine mesylate, as well as certain prostaglandin inhibitors.[47–49] Intravesical administration of several agents has also been studied as an alternative to conventional oral medications. This route offers the possibility of obtaining a high concentration of drug at the detrusor muscle and preventing systemic side effects. Agents studied thus far include emepronium bromide,[50] lignocaine hydrochloride,[51] oxybutynin,[52] and verapamil.[53]

Behavior Modification

The intent of behavior therapy is to cure urinary incontinence by teaching the patient to regain control of her bladder and sphincter. The general principles include titrating oral fluid intake; performing specific pelvic floor–training techniques, including the time-honored Kegel's exercises; applying relaxation and avoidance techniques; instituting programmed voiding by the clock; and keeping a detailed voiding diary. Behavior therapy generally consists of eight to twelve weekly sessions with a therapist who has been specially trained in both behavior techniques and lower urinary tract physiology.

The concept of behavior therapy was first popularized by Frewen.[11] He coined the term *bladder drill* to describe his technique for treatment of the unstable bladder. His methods were simple, involving primarily keeping a voiding diary and performing timed voiding. The patient was instructed to increase gradually the time between voidings. With the use of this method, he reported an 80% success rate. With a much simplified behavior approach, Fantl and co-workers[54] reported a 10% cure rate in patients with urinary incontinence related to either DI or sphincteric abnormalities. Nevertheless, 60% of the women derived enough improvement that they believed that further therapy was not necessary.

Biofeedback

Biofeedback is a technique that is designed not only to strengthen the sphincter, but also to teach the patient to regain control. A number of techniques are available, all of which attempt to measure the strength of the muscle contraction and record the intensity of the contraction by using a series of light or sound signals or by displaying the actual recordings on a screen for the patient to visualize. The biofeedback sessions are usually performed once a week. Although this method of treatment has received a fair amount of publicity in the lay press, there is little documentation of its efficacy in prospective controlled studies.[55]

Electrical Stimulation

Electrical stimulation of the sphincter muscle has been advocated by some as a method of treatment for urinary incontinence. The principle is that, by stimulating the sphincter muscle to contract, the muscle will be strengthened and its tone will be increased. Also, through a negative sacral-neural feedback system, bladder contraction will be inhibited. Beneficial results lasting from 1 week to 1 year have been reported.[56–60] Fall[57] reported on a long-term follow-up of vaginal electrical stimulation in the treatment of refractory DI and GSI. Seventy-three percent of women with DI were free of symptoms during treatment, and 45% remained free of symptoms after withdrawal of treatment. Many patients required up to 6 months of treatment before benefit was apparent.

Self-Catheterization

In some patients, the desired goal of abolishing involuntary detrusor contractions is accompanied by loss of voluntary detrusor contractions as well. This generally results in either complete urinary retention or incomplete bladder emptying. In these patients, the addition of intermittent self-catheterization to the treatment regimen is usually a satisfactory alternative.

SURGICAL TREATMENT OF DETRUSOR INSTABILITY

Surgery is indicated only occasionally in patients with DI. It should be considered only for patients with longstanding symptoms that have proved refractory to prolonged trials of more conservative therapies.

Although a number of surgical therapies are discussed in this section, almost all are designed in one way or another to circumvent the problem. With the exception of operations intended to relieve urethral obstruction, none of the therapies are purported to abolish DI and restore normal micturition. To the contrary, when DI is abolished, subsequent bladder emptying is generally accomplished either with abdominal straining or intermittent self-catheterization. If the former option is chosen, in a significant number of patients daytime and nighttime urinary frequency and enuresis develop. For this reason, we recommend that the patient strongly consider the likelihood of performing intermittent self-catheterization as a permanent means of bladder emptying before consenting to a surgical procedure.

Surgical options include operations to relieve urethral obstruction, hydrodistention of the bladder, bladder denervation procedures, augmentation cystoplasty, and urinary diversion (see Chapter 11). In general, ablative neurosurgical procedures are considered only in patients with chronic neurologic conditions, such as spinal cord injury and progressive multiple sclerosis. Ureterointestinal cutaneous diversion such as the ileal loop is truly the treatment of last resort and, with rare exception, is considered only for female quadriplegics who are unable to perform intermittent self-catheterization. Continent urinary diversion or augmentation cystoplasty with a continent abdominal stoma is recommended for female paraplegics or other patients who are physically unable to perform intermittent self-catheterization through the urethra because of physical limitations.

Procedures To Relieve Urethral Obstruction

As discussed earlier, primary urethral obstruction in women is exceedingly rare. In a personal series of more than 10,000 videourodynamic studies, primary urethral obstruction was found in only 10 patients. Eight had primary vesical neck obstruction and 2 had obstruction of the distal segment of the urethra. Detrusor instability was found in half the patients, and it subsided in 4 of 7 who underwent surgical correction.[27]

Historically, the first line of treatment for urethral obstruction has been urethral dilation with urethral sounds or optical urethrotomy. Although there appears to be little harm from a single urethral dilation, we do not believe that there is any evidence to support its efficacy. More definitive results can be obtained from transurethral incision[27] or Y-V plasty of the vesical neck.[31] We have obtained uniformly good results with transurethral incision. Therefore, we see little reason to subject a woman to an open surgical procedure for so simple a problem.

Before considering surgical treatment of a primary urethral obstruction, the diagnosis should be confirmed by using videourodynamic studies. The exact anatomic site of obstruction also should be clearly defined. For obstruction at the vesical neck, transurethral incision is best accomplished with a Colling's knife electrocautery blade. The vesical neck is incised at the 5- and 7-o'clock positions. Great care should be taken to ensure that postoperative sphincter incontinence does not complicate the procedure. Because the obstruction is generally a functional one, there are no anatomic landmarks that guide the length and depth of incision. We begin the incision just inside the vesical neck and cut to a depth of about 1 cm for a distance of about 1 cm. The underlying tissue usually has an appearance similar to that of prostatic tissue. The most important caveat is to be sure not to cut too deeply or for too great a distance. It is quite a simple matter to repeat the procedure if there is residual obstruction. The treatment of GSI, however, is much more difficult.

Urethral obstruction is prevalent after vaginal and retropubic operations for incontinence and prolapse. In our experience, almost all women with postsurgical urethral obstruction have DI. Its development after corrective surgery for GSI is disconcerting, both to the patient and to the surgeon. When the instability is clearly accompanied by urethral obstruction, some investigators have recommended urethrolysis and performance of a second anti-incontinence operation. Webster and Kreder[61] described 15 women in whom voiding dysfunction developed after a cystourethropexy procedure. Although none of the patients had bladder instability symptoms before the bladder suspension, 13 of 15 had urgency and frequency after the original procedure. Only 5 of 13 demonstrated involuntary detrusor contractions with urodynamic studies, and the remaining 8 had sensory urgency. After retropubic takedown of the prior repair and substitution with an obturator shelf repair, all 13 women with urgency and frequency experienced resolution of their symptoms, and 6 of 7 patients with urinary retention were able to void spontaneously again.

Hydrodistention of the Bladder: Helmstein's Procedure

Hydraulic distention of the bladder has been used for decades as an empiric treatment for interstitial cystitis. In 1972, Helmstein described a new technique of hydrodistention, with the use of a balloon catheter, to treat bulky unresectable carcinoma of the bladder.[62] He theorized that hydrodistention compressed the blood vessels within the wall of the bladder, thereby compromising the blood supply to the tumor. Subsequently, hydrodistention was used in an attempt to treat DI.[63–66]

Hydrodistention is performed by distending the bladder until the intravesical pressure falls within the range between the diastolic and the systolic blood pressures. In reported clinical studies, the duration of distention and the pressure level attained varied but did not seem to affect the results. Ramsden and colleagues[65] maintained the intravesical pressure at systolic blood pressure for four consecutive 30-minute periods. Others have kept the bladder distended for 4 consecutive hours. Andersen and co-workers[67] found that prolonged overdistention resulted in interstitial and submucosal hemorrhage and subsequent deposition of collagen. In the series of Ramsden and co-workers,[65] electron and light microscopy revealed axonal degeneration in the bladder wall. They suggested that prolonged bladder distention results in denervation of the bladder wall by causing degeneration of unmyelinated nerve.[65]

The basic technique, as we perform it, is as follows. Epidural anesthesia is accomplished, and the patient is placed in the dorsal lithotomy position. For optimal effect, anesthesia should be achieved at the level of the fourth to sixth thoracic spinal cord level. If the level of anesthesia is lower than this, administration of supplementary narcotics may be necessary because of abdominal or suprapubic pain. A specially designed balloon catheter is introduced into the bladder. The catheter has two lumens. One lumen is connected to a 5-mL retention balloon, which is inflated with sterile water at the vesical neck. The second lumen is connected to a high-compliance balloon, which holds at least 1 liter of infusant. The balloon is inflated to whatever volume is necessary to attain a balloon pressure equal to systolic blood pressure. This usually requires volumes of 500 to 1000 mL. The infusant is normal saline to which radiographic contrast medium is added. The bladder is distended for 4 hours while fluid is added or removed from the balloon as necessary to maintain the desired pressure.

Whitfield and Mayo[66] reported that 14 of 20 patients had objective improvement, confirmed with cystometry findings, after undergoing Helmstein's balloon hydrodistention. Ramsden and colleagues[65] reported that 16 of 51 patients with urgency and urge incontinence were free of symptoms, 25 were substantially improved, and 10 were symptomatically unchanged 13 months after distention. Only 2 of 13 whose symptoms relapsed after a previous distention responded to a second distention. Delaere and co-workers,[63] however, failed to corroborate such a high success rate, reporting a cure or improvement in about 33% and a complication of bladder rupture in 8%. Although bladder rupture is an alarming complication, they reported that it does not adversely affect the outcome. Because the rupture is usually retroperitoneal, treatment usually consists of simply leaving an indwelling vesical catheter in the bladder for 5 to 7 days and administering broad-spectrum antibiotics. A cystogram needs to be performed before the Foley catheter is removed to ensure that the bladder has healed.

In our opinion, there is insufficient evidence to support the routine use of Helmstein's balloon hydrodistention for the treatment of refractory DI. Our own experience has been so unfavorable that we no longer offer it to women with DI. We do, however, continue to use this modality for the treatment of women with refractory symptoms related to interstitial cystitis.

Bladder Denervation Procedures

Surgical procedures intended to denervate the bladder have an extensive and innovative history, but a rather unimpressive clinical success rate. In virtually all the clinical studies cited below, excellent short-term success rates are described in most patients. None of these procedures, however, ever achieved widespread use, and most procedures were eventually abandoned by the original investigators.

From a theoretic standpoint, *denervation* implies destruction of the functional nerve supply to an organ, whereas, in *decentralization,* the peripheral neuron remains intact. The peripheral neurons innervating the bladder lie in its wall and have been designated the *urogenital short neuron system.*[68] Hence, surgical denervation procedures probably do no more than, at best, decentralize the bladder, leaving the urogenital short neuron system intact. We believe that the main problem with the denervation procedures has been that, despite an initial success lasting as long as 6 to 12 months, the long-term results are dominated by the development of low bladder compliance or detrusor hyperreflexia. It has been postulated that reflex activity of the remaining intramural neurons plays an important role in the late development of these conditions.

Bladder denervation may be attempted by ablating the spinal roots with alcohol or phenol injections[69] or by performing surgical rhizotomy.[70–74] The peripheral nerves may be approached at or near the bladder by a transvaginal approach,[3,75,76] with subtrigonal injection of phenol or alcohol,[77–84] with presacral neurectomy,[85,86] or by means of cystolysis.[87,88] Denervation has also been attempted with detrusor myotomy[89] and bladder transection.[90–92]

Learmonth[85] described an operative technique designed to transect the sympathetic chain and the presacral nerve at the level of the sacral promontory. He reported symptomatic improvement in four of five cases with a follow-up of only 4 months. No objective data were presented. Richer[86] resected the hypogastric and lumbar splanchnic nerves bilaterally for the treatment of severe pelvic pain and, for many decades thereafter, presacral neurectomy enjoyed fairly widespread popularity. No meaningful data exist with respect to DI, however, and the procedure is rarely used. Ingelman-Sundberg[75] reported on a transvaginal approach intended to accomplish partial bladder denervation (described more fully later).

There have been sporadic reports for more than four decades on the use of selective rhizotomy for patients with detrusor hyperreflexia related to well-defined neurologic conditions, such as spinal cord injury and multiple sclerosis.[71–74,93] At least since the work of Heimburger and colleagues,[93] it has been known that the third sacral root is the dominant motor nerve to the bladder. A number of investigators have reported good results after sacral nerve root section. As with most other denervation procedures, the optimistic short-term results have not been sustained over time. More importantly, in many of these patients low bladder compliance has developed. Recent experience with selective nerve root transections in patients undergoing implantable sacral nerve root stimulators for the treatment of urinary incontinence related to detrusor hyperreflexia, however, suggests that transection of the posterior roots of the sacral nerves results in prolonged detrusor areflexia without the development of low bladder compliance. We believe that this procedure may prove to be useful in certain patients with detrusor hyperreflexia, but further clinical trials are necessary.

An intrathecal baclofen infusion system has been used to reduce severe spasticity resulting from neurologic disease. Inhibition of polysynaptic spinal reflex pathways has been helpful in patients with spinal cord injury and multiple sclerosis. In addition to a reduction in spasticity, improvement in bladder capacity and a decrease in urinary incontinence has also been observed.[94,95] Results of longer trials with this technique will determine whether tolerance develops. The use of other intrathecal pharmacologic agents to inhibit the unstable bladder is a possibility for future research.

Transvaginal Denervation (Ingelman-Sundberg Procedure)

In 1959, Ingelman-Sundberg described a transvaginal technique intended to accomplish partial denervation of the subtrigonal nerve supply to the bladder.[75] He reported an 88% success rate in 34 women with urinary frequency and urgency, urge incontinence, and bladder pain. Results of a subsequent series corroborated these findings, and a 6% to 15% recurrence rate was cited in the two series.[76] Several other investigators cited success rates of about 50%.[96,97] Wan and colleagues reported that 72% of 62 patients were "either cured or significantly improved" at least 1 year after surgery.[98]

Despite these encouraging results, transvaginal partial bladder denervation has never achieved a high level of clinical utility, and there have not been enough studies to determine its efficacy. In our own experience, the procedure has rarely proved useful, and we only occasionally consider it as a last attempt at treatment before considering major surgical procedures such as augmentation enterocystoplasty.

Indications. Patient selection is of critical importance. Only patients with refractory DI who respond favorably to a temporary nerve block should be considered as candidates for the procedure. The nerve block is performed by injecting a long-acting local anesthetic beneath the trigone through either a transvaginal or a transurethral approach. One of us (MBC) generally uses a 22-gauge spinal needle and approximately 5 mL of 1% bupivacaine hydrochloride (Marcaine) on each side of subtrigonal nerve supply. The other (JGB) injects about 5 to 10 mL of 0.5% Marcaine subtrigonally with a cystoscopic needle. The patient is placed in the lithotomy position after she empties her bladder. With digital guidance the needle is inserted into the anterior wall of the vagina at the bladder neck. The needle is directed laterally toward the vaginal fornix 1 cm lateral to the cervix to a depth of 3 cm.

Cystometry is performed before and after the nerve block. If there is an improved cystometric response, or if the patient reports an overt clinical improvement, surgery may be considered. If there is no beneficial response, other options should be considered. If the patient experiences a large residual urine or is unable to void after administration of the local anesthetic, she should be warned that she has a higher than normal risk of requiring intermittent self-catheterization after surgery.

Technique. The procedure is performed with the patient in the lithotomy position. We generally perform a cystourethroscopy and insert ureteral catheters bilaterally to aid in recognizing the transmural ureters and to prevent their injury during the dissection. A Foley catheter is placed transurethrally to decompress the bladder and to assist in identifying the vesical neck. A small amount of normal saline may be injected submucosally in the anterior area of the vagina to facilitate dissection. A vertical (MBC) midline or inverted U (JGB) anterior vaginal incision is made from midurethra to approximately 2 to 4 cm proximal to the bladder neck. The anterior wall of the vagina is dissected free from the urethra and the bladder, and long scissors or a right-angled clamp is used to dissect the soft tissue between the bladder (beneath the trigone) and the anterior wall of the vagina. The tissue is excised between clamps. Care must be taken to prevent injury to the ureters at this point. In addition, it is important to confine the limits of the dissection to the lateral limits of the trigone and not to perforate the endopelvic fascia and enter the retropubic space, so that GSI does not develop after surgery. The vaginal wall is replaced and sutured with a running 2-0 absorbable suture. A gauze pack is placed in the vagina. A Foley catheter or suprapubic catheter (by means of percutaneous cystotomy) is inserted, and the patient is given a voiding trial the next day.

Subtrigonal Phenol Injection

Subtrigonal phenol injection has been used in the treatment of patients with refractory DI and sensory urgency, but lack of overall efficacy and the possibility of bladder and ureteral necrosis have all but eliminated its clinical use. Technically, subtrigonal injection of phenol is a simple, minimally invasive procedure. A test nerve block (as described earlier) should be performed to confirm the potential efficacy. The injection is done through a cystoscope with a 20- to 23-gauge needle. Approximately 10 mL of 5% aqueous phenol is injected under direct vision below and lateral to the ureteral orifices near the pelvic plexuses. I (MBC) use a finger in the vagina to palpate and guide the tip of the needle. A Foley catheter is left in the patient's bladder overnight. A second injection may be needed in some patients who show partial improvement.[82,84]

Findings in most of the initial reports suggested that the technique was effective.[77–79,82,84] Harris and coworkers[80] reported that 6 of 10 patients developed an acontractile detrusor; 3 of 10 patients experienced vesicovaginal fistula as a complication after extravesical subtrigonal injection of 50% ethanol for DI.

Subtrigonal injection has fallen out of favor because of recent disappointing outcomes. McInerney and colleagues,[81] in a long-term follow-up of 97 patients, reported only 19% long-term success, 24% short-term but unsustained benefit, and 57% failure. In addition, there was a 17% complication rate. Complications included urinary retention (transient in 1 patient; permanent, requiring intermittent self-catheterization, in 7 patients), nerve palsies (4 patients), erectile impotence (1 of 9 men), and bladder mucosal necrosis (2 patients). Many of the patients who experienced failures with the phenol injections subsequently underwent augmentation cystoplasty as the definitive treatment. The results were successful. Prior pelvic radiation therapy is an absolute contraindication to phenol injection. In our opinion, the marginal long-term success with subtrigonal phenol coupled with the sometimes disastrous complications does not justify its clinical use except in unusual circumstances.

Bladder Transection, Detrusor Myotomy, and Cystolysis

Bladder transection (cystocystoplasty) was introduced for the treatment of patients with refractory DI by Turner-Warwick and Ashken in 1967.[92] The procedure is essentially a circumferential transection of the bladder with immediate reconstruction. An incision is made through the full thickness of the bladder wall and perivesical tissue between a point 1 to 2 cm lateral to each ureteral orifice. The incision through the bladder wall is then closed in one layer with absorbable suture.[99,100]

Various modifications have been devised involving partial versus complete bladder transection and cystolysis. In 1972, Mahony and Laferte reported on the use of multiple detrusor myotomies in the treatment of detrusor hyperreflexia refractory to pharmacologic therapy.[89] The operation was performed with the patient in the supine position. The bladder was exposed, and multiple vertical and horizontal incisions were made through the detrusor, leaving the mucosa intact. Postoperative hydrodistention was used to prevent healing of the bladder muscularis. Only one patient showed improvement; the procedure has subsequently been abandoned.[89]

In cystolysis, the bladder is circumferentially dissected as if a cystectomy were to be performed, but the bladder is left in place.[90]

All these procedures are intended to result in partial denervation of the bladder. Initial report results have been quite encouraging. Essenhigh and Yeates[101] have used bladder transection in more than 100 patients and reported satisfactory results in approximately 75%.[99,100,102] Nevertheless, the detrusor myotomy, bladder transection, and cystolysis never achieved widespread acceptance, and no long-term results have been reported. In our opinion, there is no role for them in current clinical practice.

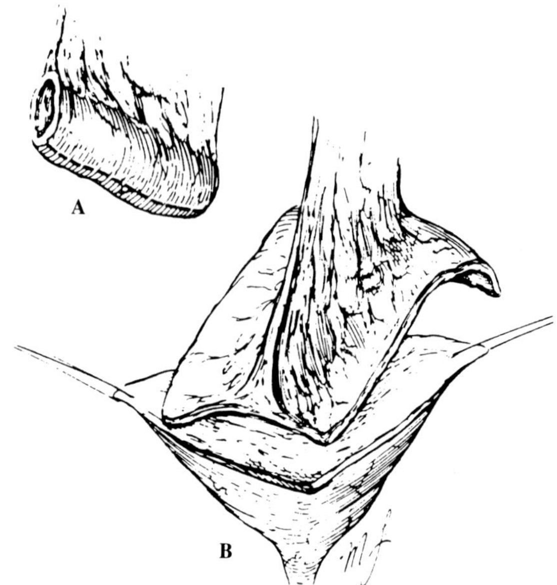

Figure 6-1 Patch-type ileocystoplasty. **A**, Anti-mesenteric border of segment of ileum is incised, and **B**, anastomosed to bladder without further reconfiguration. *Source*: Reprinted with permission from B Goldwasser and GD Webster, Augmentation and substitution enterocystoplasty, *Journal of Urology* (1986;135:215). Copyright © 1986, Williams & Wilkins Company.

Augmentation Cystoplasty

We believe that augmentation cystoplasty is the treatment of choice for patients with refractory incontinence or urinary frequency related to DI, detrusor hyperreflexia, or low bladder compliance. It should be considered, however, only when all conservative treatment measures in the patient have failed. Also, patients who consent to augmentation cystoplasty should be able and willing to accept permanent intermittent self-catheterization should this technique prove to be necessary after surgery.

Historical Considerations

Augmentation enterocystoplasty was first reported by Mikulicz in 1899.[103] He used a segment of ileum to enlarge a small contracted bladder. A number of case reports appeared sporadically in the European literature, but it was not until the 1950s that any meaningful series were reported.[104–106] Until the publication of Goodwin's "cup-patch" technique of ileocystoplasty,[106] in all previous series an intact segment of ileum, cecum, or sigmoid was used. The segment was anastomosed to the bladder. As will be discussed in more detail later, the use of intact bowel segments has been all but completely abandoned because of problems with persistent high-pressure bladder contractions, low bladder compliance, consequent upper tract damage, persistent incontinence, and enuresis.[107–114]

Goodwin recognized the need to detubularize completely the intestinal segment to prevent unwanted contractions and to provide for the best possible bladder compliance[106] (Figure 6-1). His original description encompasses all the important principles in use today (Figure 6-2).

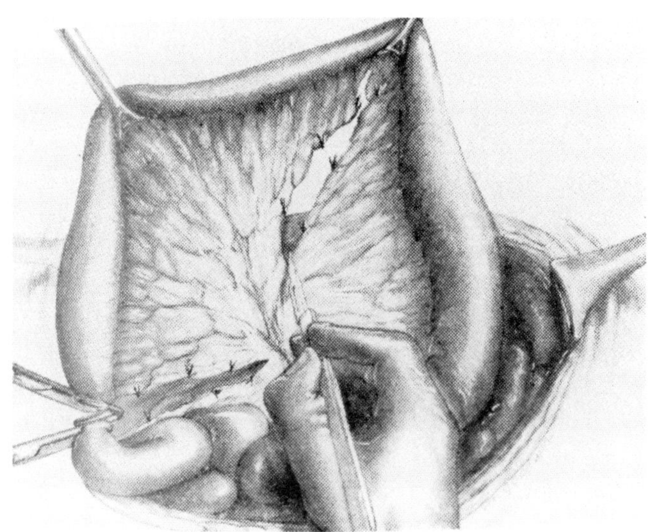

A

Figure 6-2 Goodwin's original description of "cup-patch" cystoplasty encompassing all principles used in current practice. **A**, Isolation of an ileal segment. **B**, Reestablishment of ileal continuity. **C**, Detubularization of ileal segment. Inset A depicts tubular ileus opened along antimesenteric border and cup-patch made from detubularized ileum. **D**, Inset A depicts bladder opened with "clam" incision, anastomosis of ileal "cup-patch," and bladder. Ureters are cannulated with 6F ureteral stents to prevent ureteral injury. **E**, Construction of "cup-patch" from detubularized bowel segment. After detubularized ileum patch is sewn together in "U" fashion, reconfigured bowel segment is curved again on itself from top to bottom to form a cup (arrows) (inset). **F**, Anastomosis of bowel "cup-patch" and bladder with running absorbable sutures. *Source*: Reprinted with permission from WE Goodwin, CC Winter and WF Barker, Cup-patch technique of ileocystoplasty for bladder enlargement or partial substitution, *Surgery, Gynecology, and Obstetrics* (1959;108:240), Copyright © 1959, Surgery, Gynecology, and Obstetrics.

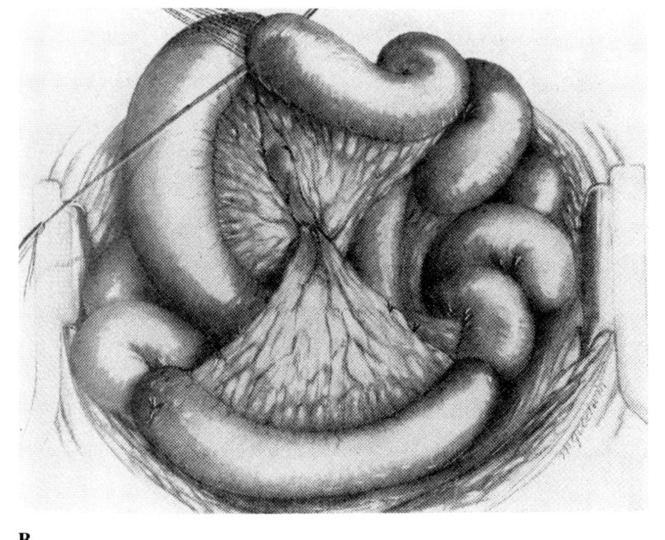

B

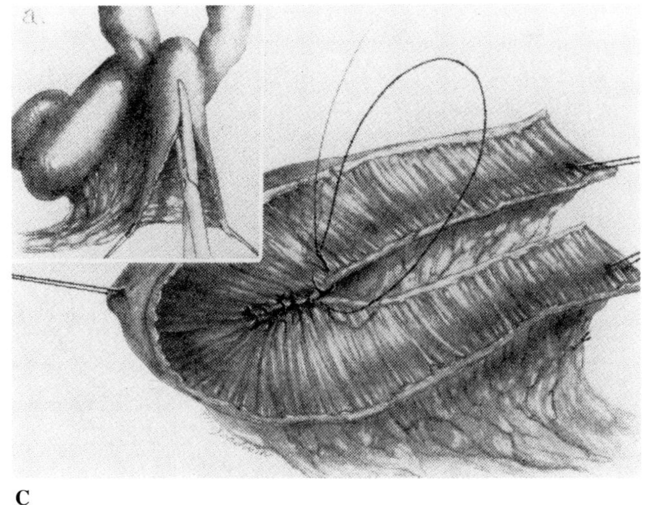

C

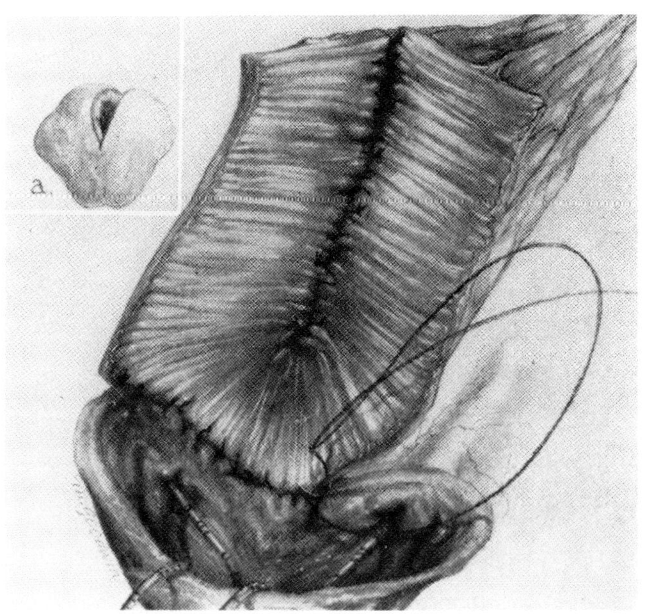

D

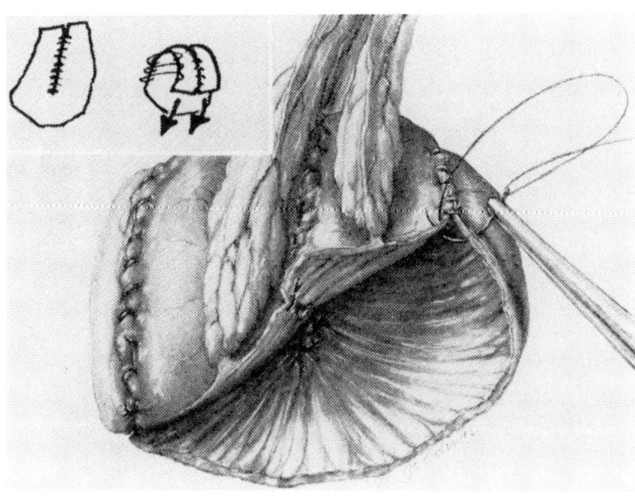

E

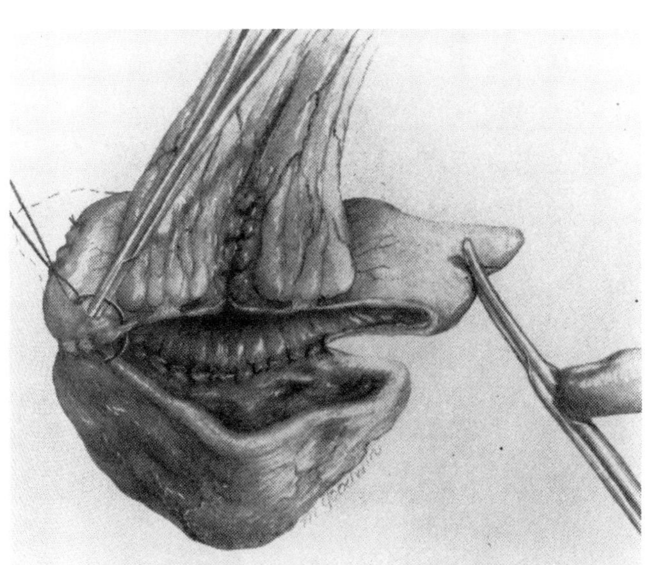

F

> After the ileum has been opened widely, it is placed in a U-shape; and adjacent margins of the cut ileum are anastomosed to each other. . . . An attempt is made to secure mucosa-to-mucosa approximation . . . but it is not presumed that this will be completely watertight. After the flattened loop of ileum has formed a U, it is in some cases curved again on itself from top to bottom to form a cup or cap which will fit on the dome of the bladder.[106]

For the next several decades enterocystoplasty appears to have been used more widely in Europe than in the United States. The procedure was associated with considerable morbidity and mortality, related, in no small part, to the fact that the usual indications were tuberculosis and bladder cancer. Its utility for treating refractory DI was not recognized, except for the occasional use in patients with neurogenic bladder.

In 1965, Gil-Vernet reported his technique of enterocystoplasty with the use of the ileocecal segment (Figure 6-3).[105] In that article, he alluded to his prior experience with 158 patients in whom the intact sigmoid colon was used. He cited his previous European publications wherein "we started a controversy about which of the two intestinal segments (ileum or sigmoid) would be more appropriate for enterocystoplasty."[105] He concluded that sigmoid colon was superior to ileum for cystoplasty, but that ileum was superior for ureteral replacement. Postoperative morbidity and mortality was considerable, primarily related to urosepsis, intestinal obstruction, and urinary or fecal fistula. He cautioned surgeons on the need for meticulous surgical technique:

> The first stage of the operation . . . is extraperitoneal. One must avoid entering the peritoneal cavity during the bladder detachment maneuver. This permits working under strict aseptic conditions . . . and prevents leakage of urine and blood into the peritoneal cavity which is one of the causes of intestinal obstruction. Defunctionalization of the colon by cecostomy or cutaneous appendicostomy is a must in cases of extremely obese patients and those in poor general condition.[105(p373)]

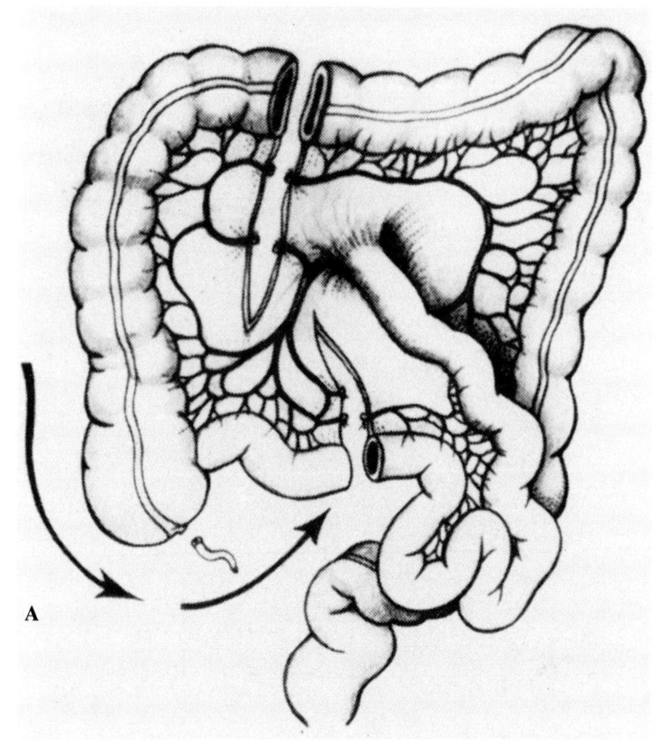

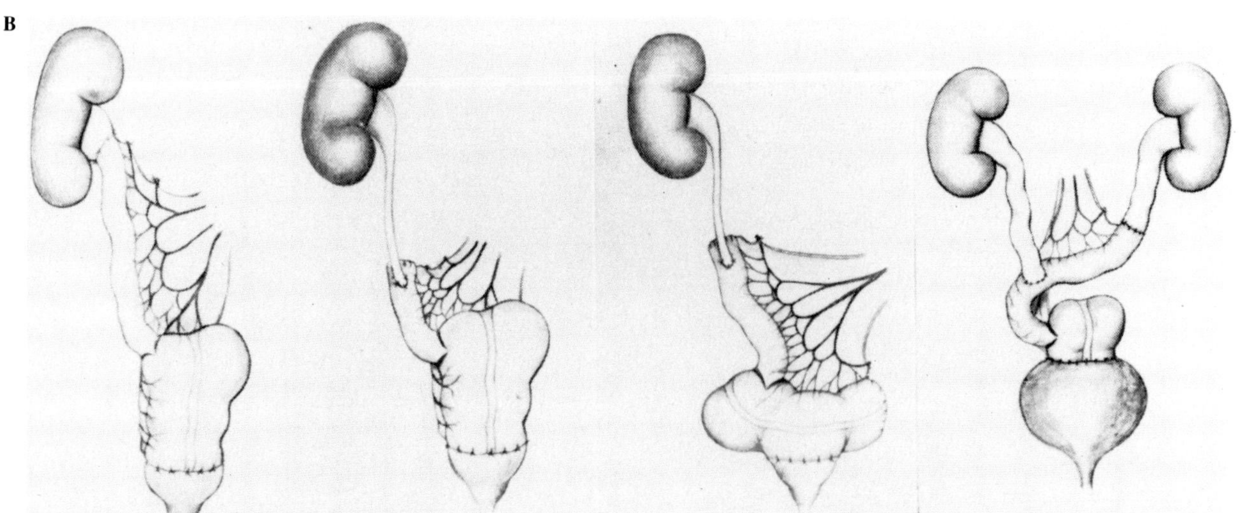

Figure 6-3 Gil-Vernet's description of various techniques with use of ileocecal segment. **A**, Isolation of ileocecal segment and appendectomy. **B**, Configurations of various techniques with use of ileocecal cystoplasty. *Source*: Reprinted with permission from JM Gil-Vernet, The ileocolic segment in urologic surgery, *Journal of Urology* (1965;94:419), Copyright © 1965, Williams & Wilkins Company.

Gil-Vernet favored the ileocecal segment because he believed it offered the advantages of both ileum (for ureteral substitution or reimplantation) and cecum (to achieve a large-capacity bladder), which "made possible voiding intervals from 4 to 5 hours, satisfactory bladder emptying and a normal forceful stream."[105] In this article, however, he does not say exactly how often these lofty goals were achieved.

Also in 1970, Kuss and colleagues[109] reported a meticulous long-term evaluation of 185 patients who underwent "intestino-cystoplasty" from 1951 to 1967. In this series, ileum was used in 55 patients, sigmoid in 122, and ascending colon in 8. The most common indication was tuberculous cystitis (97 patients), followed by bladder cancer (57 patients) and bilharziasis (11 patients). Of note, 7 patients had neurogenic bladder, and 3 had interstitial cystitis. In that series, septicemia and venous thrombosis accounted for eight postoperative deaths, and complications of intestinal obstruction were responsible for three other deaths. Prolonged urinary drainage was seen in 32 patients, 12 of whom required second operations for cutaneous fistula. In addition, fecal and urinary fecal fistulas were encountered in another 23 patients.

Eighty-nine patients were monitored for 2 to 16 years. In about half these patients, renal function either improved or remained stable. In the remainder, renal function deteriorated over time, but almost all patients had either bladder cancer or renal tuberculosis. The investigators attributed deterioration in renal function primarily to infection and urolithiasis. (In more than 11% of patients renal or bladder stones developed.) After cystoplasty, micturition was accomplished by "abdominal straining and true contraction of the bowel." The average intervoiding interval was about 2 hours, being less after ileocystoplasty and greater after sigmoidocystoplasty. Nocturia averaged four times per night after ileocystoplasty and two times after sigmoid augmentation. Approximately 25% of patients had incontinence both during the day and at night.

The investigators made the astute observation that

> as far as neurourology is concerned, one should consider complete traumatic lesions of the cord . . . because they leave a tonic or sometimes spastic perineum and external sphincter capable of maintaining continence. On the contrary, patients with complete autonomous bladders due to lower cord or cauda equina lesions are unsatisfactory candidates [because they will be unable to void satisfactorily]. . . . A funnel-shaped urethra or a prior large bladder neck resection might impair the expected continence . . . and satisfactory renal function.[109]

In the 1970s, although tuberculosis remained a common indication, many more procedures were performed on "the small contracted bladder" because of radiation or chemical injury, because of interstitial cystitis, and as part of urinary diversion for children and adults who had previously undergone supravesical diversion.

Before 1980, most urologists considered neurogenic bladder a contraindication to augmentation enterocystoplasty. This was primarily because intermittent self-catheterization was not yet in vogue, and, without this technique, bladder emptying was generally not possible. After augmentation cystoplasty, many patients with neurogenic bladder experienced serious urinary tract infections and upper tract deterioration. Smith recommended that "because of the low voiding pressure that results from this procedure a limited Y-V plasty of the bladder neck is always advisable."[113] With the advent of routine intermittent self-catheterization, neurogenic bladder has become one of the most common indications.[26,107,112,115] Y-V plasty is no longer considered because of the almost inevitable GSI that would ensue if the procedure achieved its desired goal. There have been few reports in the literature that specifically evaluate augmentation cystoplasty in patients with refractory DI.[116] It appears, however, that a number of patients with refractory DI have been misdiagnosed and categorized in previous studies as having neurogenic bladder.

General Principles

The purpose of augmentation cystoplasty is to abolish clinically significant involuntary detrusor contractions and to allow the bladder to accept large volumes of urine at low filling pressures without pain. This goal is best accomplished by using a detubularized segment of intestine for the augmentation. If sphincter function is intact, no further operative procedure is necessary. When sphincteric incontinence is present, however, concomitant pubovaginal sling[115] or sphincter prosthesis may be required.[107] To prevent a contraction ring at the anastomosis between the bladder and the bowel segment (the hourglass deformity), which can sometimes occur after enterocystoplasty, we usually create a posterior bladder flap and bilateral psoas hitch.[115] This ensures the widest possible anastomosis and, we believe, helps to prevent unwanted spontaneous detrusor contractions. Raz and colleagues[117] used an anterior-based bladder flap.

In our judgment, the admonition that the diseased bladder must be removed from patients with DI and neurogenic bladder[118] is groundless. We routinely do not excise any bladder segment. A number of surgeons, however, have recommended that, in patients with interstitial or tuberculous cystitis, subtotal or supratrigonal cystectomy should be performed routinely.[92,104,105,113,119] Others believe this is not necessary.[113,119]

Configuration of the Cystoplasty

Before the 1980s, most cystoplasties were accomplished by anastomosing intact bowel segments directly to the bladder. These segments retained their peristaltic and mass contraction properties, resulting in high-pressure systems that caused urinary incontinence, hydronephrosis, and vesicoureteral reflux.[107,112,114,121,123] Hinman[120] and Koff[121] reviewed the physical and physiologic characteristics of different geometric configurations and clearly demonstrated the superiority of detubularized bowel segments reconfigured into the approximate shape of a sphere. From a physiologic standpoint, they postulated that incision of the entire antimesenteric border of the intestinal segment disrupts peristalsis and prevents a coordinated muscle contraction. This maneuver effectively prevents high-pressure contractions.[107,112,115,123]

Geometric considerations clearly demonstrate that, for any bowel segment, a spheric configuration will hold a considerably larger volume than a tubular segment. This is because the volume of a sphere is calculated by using the formula $V = 4/3r^3$, whereas that for a cylinder is calculated using $V = r^2l$, where V = volume, r = radius, and l = length. Thus, if a cylindric bowel segment is opened longitudinally and folded back on itself to approximate a half sphere, its radius will increase proportionally and the volume it holds will be related to the cube of the new radius when it is anastomosed to the bladder to form a complete sphere. For example, if a 20-cm length of bowel with a 2-cm radius is anastomosed to a bladder with a capacity of 100 mL, the new capacity (exclusive of the distensibility of the bowel) will be 630 mL. A number of clinical study findings have confirmed these theoretic considerations.[110,112,120,121]

Choice of Bowel Segment

Before the widespread use of detubularized bowel segments, considerable controversy existed about which part of the intestine to use for augmentation. Purported differences in contractile properties of ileum, sigmoid, and cecum led many surgeons to favor one particular segment over another. It is now well accepted that virtually any segment of bowel may be used, reportedly with equal efficacy. Because of the propensity of the jejunum to lose salt and water, however, it should not be used.

Certain physiologic and technical considerations might affect the choice of bowel segment. Small bowel motility is peristaltic in nature, whereas the large bowel, in addition to peristalsis, also exhibits mass contraction of entire segments. These mass contractions can lead to high pressures and sustained contractions, which may likely cause incontinence or upper tract damage. After detubularization and reconfiguration, these theoretic differences do not appear to affect the outcome.

Because large intestine has a greater radius than small intestine, for any given length of bowel segment, large bowel will result in a much larger final volume. This obstacle may be overcome by selecting a longer segment of small bowel, but this requires considerably more suturing and infolding to achieve the same size sphere. Ileum is almost universally available and reaches to the bladder with ease; with this segment the need for extensive mobilization of the mesentery is eliminated. When the sigmoid colon is redundant, it can also be used without extensive mobilization; when it is not redundant, it may require mobilization of the splenic flexure. The ileocecal segment offers a good compromise. The main advantages of this segment are its reliable blood supply, ease of mobilization, and inherently large capacity. The disadvantages are the potential for malabsorption of bile salts, late requirements for vitamin B_{12}, and a small tendency for diarrhea to develop in the patient.[112,123] The ileocecal valve, after reinforcement with nonabsorbable sutures, may also be used as an antireflux mechanism for reimplantation of the ureters or as a continent stoma in patients for whom catheterization through the abdomen is preferable.

A segment of stomach, rather than small or large intestine, may be more suitable in renal-compromised patients.[124] The acidity of the stomach may also decrease risks of recurrent urinary tract infection, but it also may contribute to persistent dysuria in some patients. Currently, there are insufficient clinical data to evaluate the usefulness of stomach segments.

The choice of bowel segment depends largely on surgeon preference. The chosen segment is isolated on a well-vascularized pedicle of mesentery. The length of the bowel used will vary, but, generally, the segment should be no shorter than 20 cm to achieve an augmented capacity of at least 500 to 600 mL after detubularization. When the ileocecal segment is chosen, it may be necessary to mobilize the hepatic flexure to obtain enough length for a tension-free anastomosis to the bladder.

The single most important step in creating the augmentation cystoplasty is to disrupt the continuity of the circular smooth muscle fibers completely by opening the bowel for its entire length along the antimesenteric border. The now rectangular segment of bowel may be refashioned into a half sphere by folding the bowel into a U and suturing its sides together.

Contraindications

There are relatively few contraindications to bladder augmentation. Any form of bladder cancer is an absolute contraindication. The patient must be able to withstand the rigors of a major abdominal operation, which may last from 2 to 6 hours or more depending on the complexity of the case. The patient's bowel must be free of disease that might preclude its use, such as significant regional enteritis or ulcerative colitis. Extensive prior radiation of the abdomen is a relative contraindication, but it is usually possible to find a relatively normal segment of bowel that has not been affected by the radiation. Previously, renal failure was considered a contraindication, but we now believe that the procedure is the treatment of choice for patients in whom renal failure was caused by low bladder compliance or detrusor external sphincter dyssynergia. Vesicoureteral reflux can be corrected at the same time by using one of several techniques.[107,114,125]

Historically, refractory interstitial cystitis has been a major indication for augmentation enterocystoplasty. We believe, however, that it is only rarely indicated for this condition. Most patients' condition can be managed adequately with more conservative measures. Those who experience failure with conservative therapy will often experience failure with surgical treatment as well.

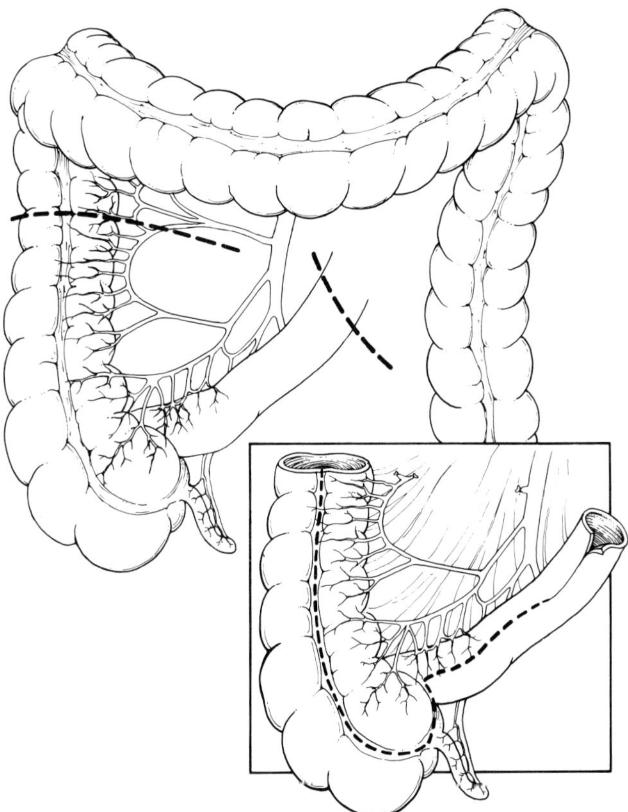

Figure 6-4 Mesentery of ileocecal segment is divided, being careful to preserve right colic artery. Entire antimesenteric border is incised with cautery. Inset depicts detubularization of ileocecal segment. Entire antimesenteric border is incised with cautery. *Source*: Reprinted with permission from R Laungkhot et al, Ileocystoplasty for the management of refractory neurogenic bladder: surgical technique and urodynamic findings, *Journal of Urology* (1991;146:1341), Copyright © 1991, Williams & Wilkins Company.

Preoperative Preparation

The patient is admitted to the hospital the day before surgery. She is given a 1-day oral bowel preparation and nonabsorbable oral antibiotics. Parenteral antibiotics are also prescribed perioperatively.

Technique

The patient is placed in the supine position, and a midline incision is made. After the peritoneal cavity is entered, a self-retaining retractor is placed. The ileocecal segment is identified, and the peritoneum is incised over the avascular white line of Toldt. The ascending colon is mobilized. If there is not enough length of bowel or insufficient mobility, the hepatic flexure can be taken down. The length of the ileocecal segment to be used is brought down into the pelvis to ensure that it comfortably reaches the bladder without tension.

The mesentery of the ileum is divided carefully to preserve the ileocecal blood supply (Figure 6-4). The ileum is divided 8 to 10 cm proximal to the ileocecal junction. The colon is usually divided in its ascending portion below the hepatic flexure unless more length is required to reach the bladder. A side-to-side ileocolonic anastomosis is performed. We generally use staple devices for the bowel anastomosis. An appendectomy is performed routinely before the bladder augmentation. With the use of a cautery, the entire mesenteric border of the colon and the ileum is incised (Figure 6-4). The side of the ileum is sutured to the side of the cecum with a running 0 chromic catgut suture (Figure 6-5).

The bowel is anastomosed to the bladder, which is opened in such a manner as to create the other half of the sphere. To this end, we prefer to make a U-shaped incision in the bladder. The bottom edge of the U is just above the vesical neck, and the two arms of the U extend to the posterolateral surface of the bladder. The anterior extension of the bladder incision is then reflected posteriorly, and the edges are sutured to each psoas muscle to hold the bladder open, thus forming the lower half of the sphere (Figure 6-6).

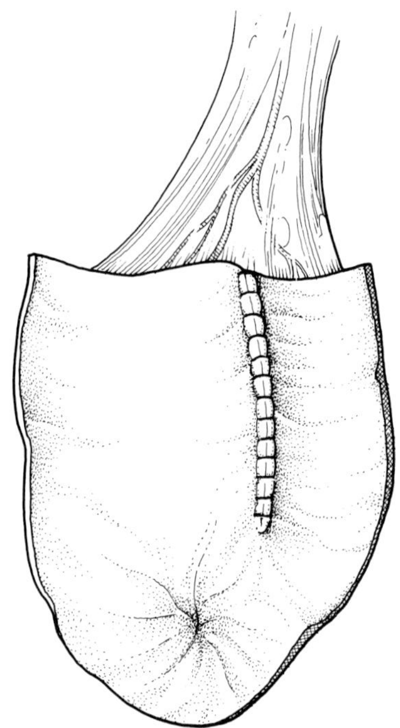

Figure 6-5 Side of ileum is sutured to side of cecum to form half sphere. If necessary, bowel is folded on itself once again to approximate better the half-sphere configuration. *Source*: Reprinted with permission from R Laungkhot et al, Ileocystoplasty for the management of refractory neurogenic bladder: surgical technique and urodynamic findings, *Journal of Urology* (1991;146:1341), Copyright © 1991, Williams & Wilkins Company.

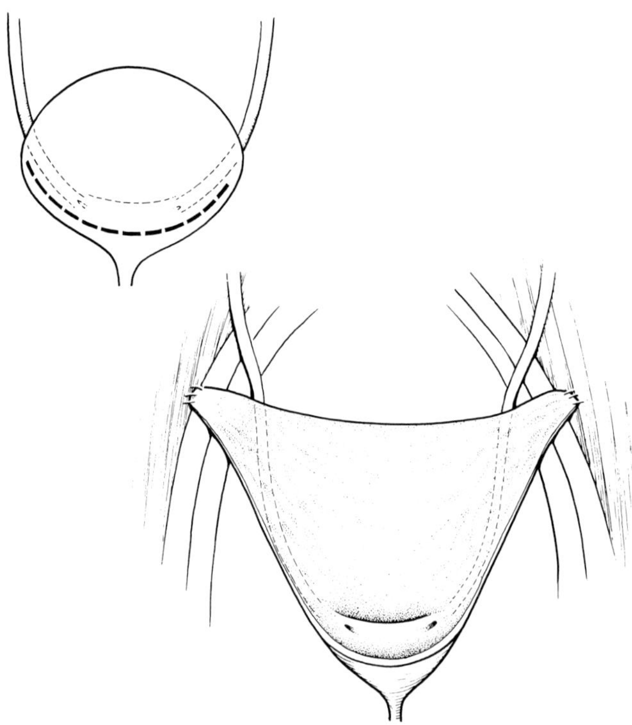

Figure 6-6 U-shaped incision is made on anterior surface of bladder extending from just above vesical neck to a point lateral to each ureteral orifice. Bladder is opened, and lateral edges of bladder flap are sutured to psoas muscle on either side. *Source*: Reprinted with permission from R Laungkhot et al, Ileocystoplasty for the management of refractory neurogenic bladder: surgical technique and urodynamic findings, *Journal of Urology* (1991;146:1342), Copyright © 1991, Williams & Wilkins Company.

The anastomosis of the bowel to the bladder is performed with absorbable sutures of at least 2-0. We prefer to use a single layer of running sutures through all layers of the bowel (Figure 6-7). In patients with interstitial cystitis, it is generally recommended that either a supratrigonal or a subtotal cystectomy be performed. In supratrigonal cystectomy, the bladder is excised just above the trigone, leaving only the trigone, the bladder neck, and the ureteral orifices. In subtotal cystectomy, the trigone and the ureteral orifices are removed with the bladder, leaving just enough vesical neck for anastomosis. In patients with DI, detrusor hyperreflexia, and low bladder compliance, it has not been necessary to resect any section of the bladder.

Both the augmented bladder and the retropubic space should be drained. The bladder is drained with a self-retaining catheter (placed by means of cystotomy) such as a Malecot (24F), which is placed through the dome of the augmentation. We do not believe that the catheter has to be placed through the remaining bladder segment. The retropubic space should be drained with a suction-type or Penrose drain.

The decision as to whether or not to reimplant the ureters into the bowel is usually straightforward. Nonrefluxing, nonobstructed ureters are not disturbed and left in situ. When significant vesicoureteral reflux or ureterovesical obstruction is present, ureteroenterostomy is necessary. The reimplantation should generally be performed with an antireflux technique, such as a modified Leadbetter-Politano or a split-cuff nipple procedure (Figure 6-8).[125]

Postoperative Care

The Foley catheter is removed as soon as the patient's urine is clear. Bladder aspiration and irrigation are instituted as necessary beginning on the third postoperative day if there is mucus build-up. A cystogram is performed on day 7 to 10. If the results indicate that there is no extravasation, the suprapubic catheter is removed, and the patient begins intermittent self-catheterization.

Complications

The most common complications are identical to those usually encountered after abdominal operations that

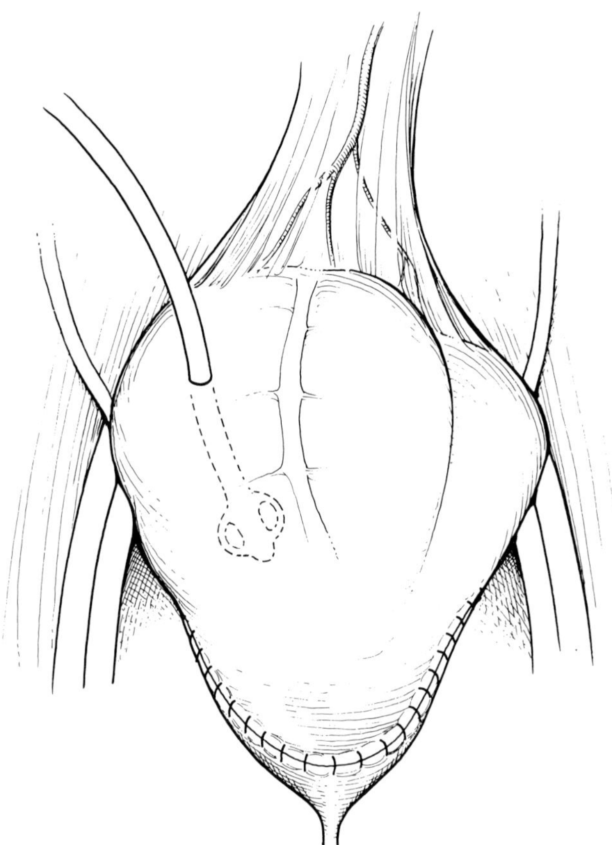

Figure 6-7 Half sphere formed by reconfigured ileocecal segment is anastomosed to half sphere of reconfigured bladder, and suprapubic catheter is placed. *Source*: Reprinted with permission from R Laungkhot et al, Ileocystoplasty for the management of refractory neurogenic bladder: surgical technique and urodynamic findings, *Journal of Urology* (1991;146:1342), Copyright © 1991, Williams & Wilkins Company.

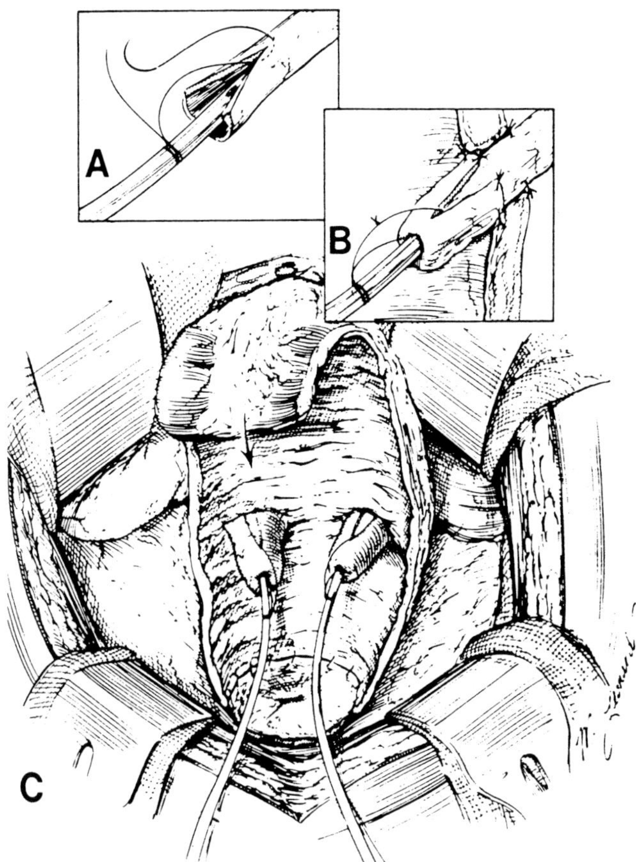

Figure 6-8 Split-cuff nipple anti-reflux ureteral reimplantation technique. **A**, Ureteral stump is incised along one wall for 1.5 to 2 cm. **B**, Split ureteral segment is pulled back over ureter forming a "nipple" and sutured with absorbable sutures. **C**, Split-cuff nipple ureters are sutured to bladder walls and intubated with ureteral stents for drainage. *Source*: Reprinted with permission from B Goldwasser and GD Webster, Augmentation and substitution enterocystoplasty, *Journal of Urology* (1986;135:215), Copyright © 1986, Williams & Wilkins Company.

involve a bowel anastomosis. These include atelectasis, pneumonia, wound infection, urinary tract infection, and intestinal obstruction. An uncommon, but severe, complication of bladder augmentation is delayed spontaneous rupture.[126,127] The few reported cases of spontaneous rupture have occurred in myelodysplastic and spinal-injured patients who have impaired sensation of filling. Spontaneous rupture is unlikely in women with normal sensation. Depending on the segment of bowel used, the risk of colon cancer may exist after augmentation, and periodic cystoscopy to rule out intestinal polyp and adenocarcinoma is prudent.[128]

Persistent diarrhea is an occasional, but troublesome, complication. In patients with neurogenic bladder and bowel disease, this often leads to fecal incontinence. Although it has been suggested that diarrhea is more common when the ileocecal segment is used for the augmentation, this has not been our experience. There exists a long-term potential for malabsorption of vitamin B_{12} and subsequent vitamin B_{12} deficiency when the ileum and ileocecal valve are used for the augmentation, but this complication has not been a recognized clinical problem. Although clinically relevant electrolyte disturbances are rare in adults with normal renal function, hyperchloremic metabolic acidosis may occur in patients with impaired renal function. In an important study of 48 consecutive patients who had bowel segments incorporated into the urinary tract, Nurse and Mundy[129] demonstrated that in all patients abnormal blood gas values occurred. This usually was manifest as a metabolic acidosis with respiratory compensation. Approximately one third of the patients also had hyperchloremia. The respiratory compensation was invariably complete, so that the pH remained within the normal range, and there were no clinical ramifications in the short term. Nevertheless, the investigators warned about the long-term sequelae of skeletal demineralization, particularly in women and children.

Results

In no reports have the long-term results of augmentation cystoplasty for the treatment of refractory DI been evaluated specifically. In most of the previous studies, investigators have grouped together all the usual indications, including tuberculous, radiation, and interstitial cystitis; low bladder compliance; bladder cancer; and neurogenic bladder. Furthermore, in almost all long-term studies, intact bowel segments were used. There are few long-term studies in which detubularized bowel was used. Nevertheless, results of our own experience (with follow-up as long as 10 years) and that of several other investigators suggest that, when a detubularized, reconfigured intestinal segment is used, an excellent result can be expected in at least 80% of patients.[107,112,113,115,116,122,130] Bladder capacity and bladder compliance are remarkably improved in almost all patients. The incidence of postoperative detrusor overactivity is no more than 15%, and, in only a small percentage of these cases, is this finding clinically important. When intermittent self-catheterization is used, recurrent incontinence is uncommon and almost exclusively related to sphincteric abnormalities.

REFERENCES

1. Turner-Warwick RT. Observations on the function and dysfunction of the sphincter and detrusor mechanisms. *Urol Clin North Am*. 1979;6:13–30.

2. Farrar DJ, Osborne JL, Stephenson TP, et al. A urodynamic view of bladder outflow obstruction in the female: factors influencing the results of treatment. *Br J Urol*. 1975;47:815–822.

3. Hodgkinson CP, Ayers MA, Drukker BH. Dyssynergic detrusor dysfunction in the apparently normal female. *Am J Obstet Gynecol*. 1963;87:717–730.

4. Hebjorn S, Andersen JT, Walter S, Dam AM. Detrusor hyperreflexia: a survey of its etiology and treatment. *Scand J Urol Nephrol*. 1976;10:103–109.

5. Blaivas JG, Olsson CA. Stress incontinence: classification and surgical approach. *J Urol*. 1988;139:727–731.

6. Arnold EP, Webster JR, Loose H, et al. Urodynamics of female incontinence: factors influencing the results of surgery. *Am J Obstet Gynecol*. 1973;117:808–813.

7. McGuire EJ, Savastano JA. Stress incontinence and detrusor instability of failed incontinence surgery in the female. *Obstet Gynecol*. 1978;51:515–520.

8. McGuire EJ. Urodynamic findings in patients after failure of stress incontinence operations. In: Zinner NR, Sterling AM, eds. *Female Incontinence*. New York, NY: Alan R Liss Inc; 1980; 351–360.

9. Hafner RJ, Stanton SL, Guy J. A psychiatric study of women with urgency and urgency incontinence. *Br J Urol*. 1977;49: 211–214.

10. Rees DLP, Wickjam JEA, Whitfield HN. Bladder instability in women with recurrent cystitis. *Br J Urol*. 1978;50:524–528.

11. Frewen WK. The management of urgency and frequency of micturition. *Br J Urol*. 1980;52:367–369.

12. Kinder RB, Mundy AR. Pathophysiology of idiopathic detrusor instability and detrusor hyper-reflexia. *Br J Urol*. 1987; 60:509–515.

13. Fihn SD, Stamm WE. The urethral syndrome. *Semin Urol*. 1983;1:121–129.

14. Moore KH, Sutherst JR. Response to treatment of detrusor instability in relation to psychoneurotic status. *Br J Urol*. 1990;66: 486–490.

15. van Duyl WA. Spontaneous contractions in urinary bladder smooth muscle: preliminary results. *Neurourol Urodynam*. 1985;4:301–307.

16. Coolsaet BRLA. Bladder compliance and detrusor activity during the collection phase. *Neurourol Urodynam*. 1985;4:263–273.

17. Coolsaet BRLA, Blaivas JG. No detrusor is stable. *Neurourol Urodynam*. 1985;4:259–261.

18. Gu J, Blank MA, Huang WM, et al. Vasoactive intestinal peptide in the normal and unstable bladder. *Br J Urol*. 1983;55: 645–647.

19. de Groat WC, Kawatani M. Neural control of the urinary bladder: possible relationship between peptidergic inhibitory mechanisms and detrusor instability. *Neurourol Urodynam*. 1985;4: 285–300.

20. Berger Y, Blaivas JG, DeLarocha ER, Salinas JM. Urodynamic findings in Parkinson's disease. *J Urol*. 1987;138: 836–838.

21. Blaivas JG, Scott M, Labib KB. Urodynamic evaluation as neurologic test of sacral cord function. *Urology*. 1979;13:682–687.

22. Blaivas JG. Management of bladder dysfunction in multiple sclerosis. *Neurourology*. 1980;30:12–18.

23. Blaivas JG. Urodynamic techniques and dysfunction. In: Yalla S, McGuire E, Elbadawi A, Blaivas JG, eds. *Principles and Practice of Urodynamics and Neurourology*. New York: MacMillan Publishing Co; 1988.

24. Blaivas JG, Sinha HP, Zayed AAH, Labib KA. Detrusor-external sphincter dyssynergia. *J Urol*. 1981;125:541–544.

25. Blaivas JG. The neurophysiology of micturition: a clinical study of 550 patients. *J Urol*. 1982;127:958.

26. Rees DLP, Whitfield HN, Islam AKMS, Doyle PT, Mayo ME, Wickham JEA. Urodynamic findings in adult females with frequency and dysuria. *Br J Urol*. 1975;47:853–860.

27. Axelrod SL, Blaivas JG. Primary vesical neck obstruction in women. *J Urol*. 1987;137:497–499.

28. O'Donnell PD, Marshall M. Telemetric ambulatory urinary incontinence detection in the elderly. *J Ambulatory Monitoring*. 1988;1:23.

29. Webb RJ, Griffiths CJ, Ramsden PD, Neal DE. Measurement of voiding pressures on ambulatory monitoring: comparison with conventional cystometry. *Br J Urol*. 1990;65:152–154.

30. van Waalwijk van Doorn ESL, Remmere A, Janknegt RA. Extramural ambulatory urodynamic monitoring during natural filling and normal daily activities: evaluation of 100 patients. *J Urol*. 1991;146:124–131.

31. Diokno AC, Hollander JB, Bennett CJ. Bladder neck obstruction in women: a real entity. *J Urol*. 1984;132:294–298.

32. Chancellor MB, Kaplan SA, Axelord D, Blaivas JG. Bladder outlet obstruction versus impaired detrusor contractility: role of uroflow. *J Urol.* 1991;145:810–812.

33. McGuire EJ, Savastano JA. Stress incontinence and detrusor instability/urge incontinence. *Neurourol Urodynam.* 1985;4: 313–316.

34. Lose G, Jorgensen L, Johnsen A. Predictive value of detrusor instability index in surgery for female urinary incontinence. *Neurourol Urodynam.* 1988;7:141–148.

35. Jorgensen L, Lose G, Molsted-Pederson L. Vaginal repair in female motor urge incontinence. *Eur Urol.* 1987;13:382–385.

36. Stanton SL. Evaluation and therapy of the unstable bladder. In: Ostergard DR, ed. *Gynecologic Urology and Urodynamics.* Baltimore, Md: Williams & Wilkins Co; 1980:229.

37. Blaivas JG, Salinas J. Type III stress incontinence: the importance of proper diagnosis and treatment. *Surg Forum.* 1984; 35:473–475.

38. Bent AE. Concurrent genuine stress incontinence and detrusor instability. *Int Urogynecol J.* 1990;1:128–131.

39. Moisey CU, Stephenson TP, Brendler CB. The urodynamic and subjective results of treatment of detrusor instability with oxybutynin chloride. *Br J Urol.* 1980;52:472–475.

40. Moore KH, Hay DM, Mirie AE, Watson A, Goldstein M. Oxybutynin hydrochloride (3 mg) in the treatment of women with idiopathic detrusor instability. *Br J Urol.* 1990;66:479–485.

41. Fisher CP, Diokno A, Lapides J. The anticholinergic effects of dicyclomine hydrochloride uninhibited neurogenic bladder dysfunction. *J Urol.* 1978;120:328–329.

42. Jensen D Jr. Terodiline treatment of detrusor hyperreflexia in sterosis multiplex. *J Oslo City Hospitals.* 1989;39:67–73.

43. Delaere KPJ, Michiels HGE, Debruyne FMJ, Moonen WA. Flavoxate hydrochloride in the treatment of detrusor instability. *Urol Int.* 1977;32:377–382.

44. Jonas U, Petri E, Kissal J. The effect of flavoxate on hyperactive detrusor muscle. *Eur Urol.* 1979;5:106–109.

45. Briggs RS, Castleden CM, Asher MJ. The effect of flavoxate on uninhibited detrusor contractions and urinary incontinence in the elderly. *J Urol.* 1980;123:665–666.

46. Chappel CR, Parkhouse H, Gardener C, Milroy EJG. Double-blind, placebo-controlled, cross-over study of flavoxate in the treatment of idiopathic detrusor instability. *Br J Urol.* 1990;66: 491–494.

47. Abrams PH, Dunn M. A double-blind trial of bromocriptine in idiopathic detrusor instability. *Br J Urol.* 1980;51:24–27.

48. Cardozo LD, Stanton SL. An objective comparison of the effects of parenterally administered drugs in patients suffering from detrusor instability. *J Urol.* 1979;122:58–59.

49. Cornella JL, Bent AE, Ostergard DR, Horbach NS. Prospective study utilizing transdermal scopolamine in detrusor instability. *Urology.* 1990;35:96–97.

50. Obrink A, Bruune G. Treatment of urgency by installation of emepronium bromide in the urinary bladder. *Scand J Urol Nephrol.* 1978;12:215–218.

51. Higson RH, Smith JC, Hills W. Intravesical lignocaine and detrusor instability. *Br J Urol.* 1979;51:500–503.

52. Mohler JL. Relaxation of intestinal bladder substitutes and neurogenic bladders by intravesically delivered pharmaceuticals. *J Urol.* 1986;137:108A.

53. Mattiasson A, Ekstrom B, Andersson K-E. Effects of intravesical instillation of verapamil in patients with detrusor hyperactivity. *J Urol.* 1989;141:174–177.

54. Fantl JA, Wyman JF, McClish DK, Bump RC. Urinary incontinence in community-dwelling women: clinical, urodynamic and severity characteristics. *Am J Obstet Gynecol.* 1990;162: 946–951.

55. Cardozo LD, Stanton SL, Hafner J, Allan V. Biofeedback in the treatment of detrusor instability. *Br J Urol.* 1978;50:250–254.

56. Janez P, Plevnik S, Suhel P. Urethral and bladder responses to anal electrical stimulation. *J Urol.* 1979;122:192–194.

57. Fall M. Does electrostimulation cure urinary incontinence? *J Urol.* 1984;131:664–667.

58. Ohlsson BL, Fall M, Frankenberg-Sommar S. Effects of external and direct nerve maximal electrical stimulation in the treatment of the uninhibited overactive bladder. *Br J Urol.* 1989;64: 374–380.

59. Plevnik S, Janez J, Vrtacnik P, et al. Short-term electrical stimulation: home treatment for urinary incontinence. *World J Urol.* 1986;4:24–26.

60. Suhel P, Kralj B, Roskar E. Treatment of incontinence relapse cases by VAGICON-X-AMFES and VAGICON-AMFES. In: *Proceedings of the Twelfth Meeting of the International Continence Society, Leiden, West Netherlands.* 1982;113–115.

61. Webster GD, Kreder KJ. Voiding dysfunction following cystourethropexy: its evaluation and management. *J Urol.* 1990; 144:670–673.

62. Helmstein K. Treatment of bladder carcinoma by hydrostatic pressure technique. *Br J Urol.* 1972;44:434–450.

63. Delaere KPJ, Debruyne FMJ, Michiels HGE, Moonen WA. Prolonged bladder distention in the management of the unstable bladder. *J Urol.* 1980;124:334–337.

64. Dunn M, Smith HC, Andran GM. Prolonged bladder distension as a treatment of urgency and urge incontinence of urine. *Br J Urol.* 1974;46:645–652.

65. Ramsden PD, Smith JC, Dunn M, Ardran GM. Distention therapy for unstable bladder: late results including an assessment of repeat distentions. *Br J Urol.* 1976;48:623–629.

66. Whitfield HN, Mayo ME. Prolonged bladder distention in the treatment of the unstable bladder. *Br J Urol.* 1975;47:635–639.

67. Anderson JD, England HR, Mollard EA, Blandy JP. The effects of overstretching on the structure and function of the bladder in relation to Helmstein's distension therapy. *Br J Urol.* 1970; 47:835–890.

68. Elbadawi A. Neuromorphologic basis of vesicourethral dysfunction. I. Histochemistry ultrastructure and function of intrinsic nerves of the bladder and urethra. *Neurourol & Urodynam.* 1982;1: 3–50.

69. Comarr AE. The practical management of the patient with spinal cord injury. *Br J Urol.* 1959;31:1–46.

70. Manfredi RA, Leal JF. Selective sacral rhizotomy for the spastic bladder syndrome in patients with spinal cord injuries. *J Urol.* 1968;100:17–20.

71. Meirowsky AM, Scheibert CD, Rose DK. Indications for the neurosurgical establishment of bladder automaticity in paraplegia. *J Urol.* 1952;67:192–196.

72. Misak SJ, Bunts RC, Ulmer JL, Eagles WM. Nerve interruption procedures in the urologic management of paraplegic patients. *J Urol.* 1962;88:392–401.

73. Rockswold GL, Bradley, WE. The use of sacral nerve block in the evaluation and treatment of neurologic bladder disease. *J Urol.* 1978;18:415–417.

74. Torrens M, Hald T. Bladder denervation procedures. *Urol Clin North Am.* 1979;6:283–293.

75. Ingelman-Sundberg A. Partial denervation of the bladder. A new operation for the treatment of urge incontinence and similar conditions in women. *Acta Obstet Gynecol Scand.* 1959;38:487–502.

76. Ingelman-Sundberg A. Partial bladder denervation for detrusor dyssynergia. *Clin Obstet Gynecol.* 1978;21:797–805.

77. Blackford HN, Murray K, Stephenson TP, et al. Results of transvesical infiltration of the pelvic plexuses with phenol in 116 patients. *Br J Urol.* 1984;56:647–649.

78. Cameron-Strange A, Millard RJ. Management of refractory detrusor instability by transvesical phenol injection. *Br J Urol.* 1988;62:323–325.

79. Ewing R, Bultitude MI, Shuttleworth KED. Subtrigonal phenol injection for urge incontinence secondary to detrusor instability in female. *Br J Urol.* 1982;54:689–692.

80. Harris RG, Constantinou CE, Stamey TA. Extravesical subtrigonal injection of 50 percent ethanol for detrusor instability. *J Urol.* 1988;140:111–116.

81. McInerney PD, Vanner TF, Matenhelia S, Stephenson TP. Assessment of the long-term results of subtrigonal phenolisation. *Br J Urol.* 1991;67:586–587.

82. Parkhouse HF, Gilpin SA, Gosling JA, et al. Quantitative study of phenol as a neurolytic agent in the urinary bladder. *Br J Urol.* 1987;60:410–412.

83. Rosenbaum TP, Shaw PJR, Worth PHL. Trans-trigonal phenol failed the test of time. *Br J Urol.* 1990;66:164–169.

84. Wall LL, Stanton SL. Transvesical phenol injection of pelvic nerve plexuses in female with refractory urge incontinence. *Br J Urol.* 1989;63:465–468.

85. Learmonth JR. Neurosurgery in the treatment of diseases of the urinary tract. *J Urol.* 1931;26:13–24.

86. Richer V. La résection des nerfs érecteurs et des ganglions hypogastriques. *J Chir (Paris).* 1935;45:54.

87. Freiha FS, Stamey TA. Cystolysis: a procedure for the selective denervation of the bladder. *J Urol.* 1980;123:360–363.

88. Worth PHL, Turner-Warwick RT. The treatment of interstitial cystitis by cystolysis with observation on cystoplasty. *Br J Urol.* 1973;45:65–71.

89. Mahony DT, Laferte RD. Studies of enuresis. IV. Multiple detrusor myotomy—a new operation for the rehabilitation of severe detrusor hypertrophy and hypercontractility. *J Urol.* 1972;107: 1064–1067.

90. Hindmarsh JR, Essenhigh SM, Yeates WK. Bladder transection for adult enuresis. *Br J Urol.* 1977;49:515–521.

91. Parson KF, O'Boyle PJ, Gibbon NOK. A further assessment of bladder transection in the management of adult enuresis and allied conditions. *Br J Urol.* 1977;49:509–514.

92. Turner-Warwick RT, Ashken MH. The functional results of partial, subtotal and total cystocystoplasty with special reference to ureterocaecocystoplasty, selective sphincterotomy and cystocystoplasty. *Br J Urol.* 1967;39:3–12.

93. Heimburger RF, Freeman LW, Wilde NJ. Sacral nerve innervation of the human bladder. *J Neurosurg.* 1948;5:154–164.

94. Penn RD, Kroin JS. Long-term intrathecal baclofen infusion for treatment of spasticity. *J Neurosurg.* 1987;66:181–185.

95. Nanninga JB, Frost F, Penn R. Effect of intrathecal baclofen on bladder aand sphincter function. *J Urol.* 1989;142:101–105.

96. Hodgkinson CP, Drukker BH. Intravesical nerve resection for detrusor dyssynergia. *Acta Obstet Gynecol Scand.* 1977;56: 401–408.

97. Warrel DW. Vaginal denervation of the bladder nerve supply. *Urol Int.* 1977;32:114–116.

98. Wan J, McGuire EJ, Wang S, Ingelman-Sundberg A. Bladder denervation for detrusor instability. *J Urol.* 1991;145: 358A.

99. Mundy AR. Bladder transection for urge incontinence associated with detrusor instability. *Br J Urol.* 1980;52:480–483.

100. Mundy AR. The surgical treatment of urge incontinence of urine. *J Urol.* 1982;128:481–483.

101. Essenhigh DM, Yeates WK. Transection of the bladder with particular reference to enuresis. *Br J Urol.* 1973;45:299–305.

102. Janknegt RA, Moonen WA, Schreinemachers LMH. Transection of the bladder as a method of treatment in adult enuresis nocturna. *Br J Urol.* 1979;51:275–277.

103. Mikulicz J. Zur Operation der angeborenen Blasenspalte. *Zentralbl Chir.* 1899;26:641.

104. Couvelaire R. La "petite vessie" des tuberculeaux genito-urinaires. Essai de classification de place et variantes des cysto-intestino-plasties. *J d'Urol.* 1950;56:381.

105. Gil-Vernet JM Jr. The ileocolic segment in urologic surgery. *J Urol.* 1965;94:418–426.

106. Goodwin WE, Winter CC, Barker WF. "Cup-patch" technique of ileocystoplasty for bladder enlargement or partial substitution. *Surg Gynecol Obstet.* 1959;108:240–241.

107. Goldwasser B, Webster GD. Augmentation and substitution enterocystoplasty. *J Urol.* 1986;135:215–224.

108. Kuss R. Colo-cystoplasty rather than ileo-cystoplasty. *J Urol.* 1959;82:587–589.

109. Kuss R, Bitker M, Camey M, Chatelain C, Lassau JP. Indications and early and late results of intestino-cystoplasty: a review of 185 cases. *J Urol.* 1970;103:53–63.

110. Kvarstein B, Mathisen W, Steinsvik E. Sigmoidocystoplasty: a follow-up study. *Eur Urol.* 1980;6:18–20.

111. Reddy PK, Lange PH, Fraley EE. Bladder replacement after cystoprostatectomy: efforts to achieve total continence. *J Urol.* 1987;138:495–499.

112. Sidi AA, Reinberg Y, Gonzalez R. Influence of intestinal segment of configuration on the outcome of augmentation enterocystoplasty. *J Urol.* 1986;136:1201–1204.

113. Smith RB. Use of ileocystoplasty in the hypertonic neurogenic bladder. *J Urol.* 1975;113:125–127.

114. Whitmore WF, Gittes RF. Reconstruction of the urinary tract by cecal and ileocecal cystoplasty: review of a 15-year experience. *J Urol.* 1983;129:494–498.

115. Laungkhot R, Peng BCH, Blaivas JG. Ileocecocystoplasty for the management of refractory neurogenic bladder: surgical technique and urodynamic findings. *J Urol.* 1991;146:1340–1344.

116. Bramble FJ. The treatment of adult enuresis and urge incontinence by enterocystoplasty. *Br J Urol.* 1982;54:693–696.

117. Raz S, Ehrlich RM, Zeidman EJ, Alarcon A, McLaughlin S. Surgical treatment of the incontinent female patient with myelomeningocele. *J Urol*. 1988;139:524–527.

118. Stephenson TP, Mundy AR. Treatment of the neuropathic bladder by enterocystoplasty and selective sphincterotomy or sphincter ablation and replacement. *Br J Urol*. 1985;57:27–31.

119. Dounis A, Abel BJ, Gow JG. Cecocystoplasty for bladder augmentation. *J Urol*. 1980;123:164–167.

120. Hinman F. Selection of intestinal segments for bladder substitution: physical and physiological characteristics. *J Urol*. 1988; 139:519–523.

121. Koff SA. Guidelines to determine the size and shape of intestinal segments used for reconstruction. *J Urol*. 1988;140: 1150–1151.

122. Goldwasser B, Barrett DM, Webster GD, Kramer SA. Cystometric properties of ileum and right colon after bladder augmentation, substitution or replacement. *J Urol*. 1987;138: 1007–1008.

123. Mundy AR, Stephenson TP. ''Clam'' ileocystoplasty for the treatment of refractory urge incontinence. *Br J Urol*. 1985;57: 641–646.

124. Adams MC, Mitchell ME, Rink RL. Gastrocystoplasty: an alternative solution to the problem of urological reconstruction in the severely compromised patient. *J Urol*. 1988;140:1152–1156.

125. Stone AR, MacDermott JPA. Split-cuff nipple reimplantation technique: reliable reflux prevention from bowel segments. *J Urol*. 1989;142:707–709.

126. Rushton HG, Woodard JR, Parrott TS, Jeff RD, Gearhart JP. Delayed bladder rupture after augmentation enterocystoplasty. *J Urol*. 1988;140:344–346.

127. Shiner JR, Kaplan GW. Spontaneous bladder rupture following enterocystoplasty. *J Urol*. 1988;140:1157–1158.

128. Filmer RB, Spencer JR. Malignancies in bladder augmentation and intestinal conduits. *J Urol*. 1990;143:671–678.

129. Nurse DE, Mundy AR. Metabolic complications of cystoplasty. *Br J Urol*. 1989;63:165–170.

130. Linder A, Leach GE, Raz S. Augmentation cystoplasty in the treatment of neurogenic bladder dysfunction. *J Urol*. 1983;129: 491–493.

7

Total Incontinence—Corrective Approaches

7-1

Management of Genitourinary Fistulas

Raymond A. Lee

A fistula originating from the genitourinary tract with its constant malodorous, irritating, unimpeded leakage is one of the most devastating complications that can occur in women. In 1920, Judd, from the Mayo Clinic, stated:

> Better obstetric management has greatly reduced the number of fistulae which occur as the result of difficult labor, but there has been a great general wave for the radical extirpation of cancer both by operative procedure and by cautery and large doses of radium.[1(p447)]

Subsequent descriptions of Mayo Clinic patients by Massee and co-workers[2] and Symmonds[3] revealed a continuation of this trend.

Although it is impossible to determine accurately the frequency of genitourinary fistulas, currently, in the United States, most of these fistulas result from a gynecologic operation (mainly total abdominal hysterectomy). Fistula complications of the ureter, the bladder, or the urethra have different clinical presentations, each type requiring inherently separate diagnostic procedures to identify the fistula and each requiring a separate surgical approach in its management. Possibly because of differences in surgical training and experience, considerable differences of opinion exist regarding the timing, surgical approach, specific operative techniques, and postoperative management in the correction of these fistulas.

Note: Portions of this chapter are reprinted with permission from RA Lee, "Surgical Management of Ureteral, Vesical, and Rectovaginal Fistulas," in *Surgical Gynecologic Oncology* by E Burghardt (ed), Georg Thieme Verlag (in press).

URETHROVAGINAL FISTULA

Prolonged labor continues to be a common cause of destruction of the urethra and the base of the bladder in patients in medically deprived countries,[4–6] whereas elective urethral and vaginal operation is a leading factor in the development of these low-lying fistulas in the United States.[7,8] The excision of friable, infected urethral diverticulum can be tedious and inexact.[9] Despite meticulous efforts to reconstruct the urethral floor accurately, infection and edema may lead to imperfect healing and fistula formation. In addition, overzealous plication of the urethra or the inadvertent intramural placement of a suture (vaginal or retropubic needle suspension) may produce a fistula of the urethra or a greater calamity—actual slough of the entire floor and bladder neck.[8]

Clinical Presentation

Patients who experience trauma to the urethra from forceps delivery or automobile accidents have leakage immediately or within the first 24 hours after damage. If a urethral catheter was in place temporarily, either after delivery or trauma, catheter removal is generally followed promptly by leakage of urine. In my experience, most urethrovaginal fistulas occur after an operation for diverticulum or an anterior colporrhaphy done for urinary stress incontinence or cystocele. Patients who have undergone these operations generally have a catheter in place for 2 to 7 days. Some of these patients may have an unrecognized suture through the wall of the urethra, which generally results in necrosis of the tissue and possibly associated hematoma formation or some degree of infection, the combination of which results in fistula formation and leakage of urine. The patient may initially be continent, only to experience leakage some 1 to 2 weeks after surgery. Patients who have had irradiation generally note the leakage some time after the treatment, generally within 2 to 4 weeks after therapy.

Simple urethrovaginal fistula, depending on its location relative to the bladder neck, may not produce urinary incontinence and may not require operative repair. Fistulas located near the bladder neck may be technically more difficult to repair. Even after what appears to be a successful repair, the patient may experience stress urinary incontinence related to fibrosis, fixation, and poor contractility of the urethral musculature. A more complex problem is presented by patients who had a major slough resulting in a linear loss of the floor of the urethra and frequently involving the bladder neck and base of the bladder.

Operative Repair

The basic phases of operative reconstruction consist of a linear incision, much like that for an anterior colporrhaphy, and mobilization of the vaginal mucosa laterally off the underlying pubocervical fascia. This procedure must be accomplished in the proper bloodless tissue plane sufficiently lateral to establish mobility, so that a tension-free closure of the urethra can be accomplished.

Once the fistula is completely mobilized and the scar tissue (fistula tract) is removed, the fistula itself is closed with fine 4-0 delayed-absorbable sutures placed extramucosally, and the tissue edges are approximated free of tension and with excellent hemostasis. The presence of a small-caliber catheter within the urethra frequently assists in accurate placement of the sutures to close the fistulous tract. This initial suture line is imbricated with a second set of sutures, the most distal suture being just distal to the original suture line. Snug plication of the bladder neck by approximation, under the urethra, of the tissue (pubocervical fascia) lateral to the urethra to create a tension-free second layer of sutures is mandatory for a successful repair. A tension-free closure of the vaginal wall as a third layer, or when necessary for the obliteration of dead space and actual replacement of the anterior wall of the vagina with a pedicled skin, fibrofatty labial graft, may be indicated.

A second-stage retropubic urethrovesical suspension for patients who have a good anatomic result with an apparently intact urethra but who nevertheless remain incontinent (intact urethra with stress incontinence) may be necessary at a later date. This result cannot be predicted at the time of closure of the urethral fistula.

VESICOVAGINAL FISTULA

It is generally agreed that gynecologic operations (ie, total abdominal hysterectomy) and, specifically, operations for benign gynecologic conditions are responsible for approximately 80%[10] of vesicovaginal fistulas. The fistulas most frequently occur after surgical treatment for relatively simple gynecologic conditions, such as uterine fibroids, menometrorrhagia, uterine prolapse, and cervical intraepithelial neoplasia. Conditions associated with difficult dissections (eg, pelvic inflammatory disease, endometriosis, or invasive carcinoma) are infrequently related to fistula formation. Perhaps the surgeon has a greater degree of apprehension and concern with the more difficult dissections and dissects more carefully and identifies adjacent and contiguous structures, thus preventing injury or at least promoting recognition and prompt repair. Approximately 10% of vesicovaginal fistulas occur after obstetric procedures, such as forceps delivery, cesarean section, or cesarean hysterectomy. In my experience, 7% of fistulas are a result of radiation therapy for management of malignant disease of the cervix, endometrium, or ovary.

During a 15-year period, 24,883 patients underwent major gynecologic operations performed by members of the Division of Gynecologic Surgery at the Mayo Clinic; fistulas developed in 5 of these patients (0.02%).[10] Three of these fistulas were urethrovaginal and resulted from an anterior repair, urethral diverticulectomy, and radical hysterectomy with total vaginectomy for invasive carcinoma of the cervix. One was a ureterovaginal fistula that developed as a result of radical hysterectomy for a postirradiation, recurrent squamous cell carcinoma of the cervix. The fifth was a vesicovaginal fistula that developed after a primary radical hysterectomy. During this same period, we saw 303 women with genitourinary fistulas, of whom 182 had vesicovaginal fistulas. Ninety-one of these women had undergone one to five previous operative attempts before operation at our institution. Our initial attempt at repair was successful (98%) regardless of the size of the fistulas, number of fistulas, or number of previous operative attempts. The rest of the fistulas were successfully corrected on a second attempt.

Clinical Presentation

In a recent series,[10] I and my colleagues determined the time of leakage onset in 140 patients referred with vesicovaginal fistulas after operation. Leakage was recorded as beginning between day 1 and day 10 in 94 patients, between day 11 and day 20 in 38 patients, and between day 21 and day 30 in 6 patients. Thus, 138 of 140 patients had leakage within the first 30 days after surgery. In two patients, leakage began 3 and 5 months after the operation. When the fistula occurred after childbirth or trauma, leakage usually began within the first 24 hours.

Time and Route of Operation

There are differing opinions regarding the appropriate timing of fistula repair. In 1960, Collins and co-workers[11] suggested early repair and reported the preoperative use of cortisone to "permit resolution of inflammatory reaction" around the vesicovaginal fistula. Of 15 fistulas operated on within 8 weeks (most of them within 4 weeks) of discovery, 13 were repaired successfully transvaginally. In 1971, Collins and colleagues[12] reported a 72% success rate in 29 patients who were treated with the same approach and medications within 2 weeks of discovery of the fistula. In 1979, Persky and co-workers[13] reported the results of early repair (within 1 to 10 weeks after recognition) in 7 patients. They used a retropubic transvesical approach in all but 1 patient. They emphasized the value of placing the peritoneum and the omentum as an intervening layer between the bladder and the vaginal repair, and the procedure was successful in all patients. Although it is impossible to determine the reasons for operative failure in patients referred to me or my colleagues after one or several unsuccessful operative attempts, we are impressed with the frequency with which early operative intervention is noted. With or without preoperative administration of corticosteroids, the presence of resolving suture material, edema, and inflammation in addition to microabscess formation should have an adverse effect on the overall success rate of primary repair.

Furthermore, in a few patients, preliminary catheter drainage of the bladder for 10 to 15 days may provide spontaneous healing of the fistula, thus preventing the need for operation. In the nonirradiated patient with a postoperative vesicovaginal fistula, results of our experience have indicated that the tissues have excellent blood supply with minimal edema at about 8 to 12 weeks after the formation of a fistula or after a failed repair. Any infection has resolved with little evidence of previous suture material, and cleavage planes are readily identifiable at the time of the dissection. These conditions permit wide mobilization and adequate dissection to allow accurate approximation of tissues without tension on the suture lines. Nevertheless, we believe that some fistulas can be managed successfully with early operation (eg, obstetric lacerations and some of the fistulas diagnosed a few hours after operation).

Selection of patients is the critical factor in determining when an operative repair may be done. This decision must be based on the type and difficulty of the causative operation and on the disease for which the original procedure was done. (For example, patients who have had an operation for malignancy, abscess formation, postirradiation problems, or pelvic inflammatory disease are not candidates.) In addition, the general overall condition of the patient should be the prime consideration before operation is undertaken. The patient or the referring physician may request or even demand immediate operative intervention. The patient and her family may not be easily convinced that additional time should elapse before the operative repair. She (or her relatives) may become impatient, seek other advice, or apply other pressures in an attempt to coerce the surgeon into an operative repair before the tissues are in optimal condition.

Route of Repair

Many fistulas may be repaired successfully by using a vaginal, an abdominal, or a transvesical approach. In specific circumstances, one of these approaches may present a singular advantage. On occasion it may be necessary to incorporate a combination of all these approaches for successful management. Unfortunately, the route chosen for the repair is frequently determined on the basis of the surgeon's specialty (ie, gynecologists use a vaginal approach; urologists, transvesical; general surgeons, transperitoneal). Anyone with significant experience in dealing with these fistulas is aware, regardless of specialty, that one must be familiar and adept with all three approaches as well as with various techniques.

From the patient's viewpoint, the vaginal approach is easiest, safest, and most comfortable. The two factors that adversely affect a vaginal approach are the visibility of the fistula and the proximity of a large fistula adjacent to the ureter. The size or number of fistulas or the history of previous operative repair does not necessarily obviate the vaginal approach. The usual fistula resulting from an operation is located above the interureteric ridge on the posterior wall of the bladder, and there is adequate distance from the ureters such that a vaginal repair can be accomplished safely and effectively. Nevertheless, a gynecologist who prefers the vaginal approach should not insist on vaginal repair for a fistula high in a fixed vaginal vault, a location that makes the dissection difficult because of limited visibility, which may result in an inaccurate repair. For patients in whom exposure is inadequate or proximity to the ureter would endanger successful repair, we prefer the transperitoneal approach, which permits mobilization of the bladder and the ureter (frequently with an indwelling ureteral catheter) such that an accurate and safe repair can be accomplished under good visibility.

Technique of Repair

Regardless of the approach chosen, the basic surgical principles originally described by Sims[14] remain essentially unchanged. The bladder wall should be accurately approximated, free of tension, and have excellent hemostasis. We prefer a wide mobilization, separating the vagina from the underlying bladder wall. The fistulous tract is excised (creating a fresh injury) (Figure 7-1.1a), and the initial layer of the bladder is closed in extramucosal fashion with fine delayed-absorbable sutures placed in an interrupted fashion (Figure 7-1.1b). A second layer of sutures (extending lateral to the original suture line), inverting the initial layer, is established with a similar suture in an interrupted or a continuous fashion (Figure 7-1.1c). At this point, the bladder is filled with 200 mL of sterile infant's formula or milk to test the suture line. Usually, with either a vaginal or an abdominal approach, the peritoneum can be pulled from the back of the bladder and fixed over the previously closed suture line in such a way that it separates the closure of the vaginal wall from the bladder (Figure 7-1.1d). This is accomplished with fine (4-0) delayed-absorbable sutures. The vaginal wall is then closed with fine sutures, usually in an interrupted fashion (Figure 7-1.1e).

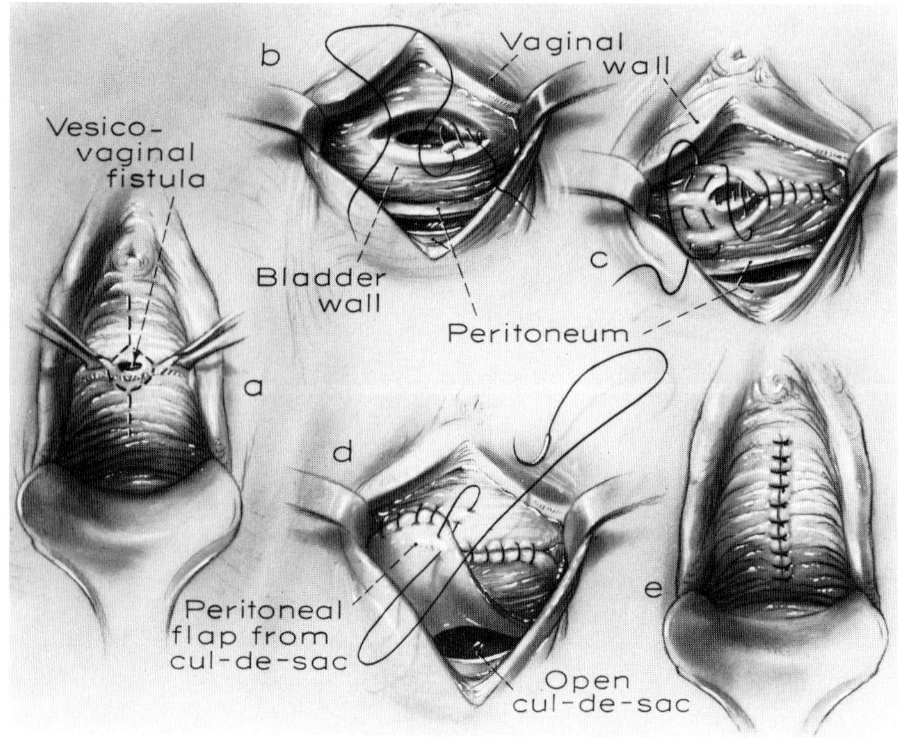

Figure 7-1.1 **a**, Initial vaginal incision with appropriate undermining of the vagina from the bladder wall. **b**, The fistulous tract is excised, creating a fresh injury; the initial layer of sutures is placed in an extramucosal fashion. **c**, The second layer of sutures is initiated just lateral to the initially closed layer and placed in a fashion that inverts the initial suture line. **d**, The peritoneum from the back of the bladder is pulled anteriorly and sutured over the two previously closed suture lines so that it separates the bladder from the underlying closure of the vaginal mucosa. **e**, The vaginal mucosa is closed. *Source:* Reproduced with permission from *Gynecology-Obstetrics Guide*, Copyright © 1962 by Commerce Clearing House, Inc, 4025 W Peterson Avenue, Chicago, IL 60646.

Latzko Technique

An alternative approach favored by many is the Latzko technique.[15] In this approach, approximately 2 cm of the vaginal mucosa encircling the fistula is excised. The denuded area is then approximated with fine absorbable interrupted sutures in such a fashion that the initial layer is invaginated toward the bladder lumen. A second layer is used to invert the initial layer, and a third layer is used to approximate the vaginal epithelium.

Postoperative Management

To ensure success of the repair, sound surgical judgment is required during and after the operation. Any tension or manipulation of the suture line must be avoided, and complete bladder drainage with a large-caliber catheter (placed urethrally, suprapubically, or both) is mandatory. Overdistention of the bladder because of obstruction of the catheter (by blood or mucus) can be prevented by hourly charting of the urinary output and by using the appropriate irrigation. Repeated urethral catheterization may potentially disrupt a well-closed bladder repair and should be avoided. To minimize infection, appropriate urine cultures are examined and antibiotics are administered. Although some surgeons have recommended early removal of the urinary catheter after treatment of simple fistulas, we are unable to predict with certainty in which patients this may be appropriate. As a result, we customarily provide catheter drainage for at least 7 days and, in specific patients, possibly for several weeks.

URETEROVAGINAL FISTULA

Surgical treatment (total abdominal hysterectomy) of benign conditions continues to be responsible for most ureterovaginal fistulas. Menometrorrhagia, uterine fibroids, and pelvic relaxation are the most frequent gynecologic conditions associated with formation of ureterovaginal fistula.

Clinical Presentation

Most patients have evidence of urine leakage within the first 14 days after operation. In approximately one third of patients, leakage begins between 15 and 30 days after surgery. Chills, fever, and various degrees of flank discomfort commonly occur during this postoperative period. It may take several days or weeks for necrosis, urinoma formation, and eventual dissection to result in a fistula through a previously closed vaginal suture line. This process is sometimes associated with relatively subtle symptoms of flank or costovertebral angle tenderness, with or without chills or fever.

Timing and Method of Repair

Factors that affect the timing of operation and the method of repair are the patient's general overall condition and the degree of obstruction of the ureter. Preservation of kidney function must be ensured by accomplishing adequate decompression of the upper renal system. This may be done by passing a ureteral catheter cystoscopically in a retrograde fashion or percutaneously down the ureter. If decompression and cessation of leakage are established, operative intervention may not be required. If any of these findings (ie, obstruction, persistent leakage) persist, operation should be undertaken. Once the patient's condition permits operation and the tissues are considered to be in optimal condition, an abdominal approach is undertaken.

The location of the injury to the ureter and its relation to the bladder will determine the choice of operative repair. Most injuries after gynecologic procedures are close to the bladder; for these we prefer to use a ureteroneocystostomy. We prefer an open technique that includes direct mucosa-to-mucosa approximation of the ureter to the bladder with fine interrupted polyglycolic acid sutures over a ureteral stent placed through the anastomosis into the renal pelvis.

Technique of Operative Repair

The end of the proximal segment of the ureter is incised in a vertical fashion in the 6-o'clock position for a distance of approximately 5 mm. A 4-0 polyglycolic acid suture is inserted through the angle of this incision. A finger is inserted inside the open bladder to tent up the bladder wall and indicate the most accessible area on the posterolateral wall for insertion of the ureter. A 1-cm opening is dissected directly through the full thickness of the bladder by means of a spreading action of the dissecting scissors. A curved forceps is then passed inside the bladder out through the opening in the bladder wall, where it is used to grasp the previously placed suture; traction on the suture delivers the ureter within the blad-

Figure 7-1.2 **A**, With the open technique and through a cystotomy incision, the ureter is delivered through the opening to the mucosa of the bladder. **B**, Full thickness of ureter is sutured to the bladder mucosa with interrupted 4-0 delayed-absorbable sutures. Three to four sutures are placed through the peritoneal flap and a portion of the wall of the ureter to fix it to the bladder. *Source:* Reprinted with permission from *Clinical Obstetrics and Gynecology* (1976;19:623–644), Copyright © 1976, JB Lippincott Company.

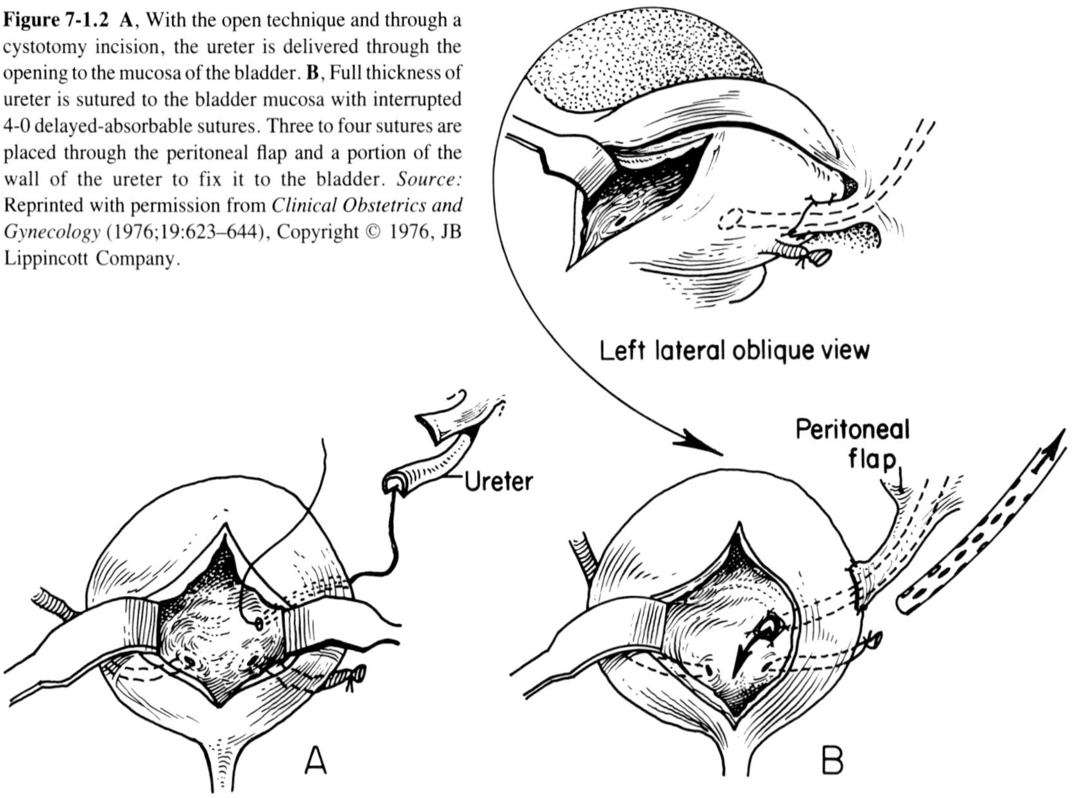

der (Figure 7-1.2A). From inside the bladder, five to six interrupted 4-0 polyglycolic acid sutures anastomose the full thickness of the spatulate ureter to near the full thickness of the bladder in a mucosa-to-mucosa approximation. Three to four interrupted sutures of the same material are placed in the peritoneum, incorporating the peritoneum of the ureter to the muscularis and serosa of the bladder to reinforce the repair and reduce any potential tension on the mucosal approximation (Figure 7-1.2B). We prefer next to pass a self-retaining ureteral catheter with its most proximal end lodged in the renal pelvis and its distal end free within the bladder. This is generally left in place for 10 to 14 days. The bladder is drained with a suprapubic Foley catheter brought out through an anterior cystotomy, which is then closed with two layers of running 3-0 polyglycolic acid suture. Appropriate suction drainage and reperitonealization are accomplished in the customary fashion.

Bladder Extension

Occasionally, a ureteral fistula will be so high that it is necessary to free the bladder from the back of the symphysis pubis and either side wall to bridge this gap without tension on the anastomosis. This technique permits a ureteroneocystostomy to be accomplished as far as the bifurcation of the iliac vessels on either side. Any tension on the anastomosis is relieved by stretching and fixing the upper lateral portion of the bladder wall to the iliopsoas fascia with several interrupted 2-0 polyglycolic acid sutures (Figure 7-1.3).

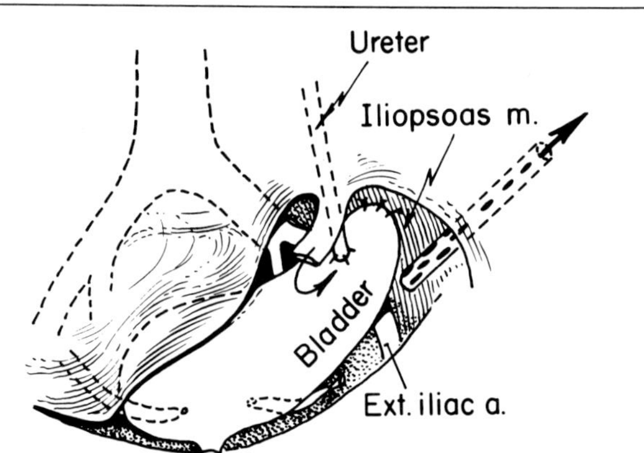

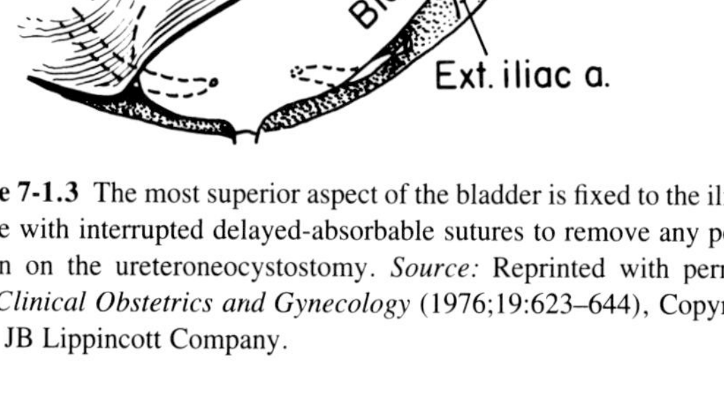

Figure 7-1.3 The most superior aspect of the bladder is fixed to the iliopsoas muscle with interrupted delayed-absorbable sutures to remove any potential tension on the ureteroneocystostomy. *Source:* Reprinted with permission from *Clinical Obstetrics and Gynecology* (1976;19:623–644), Copyright © 1976, JB Lippincott Company.

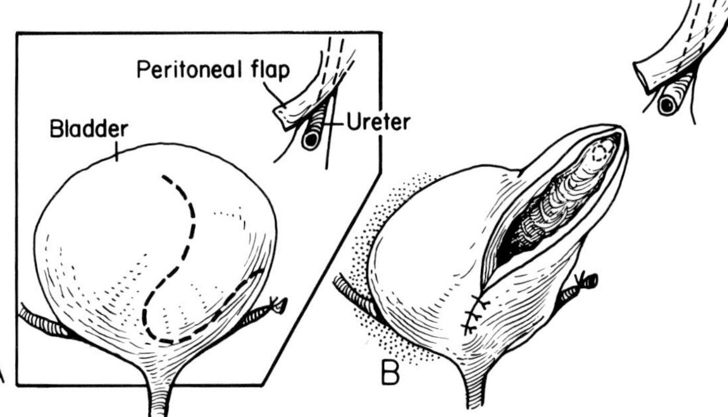

Figure 7-1.4 A widely based flap is developed from the superior aspect of the bladder (**A**) and placed in a cone-like fashion (**B**). The opening that will later accept the ureter is made through the posterior wall of the bladder. *Source:* Reprinted with permission from *Clinical Obstetrics and Gynecology* (1976;19:623–644), Copyright © 1976, JB Lippincott Company.

Bladder Flap

If the technique described earlier does not allow the bladder to reach the ureter free of tension, construction of a tube from the bladder flap to bridge the defect must be considered. Methods to accomplish this have been reported by Boari.[16] An oblique-placed flap is outlined on the outside of the bladder. This must be widely based superiorly (Figure 7-1.4); when care is taken to avoid making the flap too narrow distally, its blood supply should be excellent. Generally, an end-to-side, mucosa-to-mucosa approximation can be accomplished, as described earlier for ureteroneocystostomy (Figure 7-1.5). The anastomosis is done under direct vision before the long linear defect of the anterior wall of the bladder, produced by the creation of the tube, is closed. When a perineal flap has been preserved along with the upper end of the ureter, this flap can be brought down well over the anterior cystotomy incision and fixed in a position, so that it will additionally relieve any tension on the anastomosis.

An alternative means of dealing with the injury high in the pelvis is ureteroureterostomy. There are several rather elaborate techniques for an end-to-end ureteroureterostomy, any one of which may be the preferred route when there is disparity in the size of the upper and lower ends of the ureters. If the ureter is small, a slight spatulation of both ends will facilitate anastomosis and enlarge its diameter. To preserve ureteral blood supply and mobility, the proximal and distal segments of the ureter should be mobilized only enough to allow an accurate anastomosis. The anastomosis is accomplished with one layer of interrupted 5-0 delayed-absorbable sutures, and care is taken to avoid the tendency to overrepair. The sutures are placed to include the ureteral sheath and muscularis down to the mucosa. This step is accomplished most accurately over a ureteral catheter.

CONCLUSION

Obstetric and gynecologic operations are responsible for most of the fistula formations of the genitourinary tract. Almost 75% of genitourinary fistulas and perhaps 90% of surgical ureteral injuries result from total abdominal hysterectomy. If surgical outcome is to be improved and the incidence of fistulas decreased, surgeons must emphasize the need for dissection of contiguous tissues

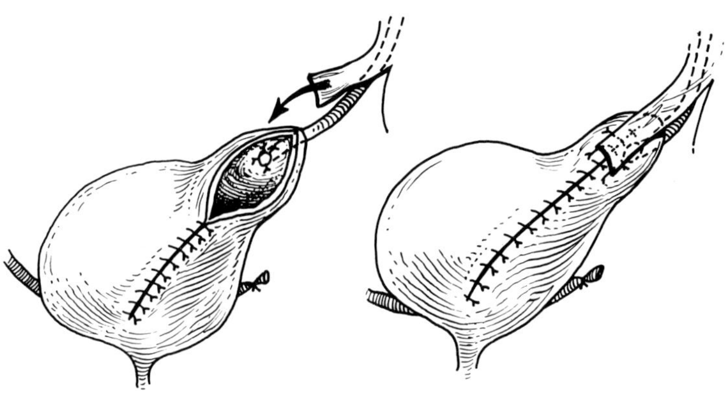

Figure 7-1.5 The ureteroneocystostomy is established with interrupted delayed-absorbable sutures (left), following which the cystotomy is closed with running or interrupted sutures in two layers of fine delayed-absorbable sutures (right). The peritoneal flap, as indicated by the arrow, is placed around the anastomosis to aid in its being a watertight closure. *Source:* Reprinted with permission from *Clinical Obstetrics and Gynecology* (1976;19:623–644), Copyright © 1976, JB Lippincott Company.

and insist on adequate mobilization and identification of the urinary tract structures. These steps will help prevent injury to the structures. Equally important, however, if injury should occur, it will be more easily recognized at the time of operation. With recognition and appropriate repair, the serious morbidity of fistula formation can be prevented.

REFERENCES

1. Judd ES. The operative treatment of vesicovaginal fistulae. *Surg Gynecol Obstet*. 1920;30:447–453.

2. Massee JS, Welch JS, Pratt JH, Symmonds RE. Management of urinary-vaginal fistula: ten-year survey. *JAMA*. 1964;190: 902–906.

3. Symmonds RE. Incontinence: vesical and urethral fistulas. *Clin Obstet Gynecol*. 1984;27:499–514.

4. Shigui F, Qinge S. Operative treatment of female urinary fistulas; report of 405 cases. *Chin Med J (Engl)*. 1979;92:263–268.

5. Vanderputte SR. Obstetric vesicovaginal fistulae: experience with 89 cases. *Ann Soc Belg Med Trop*. 1985;65:303–309.

6. Hamlin RHJ, Nicholson EC. Reconstruction of urethra totally destroyed in labour. *Br Med J*. 1969;2:147–150.

7. Gray LA. Urethrovaginal fistulas. *Am J Obstet Gynecol*. 1968;101:28–35.

8. Symmonds RE, Hill LM. Loss of the urethra: a report on 50 patients. *Am J Obstet Gynecol*. 1978;130:130–138.

9. Lee RA. Diverticulum of the female urethra: postoperative complications and results. *Obstet Gynecol*. 1983;61:52–58.

10. Lee RA, Symmonds RE, Williams TJ. Current status of genitourinary fistula. *Obstet Gynecol*. 1988;72:313–319.

11. Collins CG, Pent D, Jones FB. Results of early repair of vesicovaginal fistula with preliminary cortisone treatment. *Am J Obstet Gynecol*. 1960;80:1005–1009.

12. Collins CG, Collins JH, Harrison BR, Nicholls RA, Hoffman ES, Krupp PJ. Early repair of vesicovaginal fistula. *Am J Obstet Gynecol*. 1971;111:524–526.

13. Persky L, Herman G, Guerrier K. Nondelay in vesicovaginal fistula repair. *Urology*. 1979;13:273–275.

14. Sims JM. On the treatment of vesico-vaginal fistula. *Am J Med Sci*. 1852;23:59–82.

15. Latzko W. Postoperative vesicovaginal fistulas: genesis and therapy. *Am J Surg*. 1942;58:211–228.

16. Boari A. Contributo sperimentale alla plastica dell'uretere. *Atti Accad Sci Nat Ferrara*. 1894;68:149.

7-2

Periurethral Injections

Rodney A. Appell

The choice of the appropriate therapeutic approach for treating urinary incontinence depends to a large degree on the underlying cause of the problem. When problems with urinary incontinence originate in the urethra, the difficulty is often related to incompetence of the urethral sphincteric mechanism at the neck of the bladder. Although this incompetence may be the result of some defect in anatomic support, it may also be related to a problem in the intrinsic urethral closure mechanism itself as a result of sympathetic neurologic injury, surgical trauma, or myelodysplasia. Urodynamically, in such cases, the bladder neck and the proximal segment of the urethra are open at rest without a detrusor contraction.

Urethral sphincteric incompetence implies that the resistance to urinary outflow has been lowered to the point that it does not adequately protect the patient from urinary loss. Nearly all procedures developed to restore urinary control in this type of outflow disorder are based on the principle of enhancing urethral pressure to resist the flow of urine.

The treatment of urinary incontinence related to the incompetent urethra has been a challenging problem. Treatment frequently involves surgical augmentation of intraurethral pressures by using techniques such as sling procedures or the implantation of an artificial urinary sphincter. Another technique to treat this type of incontinence is periurethral and transurethral injection of bulk-enhancing agents to increase pressure on the urethra and reduce the urethral lumen size with resultant additional urethral resistance to the flow of urine.

HISTORICAL REVIEW

Periurethral and transurethral injection of material as a technique to increase outflow resistance in patients with urinary incontinence is not new. In 1938, Murless[1] described the injection of a sclerosing solution (morrhuate sodium) into the anterior wall of the vagina in 20 patients. An inflammatory response developed with secondary scarring and resultant compression of the incompetent urethra. Cure or improvement was reported in 17 patients; however, the complications, including pulmonary infarction and cardiorespiratory arrest, were unacceptable. In 1955, Quackels[2] described 2 patients who were treated successfully with periurethral paraffin injection without complications. In 1963, Sachse[3] described 31 patients after treatment with another sclerosing agent, dondren. Four of seven women were cured. Pulmonary complications including pulmonary emboli, however, were again the major drawbacks.

The first report of the use of polytetrafluoroethylene (Teflon, Polytef, and Urethrin) by Berg[4] appeared in 1973. He described 3 patients with surgically induced type III stress incontinence who underwent injection with this material with resolution of symptoms. Two of three required a second injection. The only complication was asymptomatic bacteriuria in 1 patient. The use of periurethral and transurethral polytetrafluoroethylene (PTFE) injection for incontinence has been promulgated for more than a decade by Politano and several associates at the University of Miami.[5–10] The use of this procedure for the treatment of urinary incontinence has not attained universal acceptance despite reports from other centers demonstrating its efficacy.[11–17] Reasons for this lack of acceptance will be addressed later.

PATIENT SELECTION

Injectables are most suitable for patients with pure sphincter incompetency and normal detrusor function. Patients with decreased detrusor contractility, however, may be candidates if intermittent self-catheterization is an option. The diagnosis of urethral incompetence and the status of the detrusor are determined with the use of urodynamic studies or fluoroscopic studies (or both). The success in attaining continence is influenced by the presence of any bladder disease. Injections in the patient with a normal bladder or poor detrusor contractility with unaltered compliance are consistently associated with a high degree of success. Detrusor hyperreflexia, if found urodynamically, must be controlled before injection. Adequate bladder capacity (greater than 125 mL) is essential, but residual urine is not a factor. Endoscopic evaluation to determine that viable tissue is present at the prospective injection site is mandatory and also helpful in determining the proximity of the ureteral orifices to the bladder neck and the posterior aspect of the urethra. As mentioned, careful urodynamic evaluation is essential to establish the bladder response to filling and the leak point pressure. This endoscopic and urodynamic evaluation of the lower urinary tract is of major importance in ensuring an optimal outcome. The only pure contraindications to injectables are uncontrolled detrusor hyperreflexia and known hypersensitivity to the injectable agent.

PREOPERATIVE PREPARATION

One of the joys of treatment with injectables is the lack of special preoperative demands. In most women, the use of a local anesthetic alone is sufficient to accomplish the procedure. I have not used preoperative antibiotics. The procedure is done with the patient in the dorsal lithotomy position with the routine povidone-iodine preparation as performed for any routine cystoscopy.

RECOMMENDED PROCEDURE

Approaches

Regardless of the material chosen, injectables may be implanted transurethrally or periurethrally. The transurethral delivery systems are designed to advance the material through the working channel of the cystoscope and are used primarily in men. The needle is advanced under direct vision into the submucosal tissues of the urethra and the periurethra (Figure 7-2.1). In this manner the suburothelial bulking of the mucosa on either side, until closure in the midline occurs, may be observed (Figure 7-2.2). Regardless of the material chosen, this is the expected end point by observation. At the time of this writing, no substance has been approved by the United States Food and Drug Administration (FDA) for use in women. The primary materials currently used for injection are PTFE and glutaraldehyde cross-linked collagen (Contigen). Both appear to be efficacious. With respect to safety and ease of application, Contigen appears to have significant advantages over PTFE.

Materials

Polytetrafluoroethylene

Polytetrafluoroethylene is a paste consisting of (1) a sterile colloidal suspension of PTFE micropolymer particles, which range in size from 4 to 100 μm and are

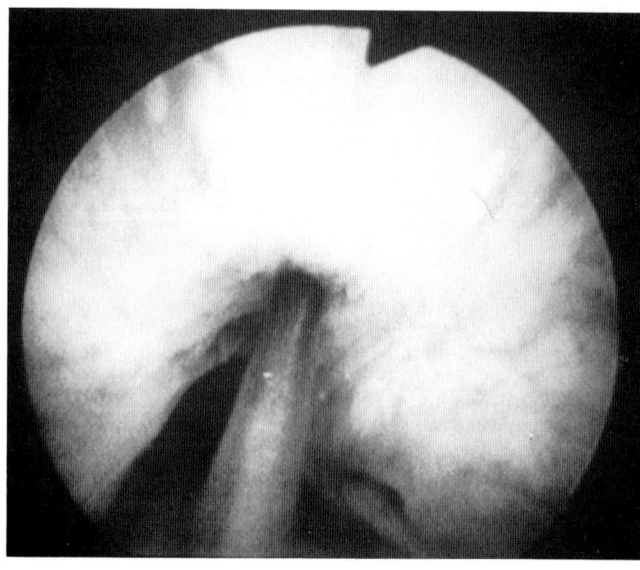

Figure 7-2.1 Endoscopic view of bladder neck during transurethral injection of Contigen.

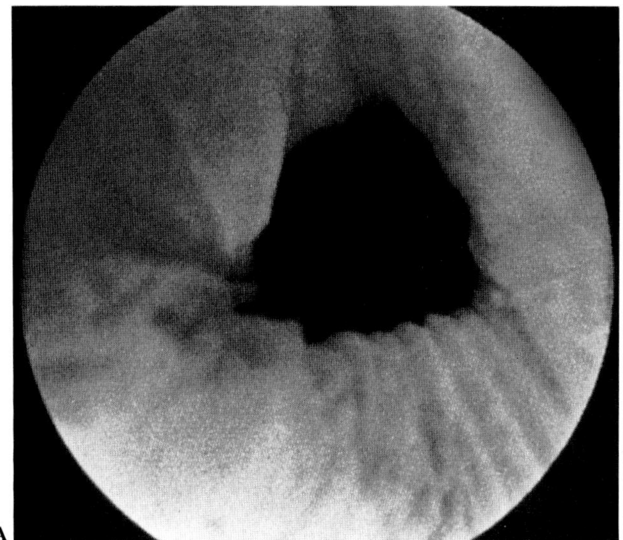

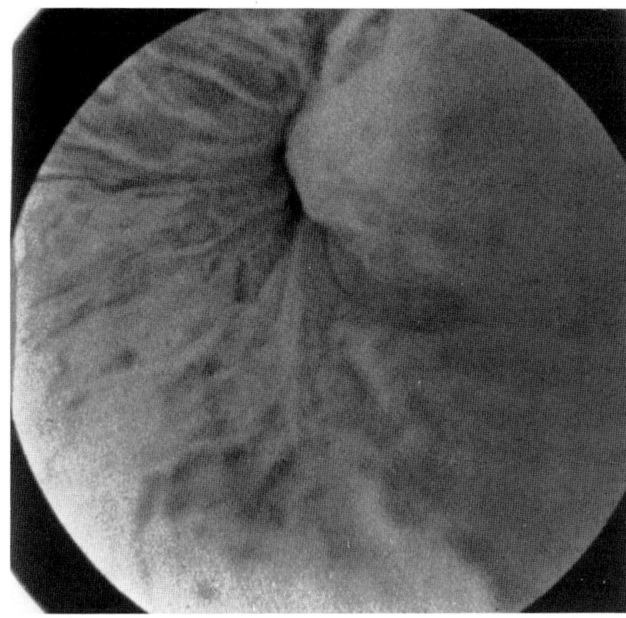

Figure 7-2.2 View of bladder neck before (**A**) and after (**B**) Contigen injection. *Source:* Reprinted with permission from *Problems in Urology* (1991;5:134), Copyright © 1991, JB Lippincott Company.

formed in irregular shapes; (2) glycerin; and (3) polysorbate. The paste is very thick and requires special instrumentation for its injection under pressure through a 16-gauge needle.

Two techniques are available. Special cystoscopic equipment allows for transurethral injections. Although this method may be more accurate in the initial placement of the material, it is difficult to prevent the paste from coming back into the urinary tract through the puncture sites. It is also difficult to wash the material out of the bladder. Additionally, the idea of violating the urinary tract in this manner is worrisome because of the potential to cause bleeding or urinary extravasation (or both). Periurethral injection (described later) can be used in women, and use of a local anesthetic is sufficient for comfort in most women. The Bruning's otolaryngologic injection device, which is similar to a caulking gun, is used to inject the PTFE. In most institutions it is readily available from colleagues in otolaryngology (Figure 7-2.3) because PTFE has FDA approval for use with several vocal cord problems. This technique requires an assistant to "pull the trigger" on the device because the surgeon must hold the cystoscope in one hand and stabilize the needle periurethrally with the other hand. Despite this drawback, this method seems far superior to transurethral methods.

Contigen

Contigen is a sterile, nonpyrogenic material composed of highly purified bovine dermal collagen that is cross-linked with glutaraldehyde and dispersed in phosphate-buffered physiologic saline. Like PTFE, Contigen can be injected transurethrally or periurethrally.

The transurethral delivery system is designed to be advanced through the working channel of a cystoscope (Figure 7-2.4). The needle of the delivery system is advanced into the urethral wall to facilitate injection of Contigen into the submucosal tissues. This delivery system consists of a beveled 20-gauge needle of approximately 1.5 cm attached to a thermoplastic catheter (5F). The Contigen is provided in a 3-mL Luer-Lok syringe that easily attaches to the long needle. Each syringe contains 2.5 mL of Contigen. In this manner, under

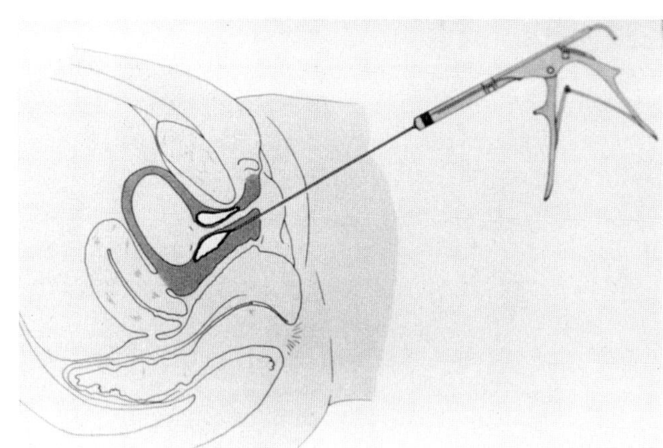

Figure 7-2.3 Periurethral injection of Urethrin with use of Bruning's injection device. *Source:* Reprinted from *Current Operative Urology* (pp 63–66) by ED Whitehead (editor) with permission of JB Lippincott Company, Copyright © 1990.

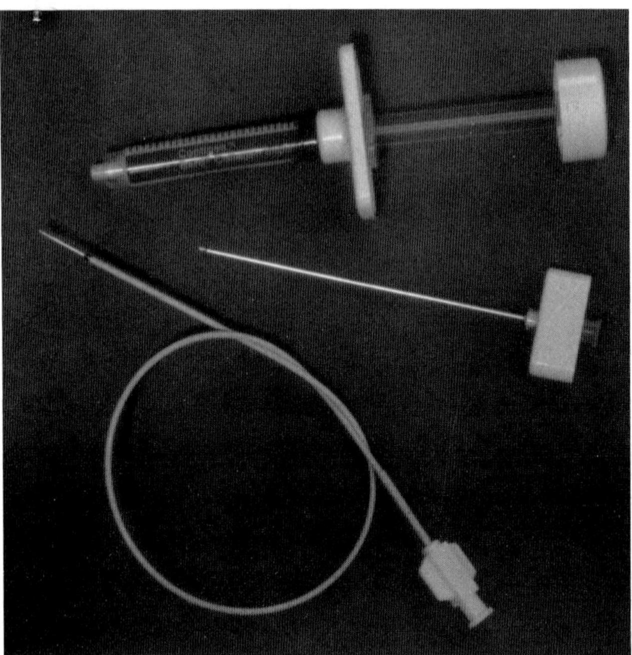

Figure 7-2.4 Injection delivery systems for Contigen.

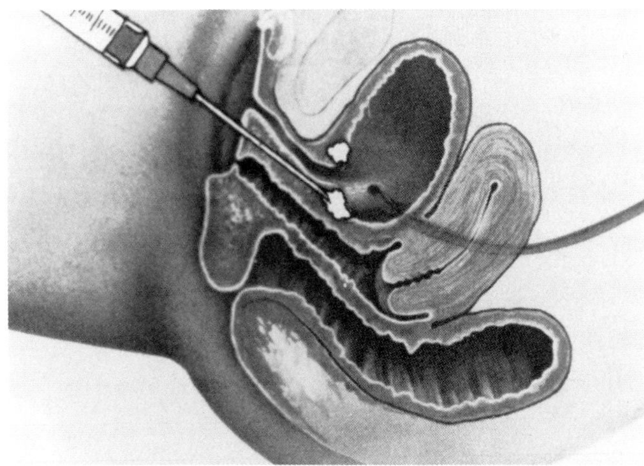

Figure 7-2.5 Periurethral Contigen injection procedure. *Source:* Reprinted with permission from *Problems in Urology* (1991;5:134), Copyright © 1991, JB Lippincott Company.

direct vision, Contigen is delivered suburothelially and one can observe the bulking of the surrounding mucosa on either side until it nearly closes in the midline (see Figure 7-2.2). As with PTFE, the possible complications of urethral bleeding and extrusion of the injectable substance are eliminated by using a periurethral rather than a transurethral approach, and the former technique is detailed below.

Technique

Preparation of the patient for the periurethral approach is identical regardless of whether PTFE (see Figure 7-2.3) or Contigen (Figure 7-2.5) is used. The introitus and the urethra are covered with 2% plain lidocaine jelly, and the anesthetic is left in place for 10 minutes before cystoscopy begins. At the 5- and 7-o'clock positions, 1% plain lidocaine is injected periurethrally up to a total of 2 mL on either side of the urethra. A 30-degree cystoscopic lens is commonly used, but I often find a 0-degree lens helpful. With Contigen, a 20- or 22-gauge spinal needle is placed periurethrally at approximately the 4-o'clock position with the bevel of the needle directed medially (ie, toward the urethral lumen). The needle is advanced slowly while the surgeon gazes through the cystoscope to notice the bulging of the tip of the needle against the lining of the urethra, so that proper positioning of the needle can be ascertained before the actual injection of Contigen. When this point is reached, the 3-mL syringe of Contigen is attached to the spinal needle. With one hand, the surgeon stabilizes the cystoscope for direct vision and, with the second hand, he or she injects the Contigen. One can actually see the material layering up outside the lining of the urethra and gradually pressing the lumen closed (Figure 7-2.5). At approximately the half way point, the needle is removed and placed in the 8-o'clock position on the opposite side, and the material is injected. Ultimately, the appearance (cystoscopically) of the posterior aspect of the urethra from the midurethra reveals what appears to be the two lateral lobes of a prostate gland "kissing" in the midline (see Figure 7-2.2). At this point, to confirm that the procedure is complete, the surgeon assists the patient to stand. The patient then performs a few provocative maneuvers in an attempt to cause urinary leakage. When both the patient and the physician are satisfied, the procedure is officially terminated. Obviously, use of a local anesthetic enables this evaluation and is one of the benefits to the success of the procedure.

An important technical point is that second injections may be necessary to accomplish total continence. This is related to the difficulty in determining the quantity of material needed for each patient. Injections may be safely repeated every 7 days to achieve total continence.

POSTOPERATIVE MANAGEMENT

An indwelling catheter is not used, so that "molding" of the collagen around the urethra does not occur. Difficulty in voiding, if present, is handled by using intermittent self-catheterization with no larger than a 14F catheter. Periurethral injection is an outpatient procedure. The patient is given oral antibiotics at the time of discharge and returns in 24 hours for evaluation, which includes determination of postvoid residual urine. Reinjections, if necessary, are scheduled appropriately.

EFFICACY AND SAFETY OF INJECTABLES IN FEMALE INCONTINENCE

Of the alternative treatments available for patients with urinary incontinence related to outlet incompetence (so-called type III stress incontinence), periurethral injections must be compared with slings and implantation of the artificial urinary sphincter. The purpose of any of these procedures is to render complete continence. Most women (and, therefore, most investigators), however, will accept a certain amount of urinary leakage. This ''social continence'' allows for urinary loss handled by the tissues or by the use of a minipad at most. If one also includes as ''cured'' those dry persons who must empty their bladder by using self-catheterization, results may appear astoundingly good. With the use of these criteria, sling surgery is successful in 81% to 98% of patients,[18] and sphincter surgery is successful in more than 90% of patients regardless of whether the abdominal[19] or the transvaginal[20] approach is used. Table 7-2.1 shows that injection with PTFE is successful in 70% to 95% of women,[17] and injection with Contigen is successful in 64% to 95% of women.[21] Because the results are comparable and therapy with injectables is less invasive than the open surgical procedures of slings and artificial sphincters, why have injectables not been universally accepted and performed? The answer involves two objectionable aspects: (1) the inability to quantify the amount of material needed in any given person and (2) the safety of the injectable substance.

With respect to the quantity of material needed for a patient, study findings with PTFE have demonstrated that the ability to judge the proper amount to render continence in a single treatment session varies between 50%[16] and 63%.[17] With Contigen, the results are similar, as continence was achieved in 55% of patients with a single treatment.[22] Once PTFE is injected it expands, whereas the bulk of Contigen is reduced as water (and local anesthetic) is resorbed. Thus urinary retention is more likely to occur after treatment with PTFE. In fact, all patients in one study[10] required intermittent self-catheterization after surgery, and, in the Louisiana State University series, 2 of 41 patients have had to use self-catheterization.[17] In the multicenter study with Contigen, only 1 of 149 women have had to use self-catheterization.[23] The total volume to achieve continence in these women injected with Contigen varied widely, from 2.5 mL to 85 mL, with 34 patients requiring less than 10 mL and 30 patients requiring greater than 30 mL.[23] An average of 2.2 injections and 19.2 mL of Contigen is necessary to attain continence.[21]

Table 7-2.1 Results of Studies with Polytetrafluoroethylene Injections in Women

Source	*No. of Patients*	*Percent Successful*
Berg[4]	3	100
Politano, Small, Harper, Lynne[6]	54	61
Politano[8]	51	71
Lim, Ball, Feneley[14]	28	53
Schulman, Simon, Wespes, Germeau[13]	56	86
Lewis, Lockhart, Politano[10]	6	100
Deane, English, Hehir, Williams, Worth[16]	28	61
Appell[17]	41	95

The second issue of safety explains the delay in approval of the use of PTFE and Contigen by the FDA. At the time of this writing, PTFE has been approved only for men with postprostatectomy incontinence (thus relegating its use to elderly men), and Contigen is still considered an investigational agent. The concerns regarding the safety of PTFE relate to particle migration[24] and granuloma formation.[25] Of course, granuloma formation signifies a chronic foreign-body reaction resulting long term in fibrosis and, possibly, carcinogenesis. Of even more importance is the fact that related polymers of PTFE have been shown to be carcinogenic in rats.[26] Despite these data, in the three-decade use of PTFE in the discipline of otolaryngology and in certain centers for urinary incontinence in the United States and Europe, there have been no reports of untoward sequelae in human beings. Also, the material may certainly be recommended for those women older than 60 years, especially since it has been approved for men in the same age category.

The concerns with the safety of Contigen are quite different from those described for PTFE. The fact that Contigen is biodegradable is both its strength and its weakness. There is no concern regarding migration and granuloma formation (as with PTFE), because Contigen begins to degrade in 12 weeks and is completely degraded in 9 to 19 months.[27] This brings to question the need for second injections later in patients rendered continent when the material degrades. Life-table analysis reveals that, once continence has been attained with

Contigen, greater than 80% of patients will not experience regression.[28]

Contigen does elicit a minimal inflammatory response (without granuloma formation), which enables replacement of the degraded bovine collagen with the patient's own collagen,[29] because there is transformation of the injected collagen into living connective tissue.[30]

The primary safety concern with Contigen is with respect to immunogenicity. Some patients who have undergone collagen injections for soft tissue augmentation have complained of symptoms, and demonstrated signs, of collagen-vascular disorders such as dermatomyositis. These complaints have resulted in litigation. Despite these claims, no evidence exists to link injection of bovine collagen with any disorder, because the patient population undergoing injection has, thus far, had a lower incidence of such disorders than would be expected in the general population.[31] The multicenter investigative study of Contigen includes skin testing to exclude any patients who may have an immunologic response. Results indicate that 5 of the first 333 patients have had a positive response to the skin test and, for this reason, were not injected periurethrally. In addition, all patients have been evaluated by using the enzyme-linked immunosorbent assay (ELISA) for humoral antibodies, and no significant anticollagen antibody responses have been found after implantation of Contigen. In fact, there appears to be a highly reduced potential to produce local immune-type reactions after collagen has been cross-linked with glutaraldehyde,[32] and none of the patients in the multicenter trials have had an adverse event related to immunogenicity. The only adverse events have been transient urinary retention in 5 patients and urinary tract infection in 12 patients and in the 1 patient apparently experiencing chronic urinary retention. Seventeen women have withdrawn from the study, but only 5 because of lack of improvement. Thus far, Contigen appears safe as well as efficacious.

CONCLUSION

The goal of treatment in women with bladder outflow incompetence related to an intrinsic defect in the continence mechanism is to compress the proximal aspect of the urethra, allowing coaptation without obstruction. In theory, this goal is best attained by using the artificial urinary sphincter, but the difficulty in the surgery in women who have had multiple failed operations has caused surgeons to search for alternative forms of management. Periurethral injections have the potential to accomplish this need. In addition, many of the patients for whom the above are indicated are unsuitable surgical candidates because of concomitant medical problems. Because therapy with injectables is less invasive than open surgery, a significant number of these patients can benefit from periurethral injection therapy because their therapeutic options are extremely limited.

The best results with periurethral injections are obtained in patients who do not have detrusor problems, who have adequate bladder capacity, and who have no anatomic abnormality. With respect to materials currently available, the injection procedure with Contigen has been easy to perform with the use of a local anesthetic and, thus far, appears free of significant complications. This procedure should be restricted to patients with clear-cut bladder outflow incompetence related to a defect in the intrinsic continence mechanism, because it will not be helpful in detrusor instability or urethral hypermobility (genuine stress incontinence).

REFERENCES

1. Murless BC. The injection treatment of stress incontinence. *J Obstet Gynaecol Br Emp*. 1938;45:67–73.
2. Quackels R. Deux incontinences après adenonectomie guéries par injection de paraffine dans le périnée. *Acta Urol Belg*. 1955; 23:259–262.
3. Sachse H. Treatment of urinary incontinence with sclerosing solutions: indications, results, complications. *Urol Int*. 1963;15: 225–244.
4. Berg S. Polytef augmentation urethroplasty: correction of surgically incurable urinary incontinence by injection technique. *Arch Surg*. 1973;107:379–381.
5. Politano VA, Small MP, Harper JM. Periurethral Teflon injection for urinary incontinence. In: *Transactions of the XVI Congrès de la Société Internationale d'Urologie, Amsterdam*. Paris: Diffusion Dion Editeurs; 1973:459.
6. Politano VA, Small MP, Harper JM, Lynne CM. Periurethral Teflon injection for urinary incontinence. *J Urol*. 1974;111:180–183.
7. Politano VA. Periurethral Teflon injection for urinary incontinence. *Urol Clin North Am*. 1978;5:415–422.
8. Politano VA. Periurethral polytetrafluoroethylene injection for urinary incontinence. *J Urol*. 1982;127:439–442.
9. Lockhart JL, Lewis RI, Politano VA. Urophysiology of persistent incontinence following periurethral Teflon injections. Read at annual meeting of American Urological Association (Abstract 469); May 1982; Kansas City, MO.
10. Lewis RI, Lockhart JL, Politano VA. Periurethral polytetrafluoroethylene injection in incontinent female subjects with neurogenic bladder disease. *J Urol*. 1984;131:459–462.
11. Heer H. Die Behandlung der Harninkontinenz mit der Teflonpaste. *Urol Int*. 1977;32:295–302.
12. Lampante L, Kaesler FP, Sparwasser H. Endourethrale submokose Tefloninjektion zur Erzielung von Harnkontinenz. *Aktuel Urol*. 1979;10:265–272.

13. Schulman CC, Simon J, Wespes E, Germeau F. Endoscopic injection of Teflon for female urinary incontinence. *Eur Urol.* 1983;9:246–247.

14. Lim KB, Ball AJ, Feneley RCL. Periurethral Teflon injection: a simple treatment for urinary incontinence. *Br J Urol.* 1983; 55:208–210.

15. Schulman CC, Simon J, Wespes E, Germeau F. Endoscopic injections of Teflon to treat urinary incontinence in women. *Br Med J.* 1984;288:192.

16. Deane AM, English P, Hehir M, Williams JP, Worth PHL. Teflon injection in stress incontinence. *Br J Urol.* 1985;57:78–80.

17. Appell RA. Commentary: periurethral polytetrafluoroethylene (Polytef) injection. In: Whitehead ED, ed. *Current Operative Urology 1990.* Philadelphia, Pa: JB Lippincott Co; 1990:63–66.

18. Blaivas JG. Treatment of female incontinence secondary to damage or loss. *Urol Clin North Am.* 1991;18:355–363.

19. Light JK, Scott FB. Management of urinary incontinence in women with the artificial urinary sphincter. *J Urol.* 1985; 134:476–478.

20. Appell RA. Techniques and results in the implantation of the artificial urinary sphincter in women with type III stress urinary incontinence by a vaginal approach. *Neurourol Urodyn.* 1988; 7:613–619.

21. Appell RA. Injectables for urethral incompetence. *World J Urol.* 1990;8:208–211.

22. Appell RA. New developments: injectables for urethral incompetence in women. *Int Urogynecol J.* 1990;1:117–119.

23. Appell RA, McGuire EJ, DeRidder PA, Bennett AH, Webster GD. Results of the multicenter study using injectable GAX-Collagen in females. Presented at 86th annual meeting of American Urological Association; June 1991; Toronto.

24. Malizia AA Jr, Reiman HM, Myers RP, et al. Migration and granulomatous reaction after periurethral injection of Polytef (Teflon). *JAMA.* 1984;251:3277–3281.

25. Mittleman RE, Marracini JV. Pulmonary Teflon granulomas following periurethral Teflon injection for urinary incontinence. *Arch Pathol Lab Med.* 1983;107:611–612.

26. Oppenheimer BS, Oppenheimer ET, Stout AP. The latent period in carcinogenesis by plastic in rats and its relation to the presarcomatous stage. *Cancer.* 1958;11:204–213.

27. Leonard MP, Canning DA, Epstein JI, Gearhart JP, Jeffs RD. Local tissue reaction to the subureteric injection of glutaraldehyde cross-linked bovine collagen in humans. *J Urol.* 1990;143: 1209–1212.

28. Bard CR. Premarket approval application submission to US Food and Drug Administration for Investigational Device Exemption # G850010, 1990.

29. Ford CN, Martin DW, Warren TF. Injectable collagen in laryngeal rehabilitation. *Laryngoscope.* 1984;95:513–518.

30. Remacle M, Marbaix E. Collagen implants in the human larynx. *Arch Otorhinolaryngol.* 1988;245:203–209.

31. Lyon MG, Bloch DA, Hollak B, Fries JF. Predisposing factors in polymyositis-dermatomyositis: results of a nationwide survey. *J Rheumatol.* 1989;16:1218–1224.

32. Griffiths R, Shakespeare P. Human dermal collagen allografts: a three year histological study. *Br J Plast Surg.* 1982; 35:519–523.

7-3

Implantation of Artificial Urinary Sphincters

Rodney A. Appell

In cases of urinary incontinence, one of the treatment goals is to establish a normal voiding pattern while allowing the patient to become dry between voidings. When incontinence is due to bladder outlet incompetence (sphincteric incontinence), procedures (eg, slings, injectables) are designed to close the outflow channel. Although this may result in the prevention of urinary leakage, these procedures may lead to an obstructive voiding pattern. Only implantation of an artificial urinary sphincter allows for the obstruction to be relieved at the time of voiding, so that the actual voiding pattern is normalized and the desired state of dryness is accomplished.

HISTORICAL REVIEW

Various models of the artificial urinary sphincter have been produced by American Medical Systems Inc. All models have a reservoir placed intra-abdominally to equalize the pressure of stress. Each model has been designed to open partially when bladder pressures exceed physiologic limits; to open fully when activated; to accept the passage of a catheter without the necessity of operating the device; and, if failure should occur, to fail in the open position. In June 1972, F. Brantley Scott, MD, of Baylor University in Houston, Texas, implanted the first artificial sphincter in a 45-year-old woman. The current device (AMS Sphincter 800) is the result of a steady evolution of design improvements (Figure 7-3.1). The rationale for each innovation improves understanding of the features of the current device.

The first hydraulic device implanted in 1972 (model AS721) consisted of a set of valves that controlled the direction of fluid flow within the system, as well as the pressure on the urethra and bladder neck by means of the cuff placed around it.[1] Placement of the fluid reservoir within the abdomen offset any stress pressures. In this way the pressure compressing the urethra could be set low enough to prevent pressure necrosis. There were separate inflation and deflation pumps, and the device was constructed of Dacron-reinforced silicone rubber. The most significant change was the use of a pressure-regulating balloon to control the pressure applied to the urethra, rather than to the valves as in the AS721. In this AS742, for the first time the cuff automatically refilled with fluid because of this active pressure in the balloon. This meant that the inflation pump could be eliminated. Thus the device became semiautomatic. Not only was the pump small enough to be used in women, the device had fewer components, thus making the surgical procedure more simple and the incidence of mechanical problems less.

The next significant change was the use of a dip-coated all-silicone rubber cuff rather than the Dacron-reinforced cuff. This change increased efficiency and

AMS Sphincter 800—
1983 to Present
The control pump combines two valves, one resistor, and a deactivation button. A surface-treated cuff helps prevent wear. Kink-resistant and color-coded tubing has also been added.

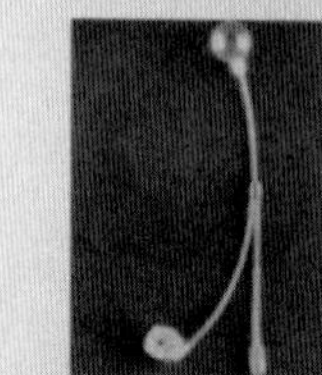

AS791/792—1979 to 1983
The control assembly which combined the valves and resistor resulted in a simpler surgery with fewer connections.

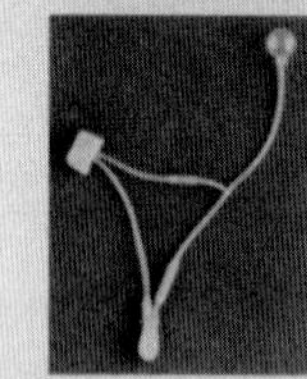

AS742—1974 to 1979
The cuff automatically refilled with fluid because of the active pressure in the regulating balloon. This was the first automatic cuff closure prosthesis.

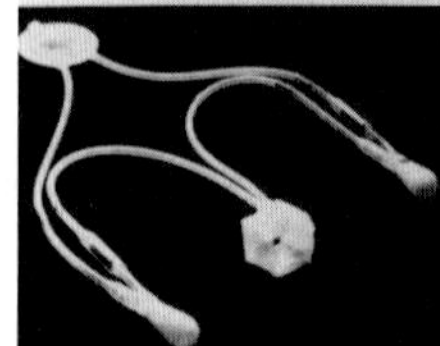

AS721—1972 to 1979
The first AMS prosthesis ever implanted in a patient. The pressure present in the cuff was mechanically regulated by valves and the separate inflation and deflation pumps.

Figure 7-3.1 Evolution of artificial urinary sphincter. *Source*: Courtesy of American Medical Systems, Inc, Minnetonka, MN.

reliability of the cuff because of increased resiliency. In addition, in this model (AS791/792) the valves and resistors were miniaturized into a single control assembly constructed of stainless steel. The fewer components (balloon, pump, cuff, and control assembly) had to be located properly at surgery to ensure function. The balloon was placed intra-abdominally beside the bladder to equalize the pressures of stress. The subcutaneous portion of the pump inside the labium allowed the patient to trap and squeeze it. The cuff surrounded the bladder neck and the posterior segment of the urethra (AS792) while the control assembly rested subcutaneously immediately adjacent to the external inguinal ring. This arrangement made the control assembly easily accessible if the need for subsequent surgical revision were to arise because the three posts of the control assembly connected the tubing from the balloon, the pump, and the cuff. The balloon controlled the pressure rendered against the urethra by the cuff, and the thickness of the wall of the balloon determined the pressure of any given balloon. Thus the pressure applied to the urethra depended on the choice made by the surgeon from a selection of balloons. The optimum pressure should, of course, close the urethra but cannot exceed the diastolic blood pressure to prevent pressure necrosis of the urethra. A radiopaque and isotonic solution filled the prosthesis because the balloon, pump, cuff, and tubing were constructed of silicone rubber, which is semipermeable. Finally, because the stress pressures were transmitted onto the bladder, the balloon, and the cuff, there was no fluid transfer inside the system with stress. Instead, an actual unstable bladder contraction of an amplitude that exceeded that of the pressure-regulating balloon would push fluid from the cuff into the balloon, resulting in urinary loss. Although automatic closure was an advantage for patients in managing the device, it created several limiting and potentially complicated problems related to the disadvantage that pressure was automatically applied even when inappropriate:

1. Pressure was placed on the bladder neck and the urethra immediately at the time of implantation without regard to tissue quality, as in patients who had undergone previous surgery or radiation treatments. In these patients the risk of tissue ischemia and ultimate cuff erosion was increased.
2. The need to activate the pump multiple times a day was problematic because the patient's labium was still tender and swollen during the early postoperative period, causing the patient considerable discomfort.
3. Prolonged need for catheterization related to tissue swelling predisposed patients to cuff erosion because the tissues were compressed between the cuff and the catheter.
4. Many patients did not need urethral compression when they were sleeping and required the compression only during activities in which they were in an upright position. Because the device could not be deactivated, the urethral and bladder neck tissue were exposed to unnecessary deterioration.

These considerations led to the concept of delaying activation or primary deactivation.[2] With the AS791/792 the concept entailed implantation of the balloon, the pump, and the cuff during one operation followed in 60 to 90 days by a second procedure to insert the control assembly and activate the device. An obvious improvement, therefore, would be a device that the surgeon could both activate and deactivate by means of external manipulation. This deactivation feature, which allows the function of the device to be suspended nonsurgically, was introduced as the AMS Sphincter 800 in 1982. It was improved in 1984 by coating the silicone rubber cuff with Teflon, which causes the silicone rubber to be 21 times more resistant to wear than silicone rubber alone.

The AMS Sphincter 800 is the artificial urinary sphincter currently in use and consists of an inflatable cuff, a pressure-regulating balloon, and a pump. The valve, the refill-delay resistor, and the deactivation button are incorporated into the pump. Squeezing the button on the pump moves a poppet valve into a locked position to prevent fluid transfer until activation by a sharp squeeze on the pump, which releases the poppet. Kink-resistant, color-coded tubing has been added recently to enhance surgical implantation and decrease mechanical failure. Faulty patient selection or surgical technique (or both) have now replaced mechanical problems as the most common cause of device failure.

PATIENT SELECTION

The AMS Sphincter 800 is most suitable for patients with pure sphincter incompetency and normal detrusor function. Patients with decreased detrusor contractility, however, may be candidates if intermittent self-catheterization can be considered. The diagnosis of urethral incompetence and the status of the detrusor are determined with the use of urodynamic studies or fluoroscopic studies (or both). The success of the artificial sphincter in attaining continence is definitely influenced by the presence of any bladder disease. The use of the device in the patient with a normal bladder or poor detrusor contractility with unaltered compliance is consistently associated with a high degree of success. Detrusor hyperreflexia, if found urodynamically, must be controlled before implantation of the device. Adequate bladder capacity (greater than 125 mL) is essential, but residual urine is not a factor. Endoscopic evaluation to determine that viable tissue is present at the prospective cuff site is mandatory and also helpful in determining the proximity of the ureteral orifices to the bladder neck and the posterior segment of the urethra. As mentioned, careful urodynamic evaluation is essential to establish the bladder response to filling. The combination of leak point pressure and voiding pressure helps to determine the pressure-regulating balloon to be chosen for an individual patient because this balloon determines the closing pressure with the cuff inflated or deflated. A pressure difference of 40 centimeters of water (cm H_2O) usually achieves continence. This endoscopic and urodynamic evaluation of the lower urinary tract is of major importance in ensuring an optimal outcome. The only pure contraindications to implanting the AMS Sphincter 800 are uncontrolled detrusor hyperreflexia and high-grade vesicoureteral reflux.

It is not sufficient to state that patients who have an incompetent urethra are therefore natural candidates for the artificial sphincter. They must also have adequate manual dexterity, mental capacity, and motivation to manipulate the pump mechanism each time they need to urinate.

PREOPERATIVE PREPARATION

Preoperative preparation is directed at reducing the chance of infection. Because the device is inserted into a closed space, the procedure can introduce organisms into that particular location. If there is infection after surgery, the entire device may have to be removed. Because of tissue viability, the operative site may not be as accessible to natural defense mechanisms and circulating antimicrobials. Therefore the device and the instruments are soaked in antimicrobials, the wound is sprayed with them, and the proper antimicrobial level is achieved in all tissues before surgery. Also, because a foreign body is being implanted, the urine must be sterile at the time of surgery. The drug, the route of administration, and the length of coverage to accomplish this are a matter of individual choice, although both aerobic and anaerobic coverage is important. Preoperative shaving and preparation are done at the time of surgery, rather than the previous night, to reduce the buildup of surface microbes.

It is advantageous to know whether the patient is right or left handed because it is much easier for the patient to operate a pump if it is placed according to her handedness.

RECOMMENDED TECHNIQUE

The AMS Sphincter 800 has four components: a pump mechanism, a cuff that encircles the bladder neck or the urethra (or both), a pressure-regulating balloon, and tubing connectors. Only a small number of women have been implanted with the device because of the fear of many surgeons regarding the difficulty in placement of the cuff around the bladder neck. The so-called urethrovaginal septum is not a true surgical plane, and this is especially challenging in women with type III stress urinary incontinence, because their urethral incompetence may occur after multiple surgical repairs for genuine stress incontinence (Figure 7-3.2). Even

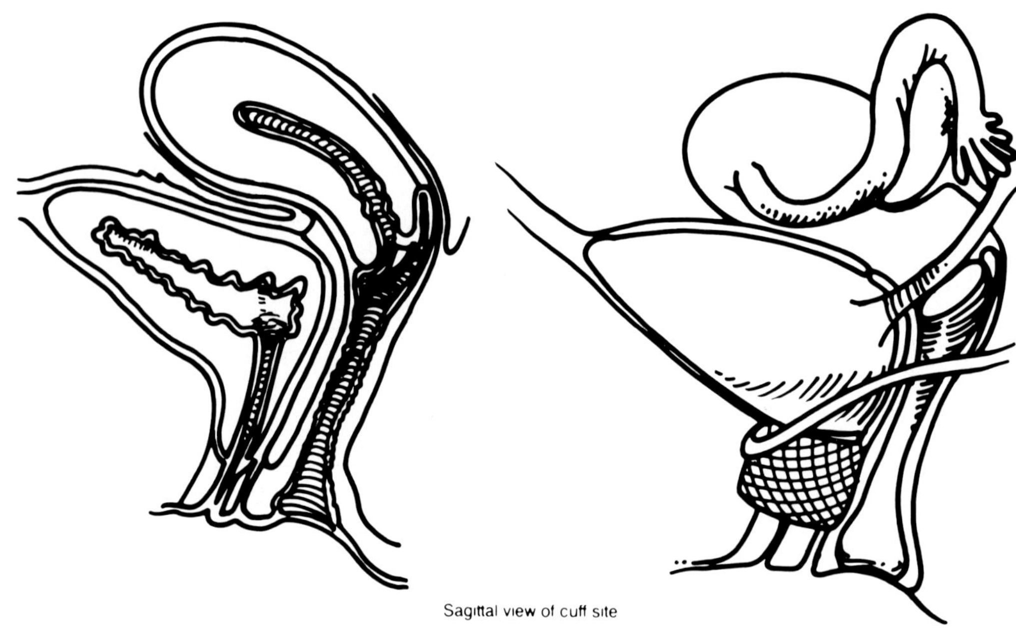

Figure 7-3.2 Cuff site in urethrovaginal septum. *Source*: Courtesy of American Medical Systems, Inc, Minnetonka, MN.

partial injury to these tissues can lead to failure related to infection or erosion of the cuff into the urethra or the vagina.

Cuff placement may be approached by means of an abdominal or a transvaginal fashion. Before describing the two approaches it is important to recognize a few general precautions that are important regardless of approach. Excessive handling of the device should be avoided. Silicone-shod hemostats are used for cross-clamping the tubing, which will prevent damage to the tubing and a potential leak. Blood must not enter the tubing because it will block the one-way valves in the pump assembly and result in device malfunction. Liberal irrigation is performed during all connections to prevent this problem. Finally, to reiterate, antibiotic spray is used liberally throughout the procedure to prevent infection.

After general or epidural anesthesia is accomplished, the patient is placed in a modified dorsal lithotomy position with her thighs abducted but minimally flexed toward the abdomen. This position is used because the surgical approach for both abdominal and transvaginal procedures requires the ability for intraoperative cystourethroscopy.

Abdominal Approach

A low transverse incision in which the rectus muscles are transected at their insertion (Cherney incision) is important for good exposure of the retropubic space. Palpation of the balloon from a Foley (16F) catheter allows identification of the bladder neck area. After the endopelvic fascia is opened adjacent to the bladder neck on each side, palpation of this catheter helps to localize the area to be dissected (Figure 7-3.3). One should not hesitate to open the bladder to see the inside as well as the outside of the bladder neck. The proper site for the cuff is

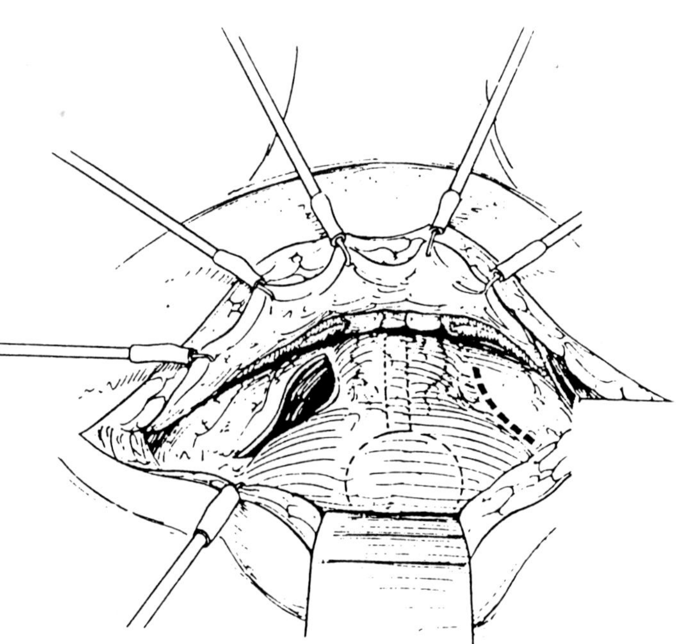

Figure 7-3.3 Anatomy of retropubic space demonstrating location of Foley catheter balloon, bladder neck, and incision of endopelvic fascia with exposure obtained by using Cherney incision. *Source*: Reprinted with permission from *Neurourology and Urodynamics* (1988;7:603), Copyright © 1988, Alan R Liss, Inc.

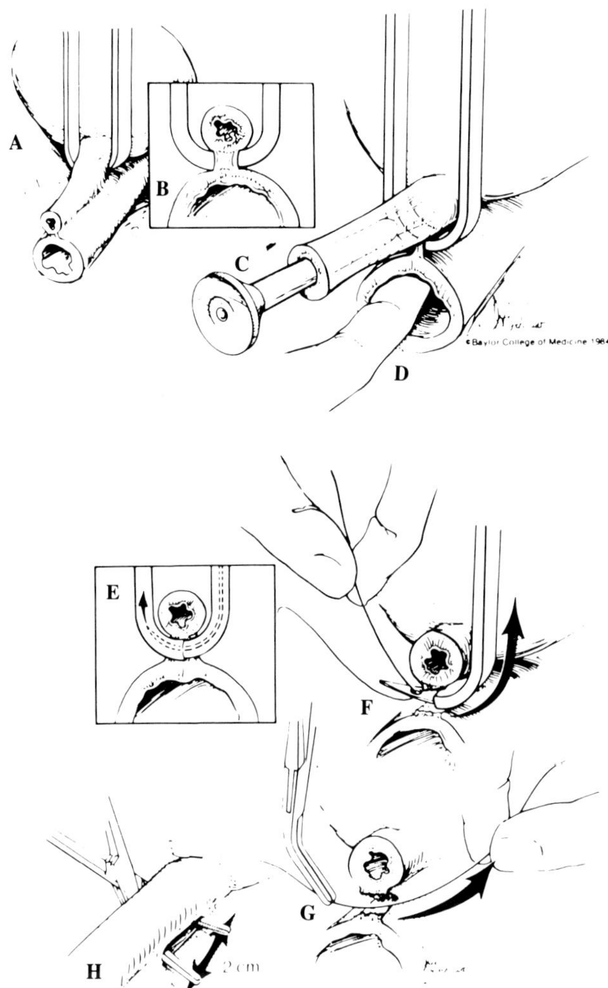

Figure 7-3.4 "Cutter clamp" pinches and holds secure the tissues for identification before it cuts (**A,B**). Cystoscopy then shows that urethra is clear (**C,D**). Cutting blade is advanced into opposite limb of device (**E**). Instrument is dismantled to expose cutting blade, which contains eye for receiving suture (**F**). Instrument is withdrawn with suture remaining in place for guidance of large right-angled clamp to dilate passage 2 cm, sufficient for cuff placement (**G,H**). *Source*: Courtesy of Baylor College of Medicine, Copyright © 1984.

inferior to the ureteral orifices and anterior to the vagina. Blunt dissection to expose the lateral margins of the bladder neck and a combination of blunt and sharp dissection to create a posterior passage are performed. The Cutter clamp (Figure 7-3.4) is extremely helpful because it is used to pinch the tissues that are to be cut. It provides a means of checking placement, cutting the tissue, and providing the passage of a suture to guide instruments for dilation and creation of the passage around the bladder neck. A large right-angled clamp is placed through this tunnel and spread to accommodate the 2-cm wide cuff. Injury to the urethra, the bladder, or the vagina may be determined by filling the wound with antibiotic solution, filling the urethra and the bladder with air through the urethral catheter, and observing for

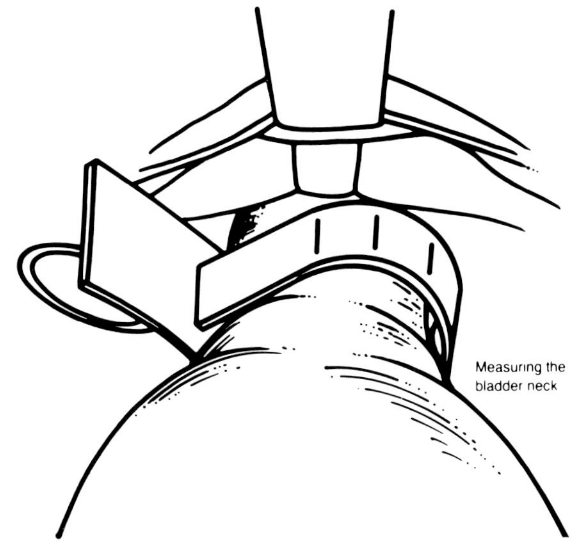

Figure 7-3.5 Flexible cuff sizer placed around bladder neck. *Source*: Courtesy of American Medical Systems, Inc, Minnetonka, MN.

bubbles. Should injury inadvertently occur, the perforation should be repaired before continuing.

Next, the flexible cuff sizer is placed around the bladder neck to measure the circumference (Figure 7-3.5). The cuff should be snug, touching the surface of the bladder neck, and not obstructive. The adult female bladder neck generally requires a 7- to 9-cm cuff. Cystoscopy is recommended at this point to ensure the integrity of the bladder neck and the urethra. Once the cuff size is selected, the surgeon slides the end of a clamp through the passage created for the cuff and pulls the cuff into position, finally threading the tubing through the adaptor hole and snapping it in position (Figure 7-3.6). (See also Figure 7-3.5.) An area is then bluntly dissected on one side of the prevesical space for placement of the pressure-regulating balloon (Figure 7-3.7).

The pressure-regulating balloon should lie in the submuscular extraperitoneal space. Several balloon pressures are available (range, 51 to 90 cm H_2O), and the closing pressure of the cuff depends on this balloon pressure. A pressure just surpassing the active leak point pressure is useful in determining which pressure-regulating balloon to use, because the least amount of pressure that is capable of preventing leakage in the individual patient is desired. Of course, as stated earlier, erosion will occur if the cuff pressure exceeds the diastolic blood pressure. Once the balloon is selected, it is filled with 22 mL of the recommended isotonic fluid and positioned. A radiopaque contrast medium is frequently added for convenience to visualize the components in the postoperative period. (Information regarding the makeup of this contrast fluid is provided by the manufacturer.)

A temporary connection is made between the pressure-regulating balloon and the cuff allowing the cuff to "charge," that is, to be pressurized to its equilibrium state. This connection is then taken down and the balloon aspirated and refilled with 20 mL of the recommended fluid. A tunnel is created into the labia for insertion of the pump mechanism into a superficial, yet dependent, position (Figure 7-3.8). All tubing is routed from the cuff and the balloon to a subcutaneous inguinal position and checked to confirm that there are no kinks present. Connections are then completed between the pump and the cuff and between the pump and the pressure-regulating balloon (Figure 7-3.9).

A functional check of the prosthesis is performed by cycling the device with cystoscopic control. At the conclusion, the prosthesis is deactivated by squeezing the control pump to deflate the cuff completely and allowing the pump to refill partially for 10 seconds before pressing the deactivation button (Figure 7-3.10). A 14F urethral catheter is inserted, and the wound is closed in standard fashion. Care is taken by the surgeon to visualize the prosthetic components during the first layer of closure to prevent inadvertent puncture. Hemostasis is exceedingly important because no drains are used.

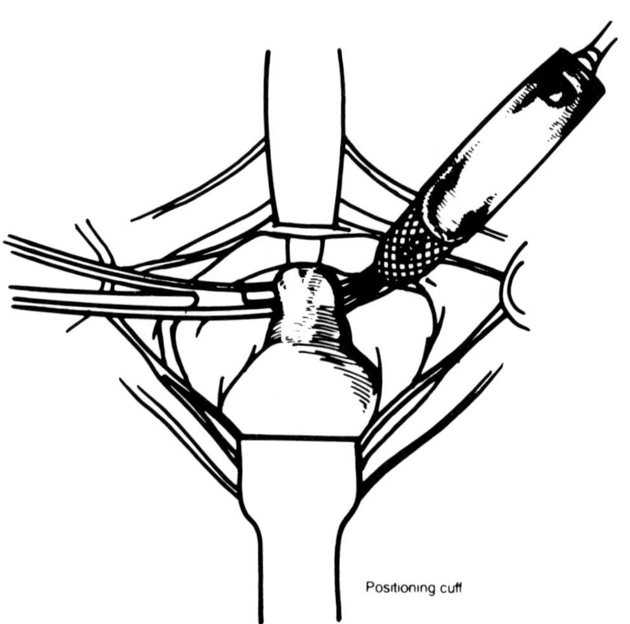

Figure 7-3.6 Positioning the cuff. *Source*: Courtesy of American Medical Systems, Inc, Minnetonka, MN.

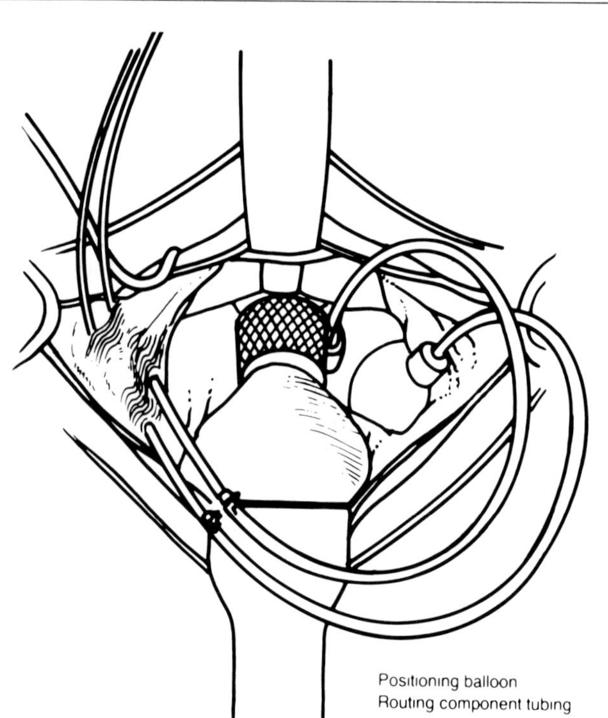

Figure 7-3.7 Positioning of pressure-regulating balloon and transfer of tubing to subcutaneous portion of abdominal incision. *Source*: Courtesy of American Medical Systems, Inc, Minnetonka, MN.

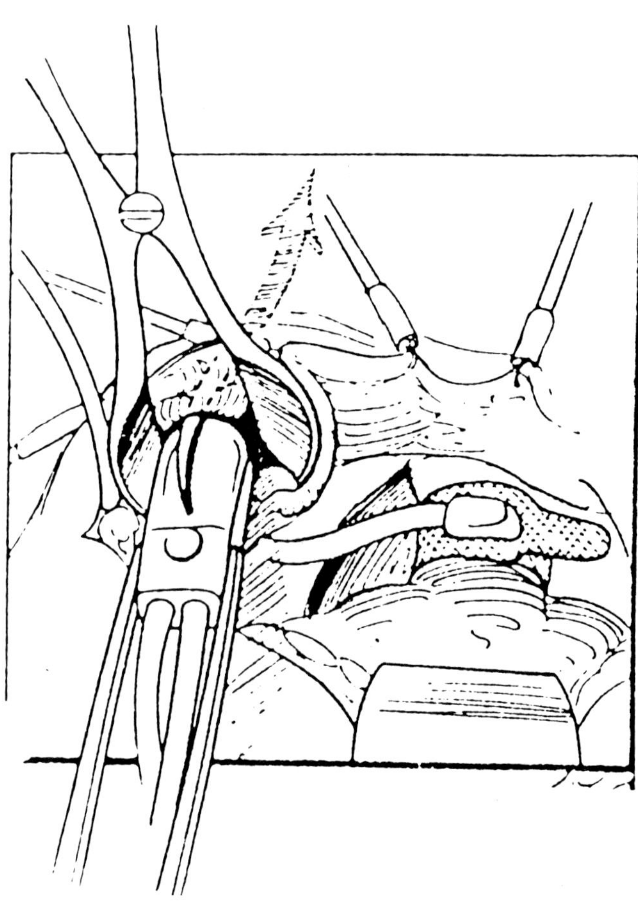

Figure 7-3.8 Implantation of pump into labium. *Source*: Reprinted with permission from *Neurourology and Urodynamics* (1988;7:603), Copyright © 1987, Alan R Liss, Inc.

Transvaginal Approach

Because of (1) difficulties in preventing injury to the urethra and the bladder neck with the abdominal approach, and (2) availability of successful alternative procedures such as the pubovaginal sling (even when the sling is made of synthetic material and placed by means of a combined abdominal-vaginal approach), a vaginal approach to cuff placement may also be considered for implantation of the AMS Sphincter 800. The patient is positioned as previously described for the abdominal approach. A posterior-weighted vaginal retractor is inserted, and the labia are sutured to the skin laterally for additional retraction to expose the anterior wall of the vagina. The urethral catheter is placed, and an inverted "U" incision (Figure 7-3.11) through the anterior wall of the vagina allows the vaginal dissection to be lateral to the urethra and the bladder neck.

The retropubic space is entered between the pubic bone and the endopelvic fascia to mobilize the urethra and the bladder neck sharply and bluntly. The endopelvic fascia is freed from its lateral attachments to the pubic bone and, in this way, bleeding is minimized and bladder or ureteral injury is very unlikely. Mobilization is extended down to the level of the ischial tuberosity by sharply dissecting the periurethral scar tissue from any previous surgical endeavors.

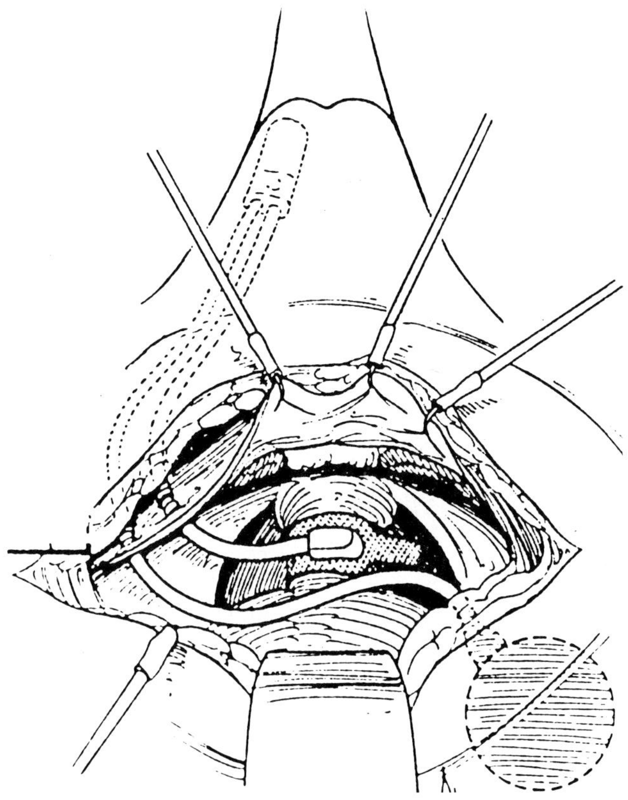

Figure 7-3.9 AMS Sphincter 800 in position. *Source*: Reprinted with permission from *Neurourology and Urodynamics* (1988;7:603), Copyright © 1988, Alan R Liss, Inc.

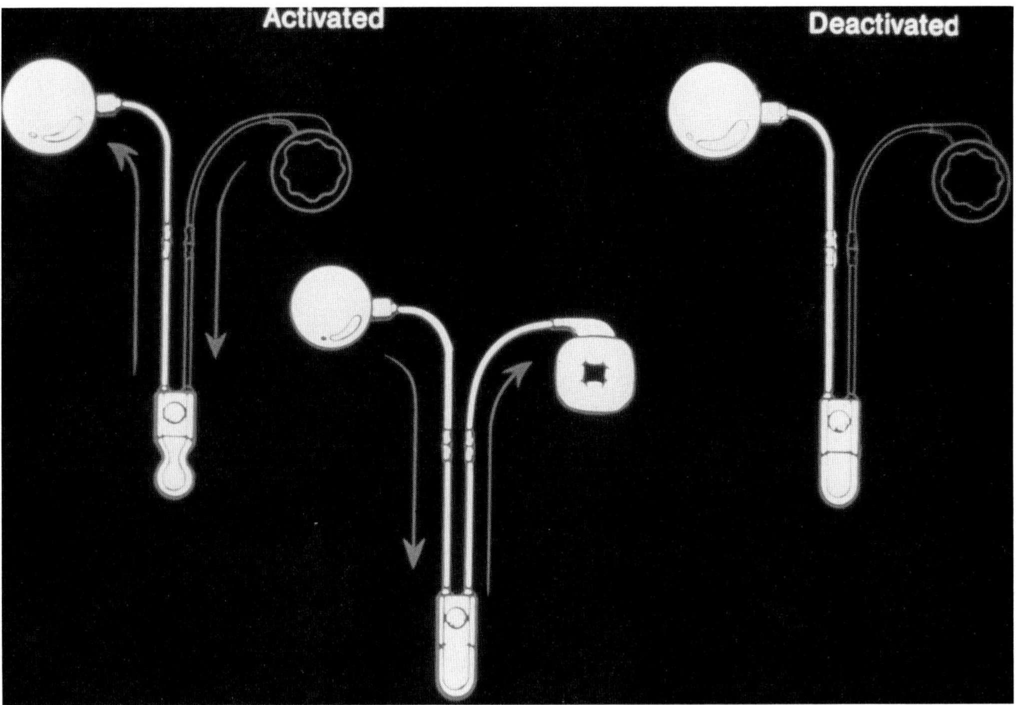

Figure 7-3.10 Primary deactivation. *Source*: Courtesy of American Medical Systems, Inc, Minnetonka, MN.

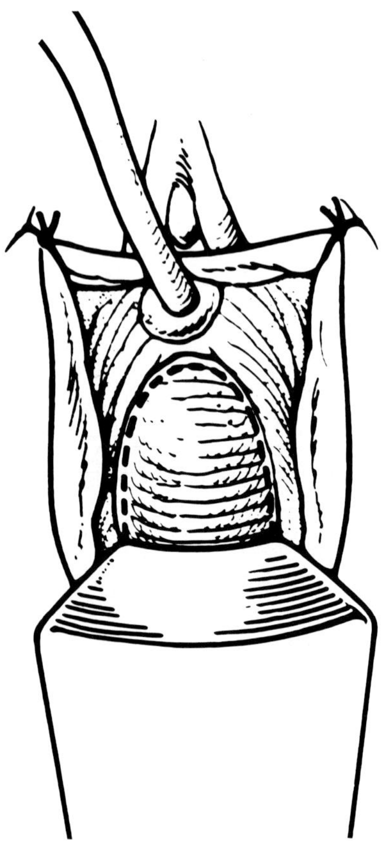

Figure 7-3.11 Inverted "U" incision in anterior wall of vagina. *Source*: Reprinted with permission from *Neurourology and Urodynamics* (1988; 7:613), Copyright © 1988, Alan R Liss, Inc.

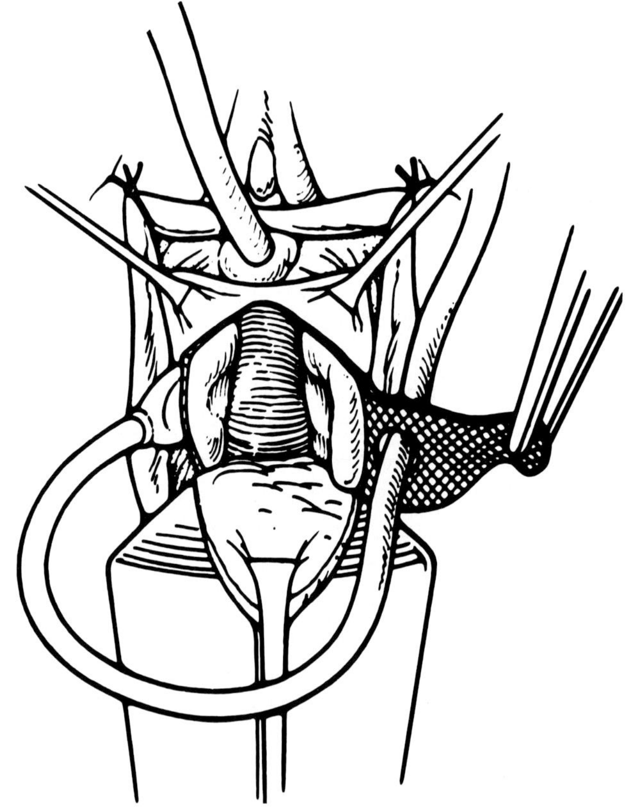

Figure 7-3.12 Passage of cuff through incision in anterior wall of vagina circumferentially around bladder neck and posterior segment of urethra. *Source*: Reprinted with permission from *Neurourology and Urodynamics* (1988;7:613), Copyright © 1988, Alan R Liss, Inc.

After the retropubic space is entered, the bladder neck and the urethra are mobilized completely from the pubic bone. Once this mobilization is complete the catheter is removed, and the calibrated cuff sizer is passed around the bladder neck to determine the size of cuff needed. This passage is facilitated by passing a curved renal pedicle clamp around the bladder neck to grasp the cuff sizer, which is then replaced with the proper-sized cuff (Figure 7-3.12). Cystourethroscopy is performed to confirm proper placement of the cuff inferior to the ureteral orifices.

At this point, attention is paid to the lower abdomen, and a small transverse lower abdominal incision is made very close to the pubis. The tubing from the cuff is passed lateral to the bladder into the abdominal incision either by using a tonsil clamp or by passing a blunt tubing-transfer needle from the abdominal wound into the vaginal wound, much the same as one would pass the needle carrier in a Pereyra-type bladder suspension. The pressure-regulating balloon and the pump are implanted through the abdominal wound, and all tubing from the three components is passed to the subcutaneous inguinal space. Filling of the system and completion of the connections are accomplished just as described in the abdominal approach.

The abdominal incision is closed in the usual fashion. The vaginal incision is closed with 2-0 absorbable suture, and a vaginal gauze pack coated with conjugated estrogen cream is left in place for 24 hours. If the integrity of the vaginal wall appears compromised, interposition of a Martius fat pad graft (from the labium not containing the pump) may be considered.

POSTOPERATIVE CARE

The urethral catheter and vaginal pack are removed on the first postoperative day. The patient receives antibiotics for 1 week, and the device is left deactivated for 6 to 12 weeks. During this period, the collateral circulation should be re-established, allowing primary healing of tissues at the cuff site. This has the added benefit of eliminating immediate postoperative pump manipulation, an inherent discomfort for the patient in this early period.

THERAPEUTIC RESULTS

The results of both the abdominal approach[3–6] and the transvaginal approach[7–9] have been excellent with greater than 90% of patients being socially continent. This is not to say that there have not been problems requiring surgical revision. Long-term results, however, have been excellent with a minimum of infection and erosion. The success is attributed to appropriate patient selection, judicious use of antibiotics, and primary deactivation. I believe that the vaginal approach facilitates cuff placement while protecting the urinary organs. Thus far, it has demonstrated no increase in infection or erosion as compared to the abdominal approach.[6,9]

CONCLUSION

The AMS Sphincter 800 provides continence in patients who fail to store urine because of an incompetent bladder outlet. It does so, in most patients, without pressure necrosis or fibrotic contraction of the bladder neck or posterior segments of the urethra (or both). The device is intended to permit intermittent urethral compression. Thus the patient can reduce urethral resistance voluntarily during voiding, as opposed to other compressive procedures in which the patient is voiding against a relative obstruction. Only a small number of women have received the device primarily because of concerns about technical difficulties encountered during the crucial part of the operation—namely, creating the space for the cuff between the bladder neck and the vagina. The results with transvaginal placement of the cuff have been most gratifying because they have been better than those of other series in which the entire procedure was approached retropubically.[6,9] With the use of either surgical technique the AMS Sphincter 800 offers a viable option in the management of bladder outlet incompetence in women because it is safe and effective.

REFERENCES

1. Scott FB, Bradley WE, Timm GW. Treatment of urinary incontinence by an implantable prosthetic sphincter. *Urology*. 1973; 1:252–259.
2. Furlow WL. Implantation of new semiautomatic artificial genitourinary sphincter: experience with primary activation and deactivation in 47 patients. *J Urol*. 1981;126:741–744.
3. Light JK, Scott FB. Management of urinary incontinence in women with the artificial urinary sphincter. *J Urol*. 1985;134: 476–478.
4. Donovan MG, Barrett DM, Furlow WL. Use of artificial urinary sphincter in the management of severe incontinence in females. *Surg Gynecol Obstet*. 1985;161:17–20.
5. Diokno AC, Hollander JB, Alderson TP. Artificial urinary sphincter for recurrent female urinary incontinence: indications and results. *J Urol*. 1987;137:778–780.
6. Parulkar BC, Barrett DM. Application of the AS-800 artificial sphincter for intractable urinary incontinence in females. *Surg Gynecol Obstet*. 1990;171:131–138.
7. Appell RA. Techniques and results in the implantation of the artificial urinary sphincter in women with type III stress urinary incontinence by vaginal approach. *Neurourol Urodyn*. 1988; 7:613–619.
8. Abbassian A. A new operation for insertion of the artificial urinary sphincter. *J Urol*. 1988;140:512–513.
9. Hadley HR. The artificial sphincter in the female. *Problems in Urology*. 1991;5:123–133.

8

Urethral Abnormalities

W. Glenn Hurt

There are three conditions involving the urethra which if symptomatic may require medical or surgical therapy: urethral diverticulum, urethral prolapse, and urethral caruncle.

URETHRAL DIVERTICULUM

The first published report on the treatment of a urethral diverticulum in women was by William Hey in 1805.[1] In his treatise, ''Of Collections of Pus in the Vagina,'' he stated that he had operated on a woman for a urethral diverticulum at The General Infirmary of Leeds (England) in 1786. He cured her by incising the overlying vagina and packing the cavity with lint. There were only a few subsequent reports on urethral diverticula in women until the middle of this century when physician awareness and improved diagnostic techniques increased its identification as a cause of lower urinary tract symptoms.

Incidence

Urethral diverticula occur rarely in infants and children but are estimated to occur in 4% to 5% of women who are 30 to 50 years of age.[2–4] The condition is more common in those who are parous and is diagnosed more frequently in those who are black. Urethral diverticula are often asymptomatic; their mere presence does not necessarily imply the need for surgery.

Causes

Urethral diverticula may be congenital or acquired. Despite a few well-documented cases of congenital urethral diverticula in newborns[5] and children, this is a rare occurrence. Congenital urethral diverticula can arise from cloacogenic cell rests, the faulty union of primordial folds, remnants of Gartner's ducts, vaginal wall cysts of müllerian origin, or dilation of paraurethral (Skene's) cysts. In each case, the wall would be almost devoid of muscle, a histologic characteristic of all urethral diverticula. When making the diagnosis of a congenital urethral diverticulum, it is important to rule out the possibility of an ectopic ureter[6] that does not enter the urethra directly but does so by means of an apparent diverticulum.

Most acquired urethral diverticula are thought to be the result of infection of the periurethral glands or of trauma to the urethra. In most cases, it is likely that an infection causes obstruction of one or more of the periurethral glands, resulting in cyst or abscess formation beneath the pubocervical (periurethral) fascia with ultimate rupture into the urethral lumen. The infectious cause of urethral diverticula is supported by the frequent history of gonorrheal infection or urethritis. Organisms commonly cultured from infected urethral diverticula include *Escherichia coli, Staphylococcus aureus, Enterococcus faecalis, Proteus* sp, *Enterobacter aerogenes, Pseudomonas aeruginosa*, diptheroids, and other gram-negative bacteria.

More than 80% of urethral diverticula are located about the distal two thirds of the urethra. The fact that this is the location of the periurethral glands and that these glands become infected lends support to the infectious cause of urethral diverticula. An occasional urethral diverticulum will be found in the proximal segment of the urethra, and it may extend beneath the trigone of the bladder. Rarely, a urethral diverticulum will be located anterior to the urethra; in more than half of these cases, a history of periurethral surgery exists.

Urethral instrumentation, urethral or periurethral surgery, and childbirth have been suggested as causative factors in acquired urethral diverticula related to trauma. Given that urethral diverticula occur in nulliparous women and that no correlation exists between parity and the incidence of urethral diverticulum, however, there is little support for the suggestion that it may be a result of the trauma of childbirth.

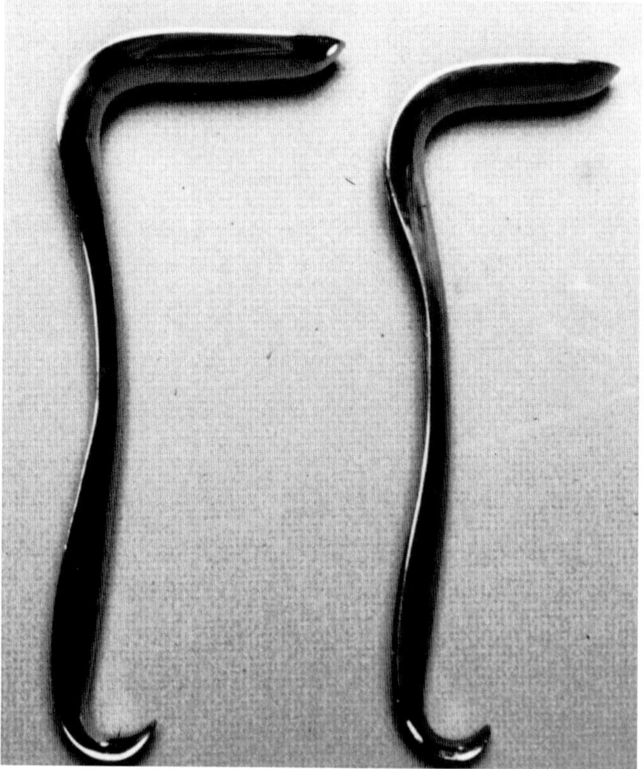

Figure 8-1 Sims' vaginal speculum.

Symptoms

Twenty percent of urethral diverticula are asymptomatic.[4] Symptomatic diverticula may be associated with the complaints listed in Table 8-1.

Half of the patients with a urethral diverticulum will have a palpable periurethral mass. The mass may be overlooked unless the physician inspects the anterior wall of the vagina with a single-blade speculum (Figure 8-1) and palpates this area as a part of the pelvic examination. It is important to differentiate the mass of a urethral diverticulum from a cystourethrocele.

Table 8-1 Complaints Associated with Urethral Diverticula

Complaint	%
Dysuria	80
Urinary Frequency	40
Urinary Urgency	25
Recurrent Urinary Tract Infection	45
Dyspareunia	20
Hematuria	15
Urethral Discharge	10
Urinary Incontinence	24
Palpable Mass	60

To increase physician awareness, it is helpful to remember the "Three Ds"—dysuria, dribbling, and dyspareunia—that suggest the diagnosis of urethral diverticula. Although many lower genitourinary tract disorders share these symptoms, when there is also a history of recurrent cystitis or urethritis (or both), it is important to examine the patient specifically for the possibility of urethral diverticula. The latter can be a cause of recurrent urinary tract infection, and surgical correction of the diverticula can eliminate this troublesome disorder. The differential diagnosis of urethral diverticula considers the disorders listed in Table 8-2.

Diagnosis

The diagnosis of urethral diverticulum is easily missed with the use of a routine pelvic examination and

Table 8-2 Disorders in the Differential Diagnosis of Urethral Diverticula

Periurethral Gland Infection
Suburethral or Vaginal Cysts
Ectopic Ureterocele
Vaginal or Urethral Tumors

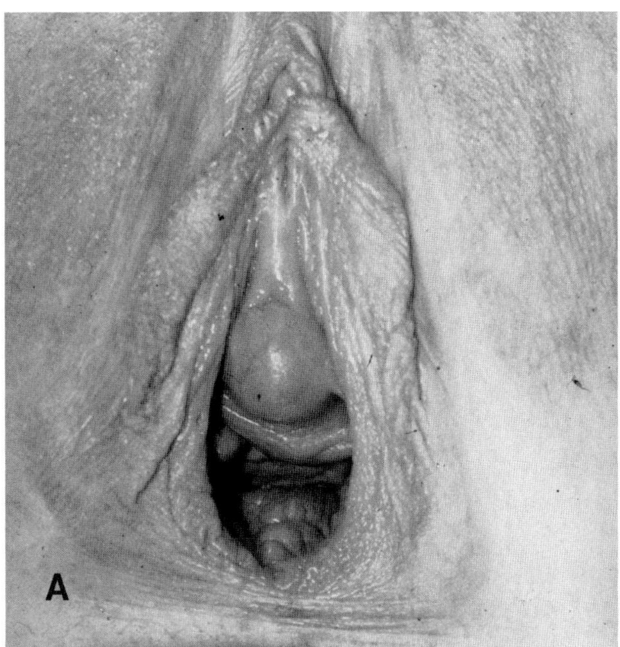

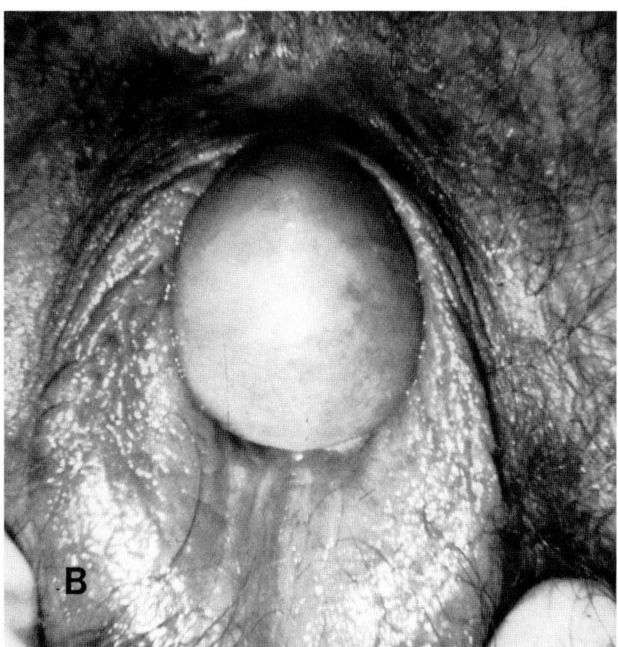

Figure 8-2 Urethral diverticulum. **A,** Diverticulum of distal segment of urethra that would be amenable to marsupialization (Spence procedure). **B,** Large urethral diverticulum.

cystoscopy. Detection may require special diagnostic techniques.

Visualization and palpation of the anterior wall of the vagina may reveal the presence of urethral tenderness or a mass (Figure 8-2). Although the average diverticulum has a diameter of 2 to 3 cm, some have been reported to have a diameter of 6 cm. Compression of the mass or urethral massage may result in the loss of urine or of a purulent exudate from the external urethral meatus. Interestingly, the symptoms associated with urethral diverticula are not necessarily related to their size, and, when there is no visual or palpable abnormality, the persistence of lower urinary tract complaints and infections suggests the need for urethroscopy and cystoscopy.

The standard cystoscope is limited in its capability for examining the female urethra. Endoscopic examination of the urethra is best performed with a female urethroscope that has a 0-degree lens and a round sheath without a terminal beak. The distending medium should be carbon dioxide or an appropriate sterile cystoscopic fluid. If, during the urethroscopic examination, the urethrovesical junction is occluded by a finger or long forceps, communicating diverticula will distend and be more easily visualized (Figure 8-3). The urethra may be massaged during the examination in an effort to open and reveal a partially occluded diverticulum.

Urethral diverticula may be single, multiple, or complex. They may have more than one opening into the urethra. All openings of multiple or complex diverticula should be located.

A urethral diverticulum can be diagnosed as a result of finding a periurethral stone on a preliminary film before performing intravenous urography or on a postvoid film

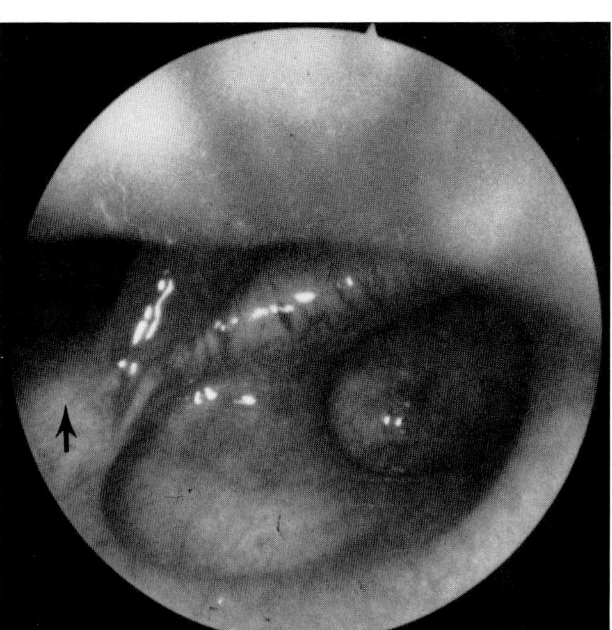

Figure 8-3 Urethroscopic examination of urethral diverticulum. *Arrow* indicates urethral lumen.

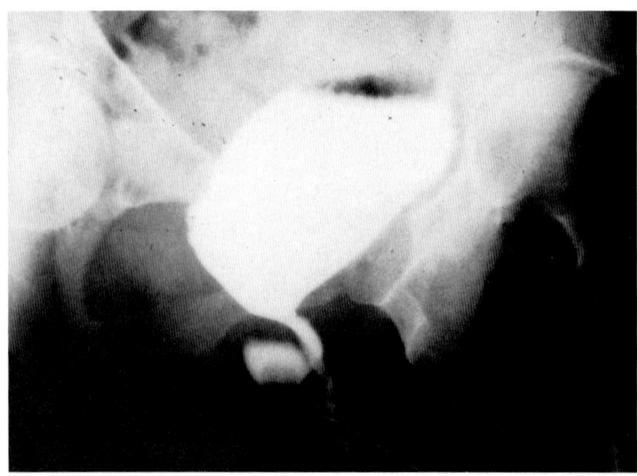

Figure 8-4 Urethral diverticulum as documented by voiding cystourethrography. Shadow within diverticulum is due to a stone.

that shows liquid contrast medium within the diverticulum. Intravenous urography may be indicated in the evaluation of patients suspected of having a urethral diverticulum to exclude the possibility of ureteral duplication or an ectopic ureterocele.

Voiding cystourethrography[2–4] is an excellent procedure to use to demonstrate communicating urethral diverticula and to differentiate them from other periurethral masses (Figure 8-4). As part of the examination, a preliminary film of the pelvis should be taken from an oblique angle with the patient in a standing position. The findings will help in detecting any stones that may be within the urethral diverticulum. The bladder should then be drained by means of a transurethral catheter and subsequently filled with 250 to 300 mL of a liquid contrast medium. Cinefluoroscopy, during voiding with the patient in the standing position, is helpful in demonstrating the openings and the positions of urethral diverticula.

Positive-pressure urethrography[7,8] was developed specifically for the diagnosis of urethral diverticula. A double-balloon, Davis or Trattner catheter (Figure 8-5) is inserted transurethrally, so that the distal balloon is just within the bladder neck. The distal and then the proximal balloon are inflated with 20 to 30 mL of water, dilute saline, or dilute liquid contrast material. After both ends of the urethra are obstructed by the balloons, 4 to 7 mL of 30% liquid contrast solution is injected through the third catheter port. This contrast material should escape the catheter by way of a slit in the lumen between the balloons. The contrast material will flow about the catheter tubing and enter communicating diverticula. The urethra is then visualized by using cinefluoroscopy, and films are made to document findings (Figure 8-6). This is a very sensitive method of diagnosing urethral diverticula. When interpreting positive-pressure urethrography findings, it is important not to overdiagnose the condition.

A pelvic ultrasound examination[9] can detect periurethral cysts and urethral diverticula. It cannot distinguish between the two conditions without visualizing the diverticula opening into the lumen of the urethra. When pelvic sonography suggests that there is a cystic mass behind or below the bladder, it is important to consider that it could be a urethral diverticulum.

Urethral pressure profilometry[10] may be used to document the location of the orifice of a communicating urethral diverticulum along the course of the urethra. A characteristic biphasic notch will be seen in the urethral pressure profile at the site of the diverticular opening (Figure 8-7). This is helpful in determining the location of the diverticular opening within the lumen of the urethra and its effect on the urethra's closure pressure and continence mechanism. If any orifice of a diverticulum opens into the proximal half of the urethra, it would be unwise to perform a marsupialization procedure. It would be better to perform diverticulectomy and, then, to provide differential support to the urethrovesical junction in an effort to prevent postoperative stress urinary incontinence (SUI).

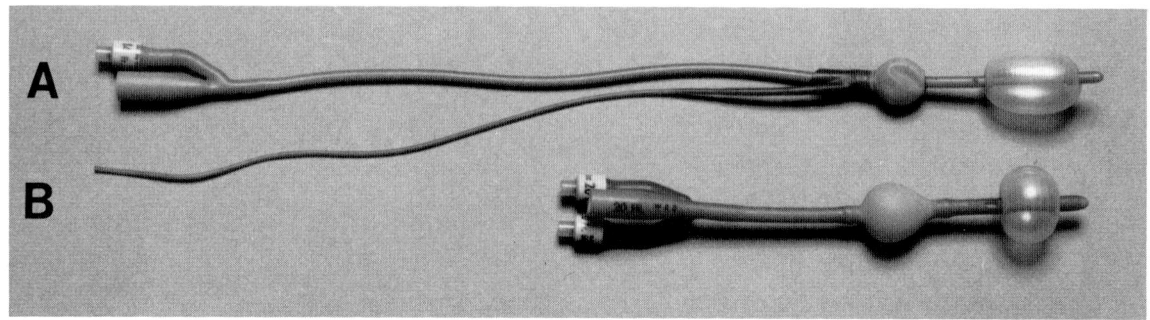

Figure 8-5 Davis (**A**) and Trattner (**B**) catheters for positive-pressure urethrography. *Source*: Courtesy of CB Bard, Covington, GA.

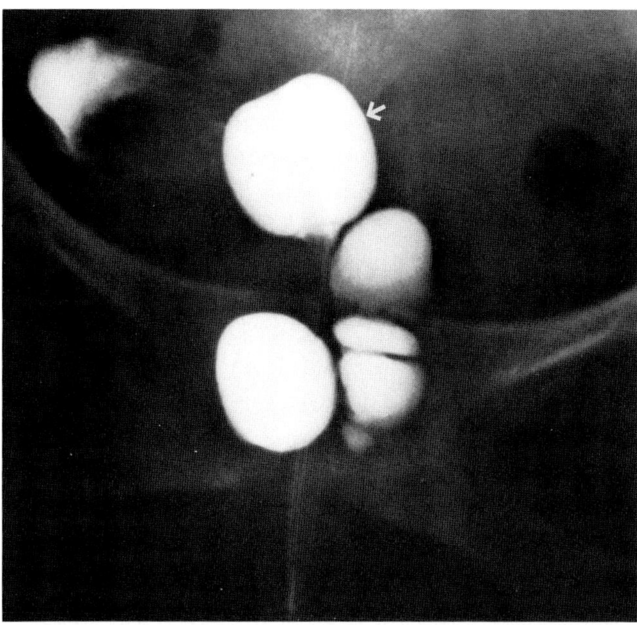

Figure 8-6 Positive-pressure, double-balloon urethrogram clearly shows four diverticula and scantly shows a fifth diverticulum. *Arrow* points to intravesical balloon. *Source*: Courtesy of Ernest I Kohorn, MD, New Haven, CT.

Urethral diverticula can be a cause of urinary incontinence. The incontinence they cause consists primarily of postmicturition dribbling. If a woman with a urethral diverticulum complains of urinary incontinence, a more in-depth urodynamic examination[11] of her lower urinary tract function is indicated to determine whether she also has SUI, incontinence related to detrusor instability, or mixed incontinence (combined genuine stress incontinence and detrusor instability). These conditions are not caused by urethral diverticula and in themselves require special attention.

Associated Findings

The main complications of untreated urethral diverticula are recurrent urinary tract infections, stone formation, and neoplastic degeneration.

Approximately 5% of urethral diverticula contain one or more stones.[12] The stones are thought to be the result of urinary stasis within the diverticulum, infection of the urine and diverticular tissues, deposition of salts, and desquamation of the epithelial lining of the diverticulum. Most of the stones are composed of magnesium ammonium phosphate.[12]

Urethral diverticula have been reported to contain foci of in situ or invasive transitional cell carcinoma,[13] adenocarcinoma,[14] or squamous cell carcinoma. Nephrogenic adenomas,[15] Paneth cell metaplasia,[16] and endometriosis[17] have been reported to occur in urethral diverticula. Herein lies the importance of the histologic examination of tissue from urethral diverticula, since diverticulectomy alone is not the treatment of choice for a urethral diverticulum containing a carcinoma.

Patients who have a urethral diverticulum and SUI should have a diverticulectomy and a continence procedure (ie, urethropexy or colposuspension).[11] If detrusor instability is diagnosed preoperatively, postoperative treatment with parasympatholytic medications may help put the bladder at rest, improve the tolerance of the bladder catheter drainage, and promote healing.

Surgical Therapy

Recommended Procedures

My preference for the treatment of an uncomplicated, unisaccular urethral diverticulum is partial diverticulec-

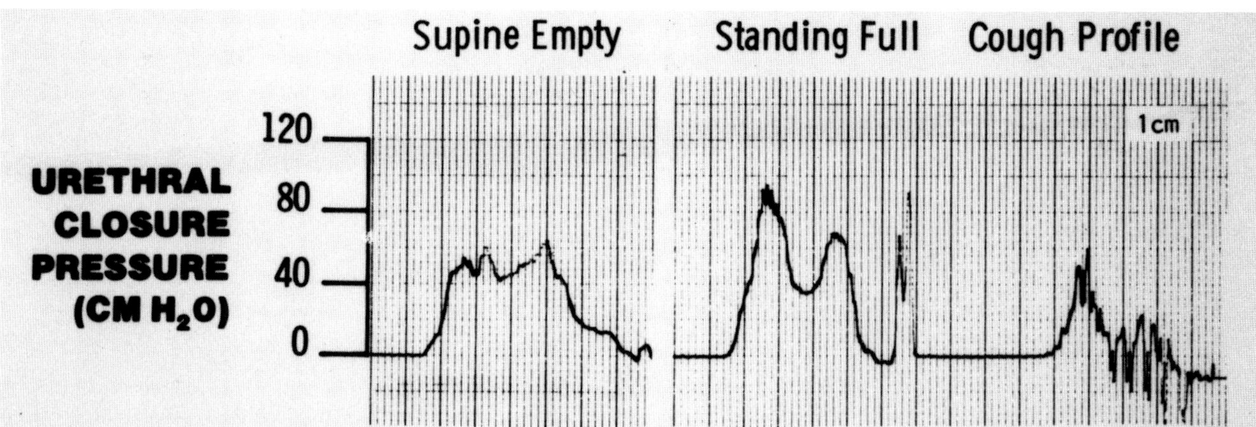

Figure 8-7 Urethral pressure profilometry with biphasic notch characteristic of communicating urethral diverticulum. *Source*: Courtesy of Alfred E Bent, MD, Towson, MD.

tomy (Figure 8-8), as described by Tancer and colleagues.[18,19] Multiple and complex urethral diverticula are best treated by performing diverticulectomy (Figure 8-9).[20,21] Marsupialization (Figure 8-10), as described by Spence and Duckett,[22,23] is reserved for diverticula of the distal segment of the urethra that do not involve the upper half of the urethra or its continence mechanism. Although I am aware that there are advocates of transurethral incision of urethral diverticulum, as described by Lapides,[24] I have had no experience with the technique.

Partial Diverticulectomy. An anesthetic is administered to the patient, who is placed in the lithotomy position, prepared, and draped appropriately for vaginal surgery. Bladder drainage is instituted by using a suprapubic or a transurethral catheter.

If a suprapubic catheter has been placed, a Foley (16F or 18F) catheter is inserted transurethrally, and its balloon is inflated. A vaginal speculum (eg, Auvard) is used to retract the perineum and the posterior wall of the vagina. A midline longitudinal incision is made through the entire thickness of the anterior wall of the vagina from within 1 cm of the external urethral meatus to the cervix or the vaginal apex. A transverse incision is made through the entire thickness of the anterior wall of the vagina in the upper aspect of the vagina perpendicular to the longitudinal incision and extending to each lateral vaginal fornix. The anterior wall of the vagina is widely dissected bilaterally from the underlying pubocervical (periurethral) fascia to expose the urethral diverticulum. The pubocervical fascia overlying the diverticulum is incised vertically and dissected bilaterally from the innermost layer of the diverticulum. The diverticulum is

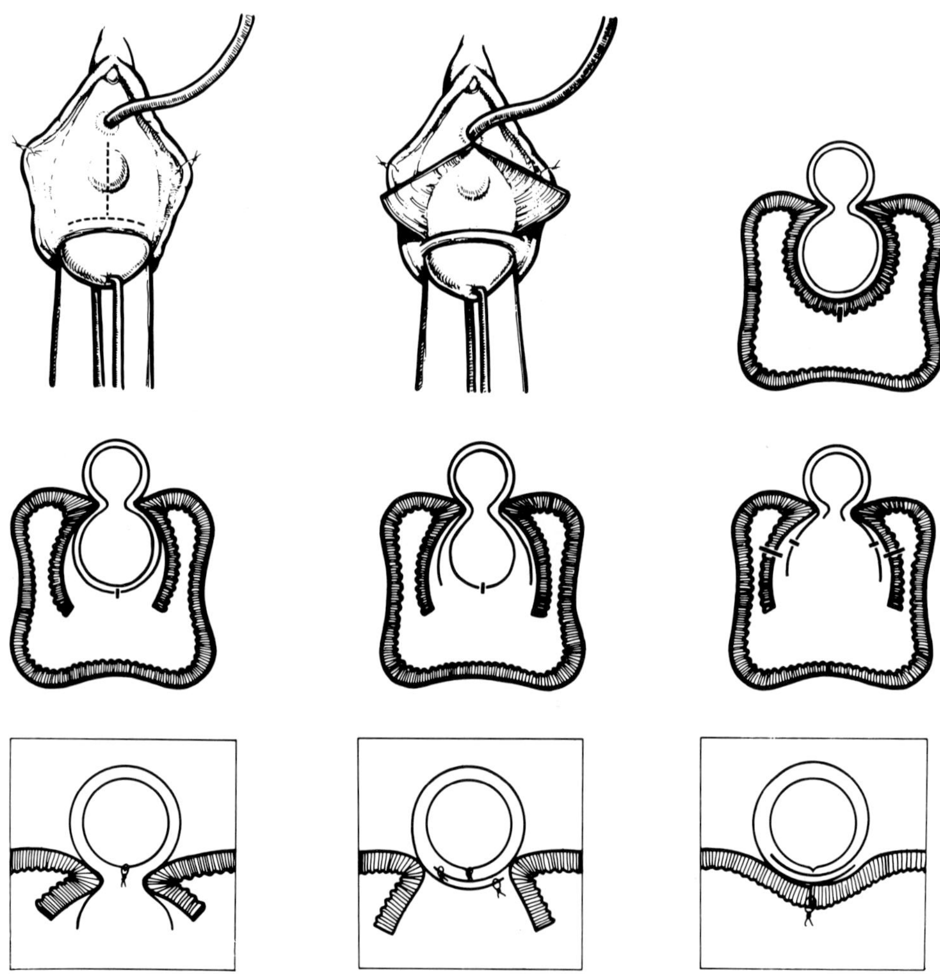

Figure 8-8 Partial diverticulectomy. From *left* to *right*: Inverted "T" incision through full thickness of anterior wall of vagina; dissection of vaginal wall from underlying pubocervical (periurethral) fascia; incision of anterior wall of vagina; dissection of anterior wall of vagina from underlying pubocervical (periurethral) fascia and incision of pubocervical fascia; dissection of pubocervical fascia and incision of diverticular wall; excision of diverticular wall and locations of excisions of pubocervical fascia and vaginal wall; suturing of diverticular wall; overlapping and suturing of pubocervical fascia in vertical vest-over-pants fashion; and suturing of vaginal wall.

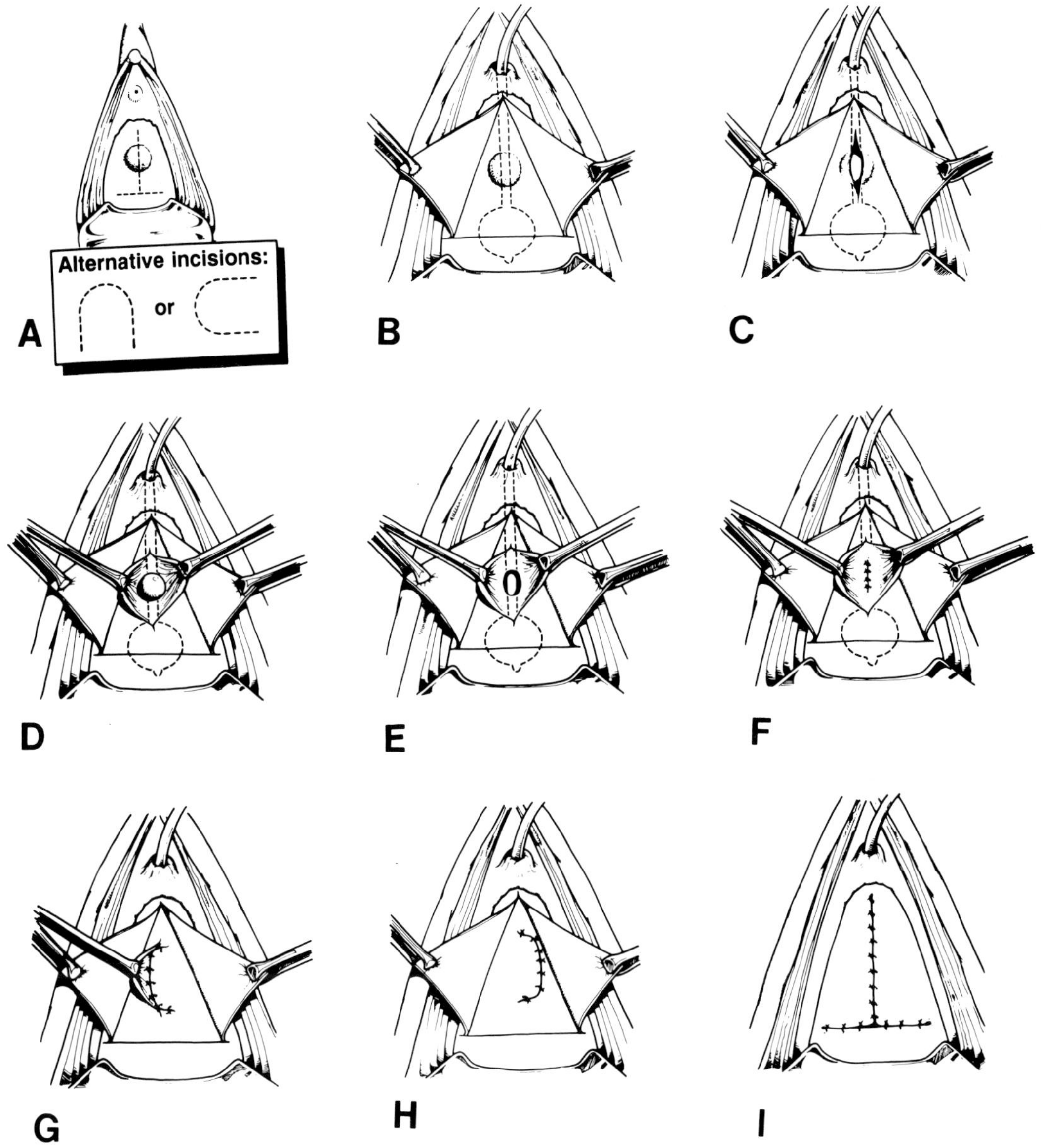

Alternative incisions:
or
A
B
C
D
E
F
G
H
I

Figure 8-9 Diverticulectomy. **A**, Alternative anterior vaginal wall incisions; **B**, dissection of anterior vaginal wall from pubocervical fascia; **C**, incision of diverticulum; **D**, dissection of diverticulum; **E**, excision of diverticulum; **F**, closure of urethra; **G** and **H**, overlapping and suturing of pubocervical fascia; **I**, closure of vaginal wall.

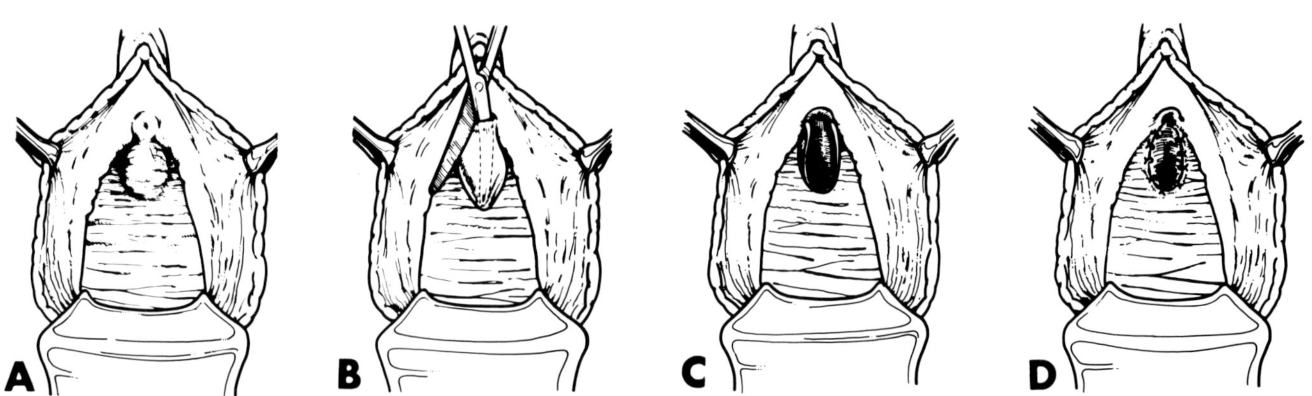

Figure 8-10 Marsupialization of diverticulum of distal segment of urethra. **A**, Visualization of anterior vaginal wall and diverticulum; **B**, insertion of tip of one blade of scissors through external urethral meatus and into diverticular sac; **C**, incised distal urethral diverticulum; **D**, approximation of urethral wall to vaginal wall.

incised vertically and resected just distal to its opening into the urethral lumen. The cut edges of the lining of the diverticulum are approximated with fine (4-0 or 3-0 chromic or delayed-absorbable polyglactin or polyglycolic acid) sutures on a small, tapered needle. The pubocervical fascia is overlapped in a vertical vest-over-pants fashion with 4-0 or 3-0 interrupted delayed-absorbable sutures. The medial margins of the anterior wall of the vagina are trimmed and approximated with 4-0 or 3-0 interrupted delayed-absorbable sutures. Perioperative antibiotic prophylaxis is recommended. Postoperative bladder drainage should be used during the initial healing phase. The patient is advised against vaginal intercourse, tampon use, douching, and vaginal examinations for at least 6 weeks.

Diverticulectomy. Anesthesia; preparation, positioning, and draping of the patient; and bladder drainage are as described for a partial diverticulectomy.

A vaginal speculum (eg, Auvard) is used to retract the perineum and the posterior wall of the vagina. The anterior wall of the vagina may be incised in an inverted "U," inverted "T," or longitudinal fashion. The anterior wall of the vagina is widely dissected bilaterally from the underlying pubocervical (periurethral) fascia to expose the urethral diverticulum. The pubocervical fascia overlying the diverticulum is incised vertically, or transversely if the surgeon is to cross suture lines, and dissected bilaterally from the innermost layer of the diverticulum. The diverticulum is carefully excised at its opening into the urethra, making certain not to remove urethral mucosa to the extent that approximation of its edges will place tension on its wall about the urethral catheter. The urethral mucosa is approximated with fine (4-0 or 3-0 chromic or delayed-absorbable polyglactin or polyglycolic acid) interrupted or continuous sutures on a small, tapered needle. The cut edges of the pubocervical fascia are overlapped in a vest-over-pants fashion with interrupted 4-0 or 3-0 delayed-absorbable sutures. The anterior wall of the vagina is trimmed and closed with interrupted 4-0 or 3-0 delayed-absorbable sutures. The use of perioperative antibiotic prophylaxis and postoperative bladder drainage, as well as the recommended limitations of postoperative activities for the patient 6 weeks after surgery, are as indicated for a partial diverticulectomy.

In patients with SUI, a plication of the urethrovesical junction or a needle urethropexy or colposuspension may be performed to elevate and stabilize the urethrovesical junction. If a needle urethropexy or colposuspension is to be part of the procedure, the retropubic dissection, abdominal skin incision, suture placement, and abdominal wall suture retrieval should be accomplished after dissection of the vesicovaginal space and before dissection and opening of the urethral diverticulum. This, at least theoretically, should reduce the incidence of infection in the retropubic space and the abdominal incision.

In a heavily scarred or radiated vagina, a Martius bulbocavernosus fat pad transplant may be used to reinforce the repair. Numerous methods of distending urethral diverticula have been described as aids to diverticulectomy. The methods include instillation of fluid by means of a urethrography catheter; passage of transurethral sound, coiling of ureteral catheter, inflating the balloon of a Fogarty or pediatric catheter, or gauze packing; and injection of silicone or a cryoprecipitate coagulum.

Marsupialization of Diverticulum of the Distal Segment of the Urethra. An anesthetic is administered to the patient, who is placed in the lithotomy position, prepared, and draped appropriately for vaginal surgery. The bladder is drained with a straight catheter, which is then removed.

A vaginal speculum is used to retract the perineum and the posterior wall of the vagina. The tip of one blade of the Metzenbaum scissors is placed through the external urethral meatus and into the depth of the urethral diverticulum. With the tips of the scissors at the 6-o'clock position, the diverticulum is deeply incised. Interrupted 4-0 chromic sutures are used to marsupialize the urethral diverticulum. Postoperative bladder catheter drainage is usually not necessary.

Complications

The overall complication rate associated with diverticulectomy is 20% to 25%.[4,20] Complications of this surgery are listed in Table 8-3.

Persistent or recurrent urethral diverticula have been reported in 25% of cases involving diverticulectomy. Most are detected within 3 years of surgery. Such cases may be due to failure to recognize and treat all sacculations of a diverticulum at the time of diverticulectomy. Compound or multiple diverticula occur in more than

Table 8-3 Complications of Urethral Diverticulectomy

Recurrent Urinary Tract Infection
Recurrent Diverticulum
Urinary Incontinence
Urethrovaginal Fistula
Urethral Stricture
Urethral Slough
Urethral Pain Syndrome

20% of cases. It is important to determine preoperatively the number of diverticula, the location of their orifice(s) with respect to the urethral lumen, and the distribution of their sacs. All openings into the urethra must be closed, and all sacs must be removed.

Postoperative SUI occurs in 5% of patients undergoing surgical treatment of urethral diverticula. Diverticula that involve the proximal half of the urethra are likely to affect the urethra's continence mechanism. If this is the case or if the patient is known to have SUI preoperatively, it may be treated by performing an anterior colporrhaphy or suspension procedure at the time of diverticulectomy.

Postoperative urethrovaginal fistulas develop in 4% of the patients who have surgery. The incidence of such fistulas, however, is reduced by meticulous surgical techniques, absolute hemostasis, the use of fine absorbable suture, the crossing of suture lines, and the use of vaginal wall flaps. A Martius bulbocavernosus fat pad transplant will help prevent fistulas in the scarred or radiated vagina.

Care should be taken to excise all of the diverticula lining, but not to remove normal urethral mucosa that must be approximated after excision of the diverticular sac. Closure over a 16F or 18F Foley catheter helps prevent urethral stricture.

URETHRAL PROLAPSE

Urethral prolapse was first reported by Solingen in 1732.[25] It is diagnosed when there is circumferential prolapse of the mucosa of the distal segment of the urethra through the external urethral meatus. It is more common in premenarcheal children 8 to 12 years old and postmenopausal women 60 to 70 years old.[25] Approximately half of all reported cases occur in children. It is seen more frequently in blacks than in other races.[26]

Estrogen deficiency and episodic increases in intra-abdominal pressure are contributing factors. The patient with urethral prolapse may be asymptomatic or may complain of urinary urgency and frequency, dysuria, urethral bleeding, vaginal bleeding, or a protruding mass about the external meatus.

The prolapsed urethral tissue will appear pale red, violaceous, or gangrenous and feel soft or firm and fleshy. It may measure from 0.5 to 4 cm in length and up to 5 cm in width. If often bleeds or produces a bloody serous discharge.[25] The differential diagnosis includes urethral polyps, papilloma, caruncle, condyloma, periurethral abscess, urethral cysts, prolapsed ureterocele, and malignant neoplasms. The diagnosis of urethral prolapse is usually made by finding the urethral orifice in the middle of what appears to be a circumferential prolapse of urethral mucosa (Figure 8-11). Histologic examination of the tissue will reveal edema, an inflammatory infiltrate, and vascular thrombosis. The blood vessels resemble sinuses and are separated by scant strands of connective tissue.[25]

If the patient is hypoestrogenic, she should be treated with direct applications of estrogen vaginal cream[27] and, if postmenopausal, with appropriate estrogen replacement therapy. When necessary, symptomatic urethral prolapse may be treated by using cryosurgery[28] or local excision.[25,29,30] It is believed that the retropubic procedure of Hepburn, as described by Hepburn[31] and used by others[32] in which the urethral prolapse is reduced and the urethra is sutured to the retrosymphysis, is usually unnecessary. Regardless of the method of surgical therapy, it is important to preserve urethral length and prevent postoperative stenosis.

URETHRAL CARUNCLE

Urethral caruncle was first described by Samuel Sharp in 1750.[33] The lesions may be asymptomatic, or the patient may complain of urinary urgency and frequency, dysuria, urethral bleeding, and the presence of a mass at the external urethral meatus. Urethral caruncles usually occur in patients 40 to 70 years of age, most of whom are postmenopausal and multiparous.

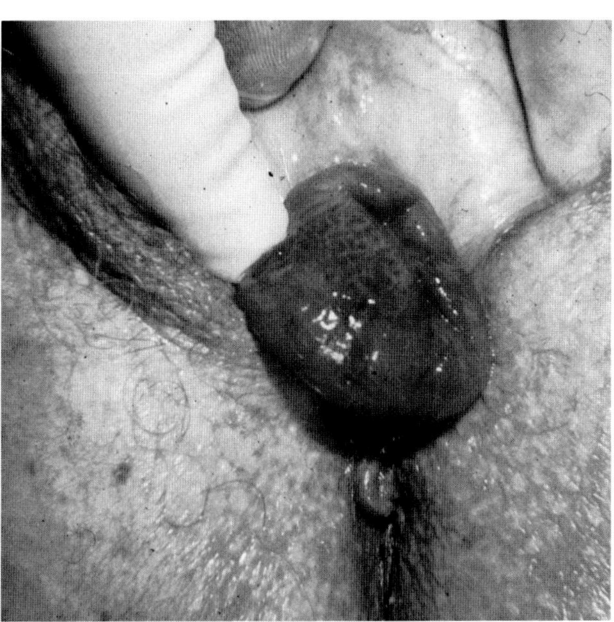

Figure 8-11 Urethral prolapse. Note that external urethral orifice is within prolapse.

Jeffcoate[34] has distinguished between true caruncles and pseudocaruncles. A *true caruncle* is a vascular papilloma that presents as a scarlet polyp with a narrow pedicle invariably arising from the posterior lip of the urethral meatus. A true caruncle may be secondarily infected but is not the result of an infection. A *pseudocaruncle* is a diffuse sessile dull red granuloma of any aspect of the urethral meatus that is the result of urethritis. The urethritis is related to or associated with an infection caused by micro-organisms such as *Trichomonas vaginalis* and *Candida albicans*.

Although Novak and Woodruff have suggested three histologic varieties[35] of urethral caruncles—granulomatous, papillomatous, and angiomatous—for the most part all caruncles show evidence of epithelial hyperplasia (transitional or squamous cell), a core of loose connective tissue containing thin-walled blood vessels, and an associated inflammatory reaction. The nondescript pathologic findings make the diagnosis a clinical one.

Evaluation of a urethral caruncle should include urethral and vaginal culture for *Trichomonas vaginalis, Candida albicans, Neisseria gonorrhoeae*, and *Chlamydia trachomatis*. If there is evidence of an infection, it must be eradicated. If the patient is hypoestrogenic, estrogen vaginal cream should be applied locally. If the patient is postmenopausal, hormone replacement should be considered.

Pseudocaruncles are more difficult to treat than are true caruncles.[36] Caruncles that do not respond to medical therapy may be successfully treated by electrosurgical cauterization or excision, cryotherapy, laser vaporization or excision, or surgical excision. Whenever surgical treatment is undertaken, a tissue specimen should be submitted for pathologic study because urethral caruncles have been associated with carcinoma in situ. Recurrent caruncles are often accompanied by recurrent urinary tract infections. Surgical therapy may be complicated by the development of a distal urethral stenosis.

REFERENCES

1. Hey W. Of collections of pus in the vagina. In: *Practical Observations in Surgery*. Philadelphia, Pa: James Humphreys; 1805: 304–305.

2. Coddington CC, Knab DR. Urethral diverticulum: a review. *Obstet Gynecol Surv*. 1983;38:357–364.

3. Ginsburg D, Genadry R. Suburethral diverticulum: classification and therapeutic considerations. *Obstet Gynecol*. 1983;61:30–33.

4. Peters WA III, Vaughan ED Jr. Urethral diverticulum in the female. *Obstet Gynecol*. 1976;47:549–552.

5. Glassman TA, Weinerth JL, Glenn JF. Neonatal female urethral diverticulum. *Urology*. 1975;5:249–251.

6. Curry NS. Ectopic ureteral orifice masquerading as a urethral diverticulum. *Am J Radiol*. 1983;141:1325–1326.

7. Davis HJ, Cian LG. Positive pressure urethrography: a new diagnostic method. *J Urol*. 1956;75:753–757.

8. Davis HJ, TeLinde RW. Urethral diverticula: an assay of 121 cases. *J Urol*. 1958;80:34–39.

9. Pliskow N, Silver TM. Ultrasonic diagnosis of urethral diverticulum. *Urology*. 1980;15:625–629.

10. Bhatia NN, McCarthy TA, Ostergard DR. Urethral pressure profiles of women with urethral diverticula. *Obstet Gynecol*. 1981;58:375–378.

11. Reid RE, Gill B, Laor E, Tolia BM, Freed SZ. Role of urodynamics in management of urethral diverticulum in females. *Urology*. 1986;28:342–346.

12. Aragonia F, Mangano M, Artibani W, Glazel GP. Stone formation in a female urethral diverticulum. Review of the literature. *Int Urol Nephrol*. 1989;21:621–625.

13. Srinivas V, Dow D. Transitional cell carcinoma in a urethral diverticulum with a calculus. *J Urol*. 1983;129:372–373.

14. Evans KJ, McCarthy MP, Sands JP. Adenocarcinoma of a female urethral diverticulum: a case report and review of the literature. *J Urol*. 1981;126:124–126.

15. Odze R, Begin LR. Tubular adenomatous metaplasia (nephrogenic adenoma) of the female urethra. *Int J Gynecol Pathol*. 1989;8:374–380.

16. Niemiec TR, Mercer LJ, Stephens JK, Hajj SN. Unusual urethral diverticulum lined by colonic epithelium with Paneth cell metaplasia. *Am J Obstet Gynecol*. 1989;160:186–188.

17. Palagiri A. Urethral diverticulum with endometriosis. *Urology*. 1978;11:271–272.

18. Tancer ML, Hyman R. Suburethral diverticulitis in the female. *Am J Obstet Gynecol*. 1962;84:1853–1858.

19. Tancer ML, Mooppan MMU, Pierre-Louis C, Kim H, Ravski N. Suburethral diverticulum treatment by partial ablation. *Obstet Gynecol*. 1983;62:511–513.

20. Lee RA. Diverticulum of the female urethra: postoperative complications and results. *Obstet Gynecol*. 1983;61:52–58.

21. Leach GE, Schmidbauer CP, Hadley HR, Staskin DR, Zimmern P, Raz S. Surgical treatment of female urethral diverticulum. *Semin Urol*. 1986;4:33–42.

22. Spence HM, Duckett JW. Diverticulum of female urethra; clinical aspect and presentation of a single operative technique for cure. *J Urol*. 1970;104:432–437.

23. Roehrborn CG. Long term follow-up study of the marsupialization technique for urethral diverticula in women. *Surg Gynecol Obstet*. 1988;167:191–196.

24. Lapides J. Transurethral treatment of urethral diverticula in women. *J Urol*. 1979;121:736–738.

25. Epsteen A, Strauss B. Prolapse of female urethra with gangrene. *Am J Surg*. 1937;35:563–569.

26. Esposito JM. Circular prolapse of the urethra in children: a cause of vaginal bleeding. *Obstet Gynecol*. 1968;31:363–367.

27. Richardson DA, Hajj SN, Herbst AL. Medical treatment of urethral prolapse in children. *Obstet Gynecol*. 1982;59:69–74.

28. Friedrich EG Jr. Cryosurgery for urethral prolapse. *Obstet Gynecol*. 1977;50:359–361.

29. Jerkins GR, Verheeck K, Noe HN. Treatment of girls with urethral prolapse. *J Urol*. 1984;132:732–733.

30. Lowe FC, Hill GS, Jeffs RD, Brendler CB. Urethral prolapse in children: insights into etiology and management. *J Urol*. 1986;135:100–103.

31. Hepburn TN. Prolapse of the urethra in female children. *Surg Gynecol Obstet*. 1927;44:400–401.

32. Devine PC, Kessel HC. Surgical correction of urethral prolapse. *J Urol*. 1980;123:856–857.

33. Kelly HA. *Gynecology*. New York: Appleton; 1928:815.

34. Jeffcoate TNA. *Principles of Gynaecology*. 3rd ed. London: Butterworths Publishers; 1967:398.

35. Novak ER, Woodruff JD, eds. *Novak's Gynecologic and Obstetric Pathology*. 8th ed. Philadelphia: WB Saunders; 1979:54.

36. Nasah BT. Urethral caruncle. *J Obstet Gynaecol Br Commonw*. 1968;75:781–783.

9

Urinary Tract Injuries

Manuel A. Penalver

This chapter is concerned with urinary tract injuries that involve the ureters and bladder and that are associated with gynecologic surgery or cancer therapy.

URETERAL INJURY

Ureteral injury has been reported to occur in 0.5% to 2.5% of gynecologic procedures.[1] In a major teaching hospital, Mann and colleagues[2] documented ureteral injury in 17 of 3185 major gynecologic cases (0.5%). Before the management of ureteral injuries is discussed, the embryogenesis, anatomy, and preoperative evaluation of the ureter will be reviewed.

The Ureter

Embryogenesis

The ureteric buds are outgrowths of the mesonephric ducts. The ureteric buds develop into the ureters, the renal pelvis, and the kidneys' collecting tubules. As the ureters elongate, the kidneys migrate in a cephalad direction. The brief understanding of the embryogenesis of the kidneys and the ureters helps explain some congenital anomalies encountered during gynecologic surgery.

A *double ureter* is found in approximately 0.5% of the population and is the result of a splitting of the ureteric bud. It is most often incomplete, giving rise to a partially duplicated (ie, double) ureter. The ascent of the kidney from the pelvis to its normal position within the posterior wall of the abdomen may be arrested by the bifurcation of the common iliac artery, giving rise to a *pelvic kidney*. A *horseshoe kidney* results from the fusion of the inferior poles of kidneys that have been mechanically obstructed by the inferior mesenteric artery.

Anatomy

The ureters are bilateral tubular urinary conduits (25 to 30 cm in length) that connect the kidneys to the urinary bladder. The ureters have an abdominal and a pelvic course. In their abdominal course, they lie on the anterior surface of the psoas muscle and receive their blood supply from the renal and the ovarian arteries and the aorta. The ureters pass over the common iliac arteries and beneath the insertions of the infundibulopelvic ligaments to enter the true pelvis. In their pelvic course, the ureters receive an additional blood supply from the internal iliac, the uterine, and the vesical arteries (Figure 9-1). The arteriolar blood supply of each ureter forms a longitudinal network within its adventitial sheath. When dissecting about the ureter, it is important to protect its blood supply by maintaining the integrity of its adventitial sheath.

At the midplane of the pelvis, the uterine arteries cross over the ureters. Each ureter then courses through its

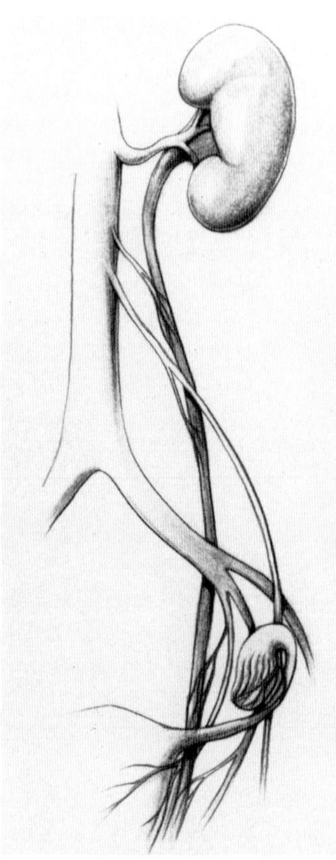

Figure 9-1 Blood supply of ureter. *Source*: Reprinted with permission from *Gynecologic Oncology* (1989;34:274–288), Copyright © 1989, Academic Press, Inc.

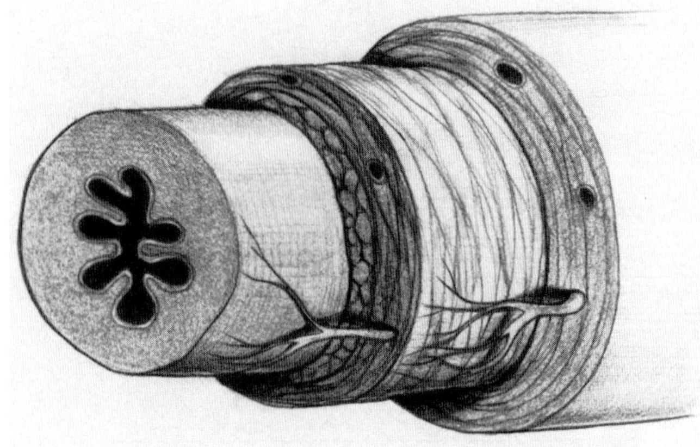

Figure 9-2 Histologic features of ureter. *Source*: Reprinted with permission from *Gynecologic Oncology* (1989;34:274–288), Copyright © 1989, Academic Press, Inc.

own parametrial tunnel to enter the urinary bladder. Within the parametrium the ureters are approximately 1.5 cm lateral to the cervix and in close proximity to the lateral vaginal fornices. When the ureters enter the bladder, their lumen expands as their muscle fibers mingle with those of the bladder. The two ureteral orifices and the internal urethral meatus form the boundaries of the trigone of the bladder.

The wall of each ureter consists of three layers (Figure 9-2). The inner layer is transitional epithelium, the middle layer consists of circular and longitudinal smooth muscle fibers, and the outer layer is an adventitial sheath.

Preoperative Evaluation

Intravenous urography (IVU) is used to document the anatomy and function of the kidneys, the ureters, and the bladder. Intravenous urographic findings provide useful information for surgery in patients with disease processes that may obstruct, displace, or otherwise involve these structures.

Intravenous urography is important in the preoperative evaluation of gynecologic malignancies. Some surgeons advocate an IVU in all patients undergoing major pelvic surgery; others advocate an IVU only in selected cases. In an effort to determine who would benefit from a preoperative IVU, Piscatelli and co-workers[3] performed the study in 493 patients who were to have a hysterectomy for a benign condition. They concluded that the only factors associated with significant abnormal IVU findings were a uterine size equal to or greater than that of 12 weeks' gestation or an ovarian cyst equal to or larger than 4 cm. There was little benefit in performing a preoperative IVU in patients with endometriosis, pelvic inflammatory disease, pelvic relaxation, and a history of previous pelvic surgery.

Preoperative retrograde ureteral catheter placement has been used by some surgeons to assist in the identification and dissection of the ureters. Unfortunately, these catheters are not always easy to palpate through thickened inflammatory or fibrotic tissue. Their presence within the ureter may traumatize its mucosa and predispose the ureter to vascular injury. Sharp dissection about the ureter is more traumatic when the ureter contains such a stent. Therefore the preoperative placement of ureteral stents is of questionable value.

Symmonds[4] has stated that the most important means of preventing ureteric injury is to identify the ureters at the time of surgery, to demonstrate their pelvic course (Figure 9-3), and to keep them out of harm's way. This will do more than preoperative IVUs or preoperative ureteral stent placement toward the prevention of ureteric injuries.

The ureters are most easily identified as they pass over the bifurcations of the common iliac arteries. If the posterior leaf of the broad ligament is incised lateral to this point and the retroperitoneal space is dissected, the

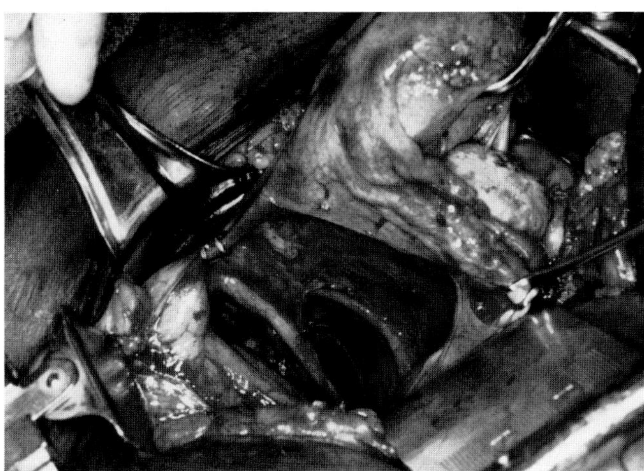

Figure 9-3 Left retroperitoneal space is opened demonstrating ureter on medial leaf of peritoneum. Surgical clamps retract left round ligament and left infundibulopelvic ligament. *Source*: Reprinted with permission from *Gynecologic Oncology* (1989;34:274–288), Copyright © 1989, Academic Press, Inc.

ureter will usually be found attached to the medial leaf of the peritoneum. If the ureter is allowed to slip between the tips of the index finger and thumb, it will render a clicking or snapping sound. Stroking or compressing the ureter will usually result in its characteristic peristalsis.

Management of the Injury

Considerations Related to Type of Injury

Ureteral injuries usually occur during attempts to secure hemostasis. Most ureteral injuries are due to kinking, sheath trauma, needle perforation, crushing injury, ligation, or transection. With minor segmental trauma, including needle perforation and sheath trauma, no treatment is usually necessary. With more extensive damage, the retrograde placement of a ureteral stent will help minimize the effects of transient edema and prevent stricture formation. When the extent of the injury suggests devitalization of the ureter, excision of the damaged segment with ureteroneocystostomy or ureteroureterostomy may be the preferred management.

If the ureter is crushed, prompt removal of the crushing instrument is usually all that is necessary. Return of peristalsis and color throughout the traumatized segment after release of the clamp signifies minimal ureteral damage. A ureteral stent should be inserted and left in place for approximately 10 days after surgery to minimize the likelihood of stricture formation. If inspection shows ischemia or necrosis, excision of the crushed segment must be considered. Ligated ureters are handled in a fashion similar to that for crush injuries. The management of ureteral transection will be described in detail later.

Considerations Related to Location of Injury

The three most common places of ureteral injuries are (1) at the pelvic brim beneath the insertion of the infundibulopelvic ligament, (2) in the cardinal ligament where the uterine artery crosses the ureter, and (3) at the cervicovaginal junction (Figure 9-4). Statistically, the most common place of ureteral injury is at the level of the uterine artery. The ureter is usually injured as a result of the placement of sutures in an attempt to obtain hemostasis. The location of the ureter must be known when taking the infundibulopelvic ligament and ovarian vessels. Clamps about the cervicovaginal junction should be placed with careful attention to preventing ureteral injury. It is important not to incorporate the ureter when suturing about the vaginal cuff.

Most ureteral injuries that are the result of gynecologic procedures involve less than 2 cm of ureteral length. When these injuries occur above the midplane of the pelvis, they are usually repaired by ureteroureterostomy (Figure 9-5). Ureteroureterostomy is performed by mobilizing the ureter about the site of injury in both a cephalad and a caudad direction in an effort to prevent tension on the subsequent anastomosis. The damaged

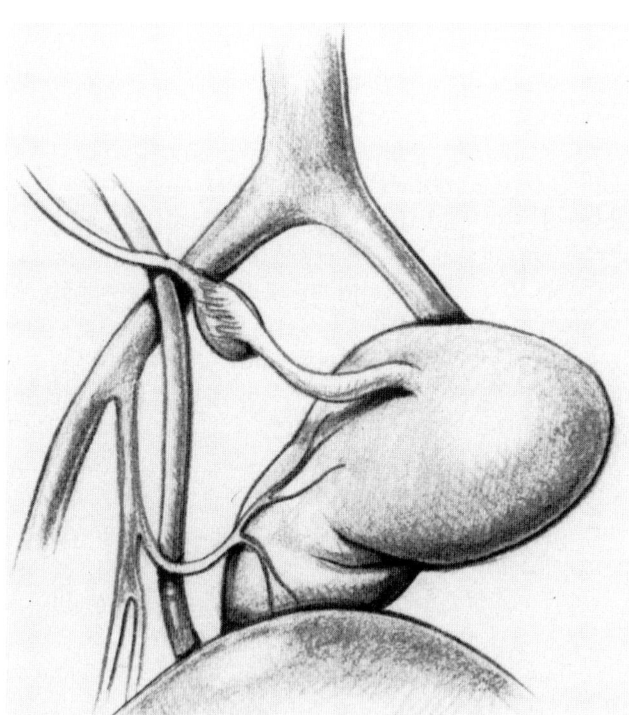

Figure 9-4 Common sites of ureteral injury in gynecologic surgery. *Source*: Reprinted with permission from *Gynecologic Oncology* (1989;34:274–288), Copyright © 1989, Academic Press, Inc.

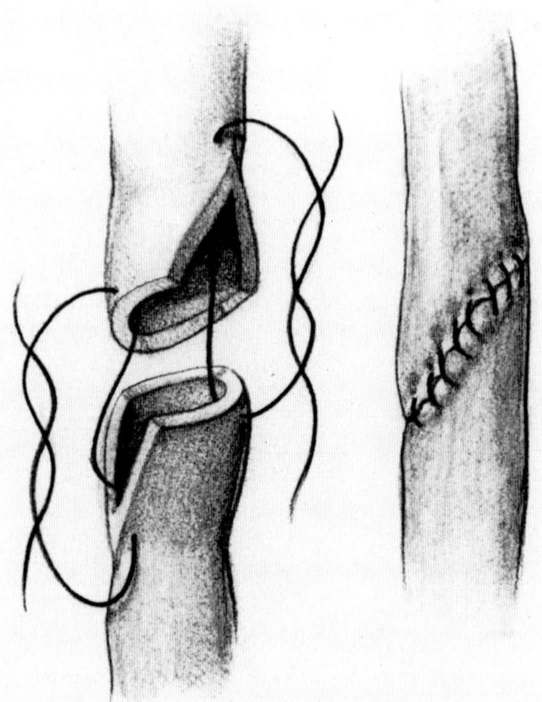

Figure 9-5 Ureteroureterostomy. *Source*: Reprinted with permission from *Gynecologic Oncology* (1989;34:274–288), Copyright © 1989, Academic Press, Inc.

segment is excised, and each end of the ureter is examined for viability. A spatulation of both ends of the ureter is performed to increase the circumference at the site of the anastomosis. A "double J" 6F or 8F ureteral catheter is inserted into both ends of the ureter as a stent. The stenting catheter should be left in place for 10 to 12 days. Four or five interrupted absorbable sutures are used to perform the end-to-end anastomosis, and a retroperitoneal perianastomotic suction drain is placed to, but not touching, the anastomotic site. This drain should be left in place for 10 to 14 days (Figure 9-6). It is important that this retroperitoneal drain not be removed as long as there is any drainage from the anastomotic site. Before removing the drain, the integrity of the anastomosis should be documented radiographically. Carlton and colleagues[5] reported excellent results in 84% of their patients who had ureteric injuries managed by ureteroureterostomy.

Ureteral injuries that are located above the midplane of the pelvis and involve more than 2 cm of the ureter may require mobilization of the ureter and the kidney, interposition of a bowel segment, transureteroureterostomy, or cutaneous ureterostomy. Most surgeons are reticent to use transureteroureterostomy because of the potential compromise of the recipient ureterorenal unit.[6]

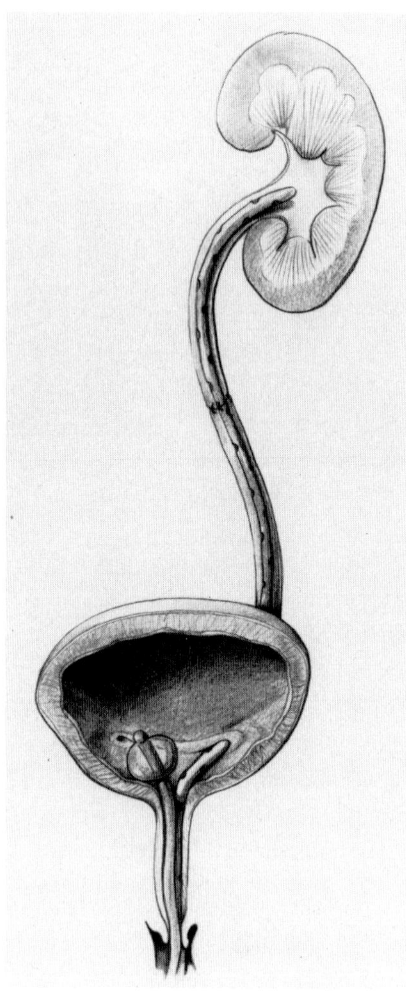

Figure 9-6 Splint in ureter after ureteroureterostomy. *Source*: Reprinted with permission from *Gynecologic Oncology* (1989;34:274–288), Copyright © 1989, Academic Press, Inc.

Injuries to the ureter that are below the midplane of the pelvis and involve less than 2 cm in ureteral length are best repaired by ureteroneocystostomy (Figure 9-7). To perform a ureteroneocystostomy the retropubic space (Retzius space) is dissected, and the bladder is mobilized toward the side of the repair. The distal segment of the ureteral stump is ligated with permanent suture, and the proximal end of the cut ureter is mobilized. A 3- to 4-cm cystotomy is performed in the extraperitoneal portion of the anterior wall of the bladder, and the trigone is identified. A Kelly clamp is introduced into the bladder, and its tips are used to tent the posterior wall of the bladder at the proposed site of ureteral reimplantation. An incision is made between the separated tips of the Kelly clamp, and the ureter is pulled into the bladder by using a traction suture. Spatulation of the tip of the ureter is performed, and four to six interrupted absorbable sutures are used to secure the end of the ureter to the mucosal and mus-

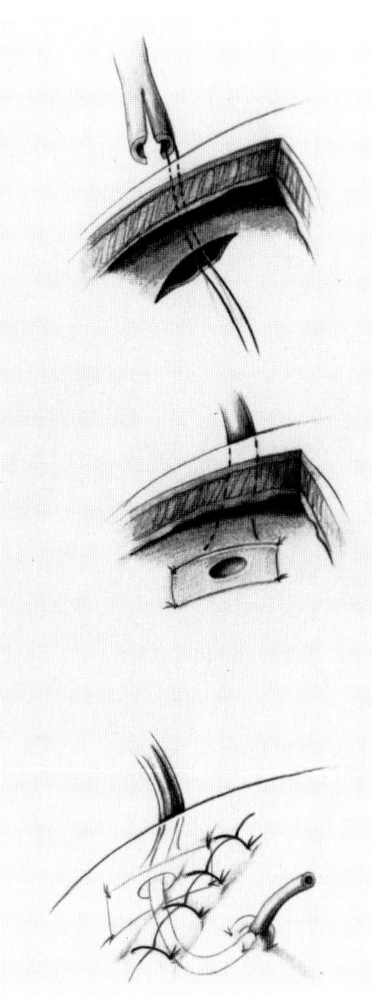

Figure 9-7 Ureteroneocystostomy. *Source*: Reprinted with permission from *Gynecologic Oncology* (1989;34:274–288), Copyright © 1989, Academic Press, Inc.

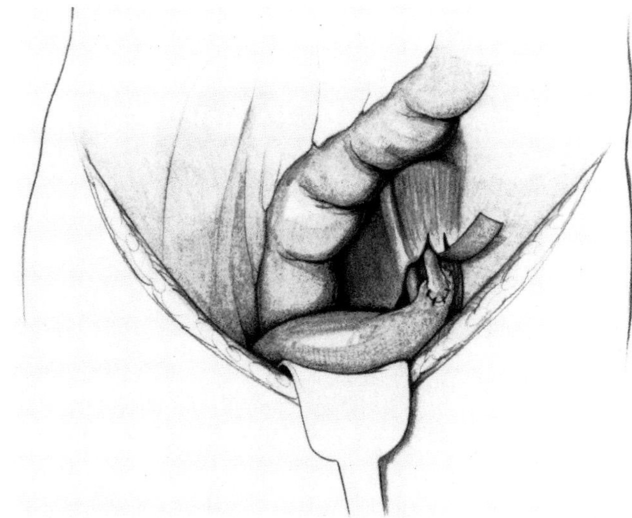

Figure 9-8 Psoas hitch procedure. *Source*: Reprinted with permission from *Gynecologic Oncology* (1989;34:274–288), Copyright © 1989, Academic Press, Inc.

cularis layers of the bladder. Submucosal tunneling, as described by Politano and Leadbetter,[7] is performed whenever possible in an effort to prevent reflux. Landau[8] and Lee and Symmonds,[9] however, have reported good long-term renal and ureteral function in patients having direct ureteral reimplantation without submucosal tunneling. This success is attributed to the fact that the bladder in the adult woman has a low pressure and, consequently, ureteral reflux is not likely to be a problem. If there appears to be tension on a ureteric anastomosis, the bladder should be extended toward the site of the anastomosis by performing a psoas hitch, by creating a Boari or Demel bladder flap, or by performing downward mobilization of the ipsilateral kidney and upper aspect of the ureter. A psoas hitch (Figure 9-8) requires retropubic mobilization of the bladder to allow its superior displacement toward the iliopsoas muscle. The outer bladder wall is anchored to the iliopsoas fascia above the iliac vessels with several interrupted absorbable sutures. It is important to prevent entrapment of the genitofemoral nerve. The Boari and Demel bladder flap procedures are methods of extending the bladder by constructing tubes out of portions of the bladder wall. In each case, the ureter is anastomosed with the most cephalad portion of the bladder. The ureterovesical anastomosis and extraperitoneal perianastomotic drainage techniques are similar to those previously described.

Considerations Related to Delayed (Postoperative) Recognition

Unfortunately, some ureteral injuries are not recognized at the time of surgery. Some become symptomatic in the early postoperative period. Symptoms may include fever, flank pain, and ileus. If ureteral injury is suspected, an IVU should be performed. Cystoscopy with retrograde ureteral catheter placement may be required.

The early postoperative diagnosis of ureteral injury is most often made 7 to 10 days after the operative procedure. At this time, there usually is a hematoma, inflammation, and infection at the site of the injury. Immediate dissection may be difficult and unrewarding. Once the location and the extent of injury have been defined, ureteral stenting or nephrostomy drainage may be of benefit in postponing the need for immediate surgery. Although some investigators advocate the immediate repair of ureteral injuries discovered during the early postoperative period, Dowling and co-workers[10] have documented the benefits of a more conservative approach. In a large proportion of their patients, the use of percutaneous nephrostomy or ureteral stents prevented surgical intervention.

BLADDER INJURY

Wheelock and colleagues[11] reported bladder injuries in 1.8% of abdominal hysterectomies and 0.4% of vaginal hysterectomies. Previous cesarean section, endometriosis, pelvic inflammatory disease, and distortion by tumors complicate bladder dissection and predispose to bladder injury.

Bladder injury occurs most often on opening the parietal peritoneum, during dissection of the bladder from the anterior surface of the cervix and the upper aspect of the vagina, and at the time of closure of the vaginal cuff. It is important to enter the peritoneal cavity in the uppermost portion of any abdominal incision in an attempt to prevent bladder injury. The separation of the posterior wall of the bladder from the cervix should be done with sharp dissection within the relatively avascular space. Excessive bleeding should alert the surgeon to the possibility of bladder injury. Care should be exercised to avoid incorporating any portion of the bladder wall within sutures that are used to secure hemostasis or to suspend or close the vaginal cuff.

If bladder injury is suspected during surgery, filling the bladder through a transurethral catheter with a solution of indigo carmine and sterile normal saline (or sterile infant's formula) will help to identify the site and the extent of injury. It is important to know the location of any injury with respect to the ureteral and the urethral orifices. It may be necessary to place a ureteral catheter in the ureter (or both ureters) to prevent ureteral injury during the repair of nearby bladder injuries.

Bladder defects should be repaired with a double layer of interrupted or running absorbable sutures. The first layer should incorporate the entire thickness of thc bladder wall. The second layer should imbricate the seromuscular layer (Figure 9-9). A suprapubic or transurethral bladder catheter should be used to drain the bladder for 7 to 10 days after the repair.

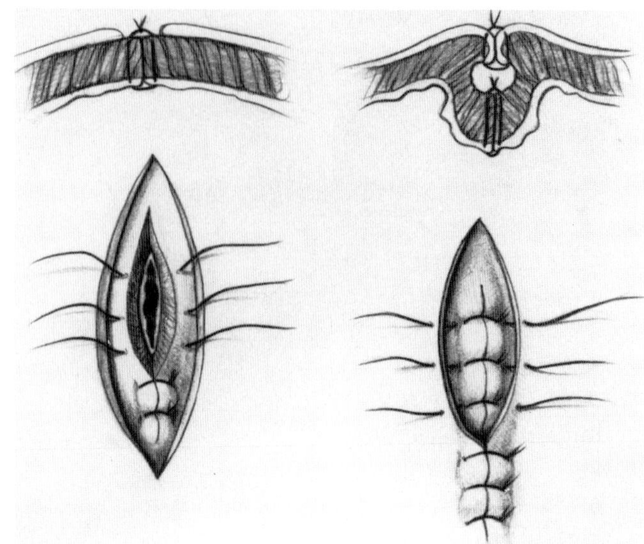

Figure 9-9 Double-layer closure of bladder. *Source*: Reprinted with permission from *Gynecologic Oncology* (1989;34:274–288), Copyright © 1989, Academic Press, Inc.

INJURIES RELATED TO CANCER THERAPY

Urologic injury may occur as a result of cancer therapy. It is most often associated with radical hysterectomy, pelvic exenteration, or radiation therapy. Radical hysterectomy requires the resection of the parametrium and the upper aspect of the vagina. To obtain adequate parametrial margins, the ureter must be dissected from below the pelvic brim to its entrance into the bladder. The ureter's longitudinal blood supply should be protected by making an effort not to damage its adventitial sheath.

The incidence of ureteric fistulas that are the result of radical pelvic surgery has decreased from 20% to less than 1%. Reasons include improved surgical technique with regard to handling of the ureter, hemostasis, irrigation, extraperitoneal drainage, prophylactic antibiotics, and continuous postoperative bladder drainage. Specific measures that have been used to reduce the incidence of ureteral fistulas include suturing the ureters to the obliterated hypogastric arteries,[12] wrapping the ureters within a layer of peritoneum,[13] and using retroperitoneal suction drains.[14] Patients in whom ureterovaginal fistulas dcvelop usually complain of total urinary incontinence, which begins 7 to 10 days after their operative procedure. Initial management of the ureterovaginal fistula should be conservative with either the placement of ureteral stents (retrograde or antegrade) or the use of percutaneous nephrostomy drainage. Spontaneous closure is rare but has been reported. Definitive repair should be delayed for 3 to 4 months. Because the site of the fistula is usually within the distal 4 to 5 cm of the ureter, a bladder extension procedure and ureteroneocystostomy are most often the procedures of choice.

With the decreasing incidence of ureteral fistulas after radical hysterectomy, the most common problem involving the lower urinary tract is neurogenic bladder dysfunction.[15] It is related to the disruption of the bladder's autonomic nerve supply as a result of the wide dissection of the cardinal and the ureterosacral ligaments. Cystometric studies of the bladder have shown hypertonic dysfunction initially with subsequent development of hypotonic dysfunction. Although most patients ultimately achieve a normal voiding pattern, intermittent self-catheterization may be necessary. The use of a routine postoperative IVU to determine the adequacy of ureteral function has been challenged. Larson and coworkers[16] showed an 18% incidence of ureteral dilation after radical hysterectomy when an IVU was performed within 15 days of surgery. Their incidence of ureteral dilation decreased to 5% if IVU was performed 31 to 60 days after surgery. In a study of 233 patients who had undergone radical hysterectomy, the postoperative IVU showed abnormal findings in 6 patients, but all patients were symptomatic and would have required an IVU on the basis of their symptoms.

Improved radiation techniques have decreased the incidence of major urologic and bowel injuries. The bladder and the ureters can tolerate radiation doses that are sufficient to cure most gynecologic cancers. Although cystitis is seen in one third of patients after pelvic radiation therapy, the incidence of major ureteric injuries (ie, obstruction or fistulas) has been reduced to less than 2% to 3%.

When there is a long delay in the development of urinary tract complications after radiation therapy, the complication (no matter what type) is often seen in association with recurrence of the cancer. Krebs and colleagues[17] reported that 83% of recurrent cancers of the cervix occur within 2 years of treatment. Muram and co-workers[18] showed a 78% recurrence within 2 years of treatment. Therefore it is likely that ureteric injuries related to radiation therapy will occur within this period.

Review of the data from the M.D. Anderson Hospital[19] from 1948 to 1964 shows a low incidence of radiation damage to the bladder. Results of this study also confirm that lower urinary tract problems after radiation therapy are usually associated with recurrent cancer.

Vesicovaginal fistulas that occur after radiation therapy are managed differently from those that develop in the absence of radiation therapy. Radiation therapy causes an obliterative endarteritis that permanently affects the blood supply to all radiated tissues. When a vesicovaginal fistula occurs in an area of radiated tissue, it may be necessary to delay definitive repair for up to 12 months, so that the likelihood of cure is improved. The repair of a vesicovaginal fistula that occurs in previously radiated tissue cannot be reliably performed by using a simple layered closure. The closure should include an attempt to provide a fresh blood supply to the site of the repair. Several techniques have been described to repair radiation-induced fistulas. They include use of the omentum (Figure 9-10),[20] bulbocavernosus fat pad,[21] and gracilis myocutaneous flaps,[22] as well as, when the situation warrants, urinary diversion.

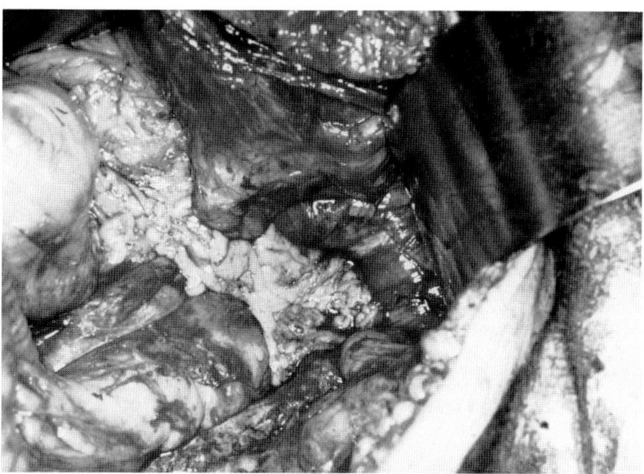

Figure 9-10 Omental flap for closure of radiated vesicovaginal fistula. *Source*: Reprinted with permission from *Gynecologic Oncology* (1989; 34:274–288), Copyright © 1989, Academic Press, Inc.

Urologic complications that occur after pelvic exenteration usually are the result of urinary diversion. (See Chapter 11.) These complications include hydronephrosis, anastomotic stenoses, and urinary leaks. The incidence of a urinary leak from a conduit is between 5% and 22%.[23] A conservative approach to these leaks is recommended because the mortality reported in the surgical literature is 30% to 50%.[24] Continent urinary diversion techniques[25] are being used. When a urinary diversion has been performed, postoperative management should include periodic IVU and retrograde dye studies.

REFERENCES

1. Halloway HJ. Injury to the urinary tract as a complication of gynecologic surgery. *Am J Obstet Gynecol.* 1950;60:30–40.
2. Mann WJ, Arato M, Patsner B, Stone M. Ureteral injuries in an obstetrics and gynecology training program: etiology and management. *Obstet Gynecol.* 1988;72:82–85.
3. Piscatelli JT, Simel DL, Addison WA. Who should have intravenous pyelograms before hysterectomy for benign disease? *Obstet Gynecol.* 1987;69:541–545.
4. Symmonds RE. Ureteral injuries associated with gynecological surgery: prevention and management. *Clin Obstet Gynecol.* 1976;19:623–644.
5. Carlton CE Jr, Scott R Jr, Guthrie AG. The initial management of ureteral injuries: a report of 78 cases. *J Urol.* 1971;105:335–340.

6. Sandoz IL, Paul DP, Macfarlane CA. Complications with transureteroureterostomy. *J Urol.* 1977;117:39–42.

7. Politano VA, Leadbetter WF. An operative technique for the correction of vesicoureteral reflux. *J Urol.* 1958;79:932–941.

8. Landau SJ. Ureteroneocystostomy: a review of 72 cases with a comparison of two techniques. *J Urol.* 1962;87:343–349.

9. Lee RA, Symmonds RE. Ureterovaginal fistula. *Am J Obstet Gynecol.* 1971;109:1032–1035.

10. Dowling RA, Corrieve JN, Sandler CM. Iatrogenic ureteral injury. *J Urol.* 1986;135:912–915.

11. Wheelock JB, Krebs H-B, Hurt WG. Sparing and repairing the bladder during gyn surgery. *Contemp Ob Gyn.* June 1984: 163–171.

12. Green TH Jr. Ureteral suspension for prevention of ureteral complications following radical Wertheim hysterectomy. *Obstet Gynecol.* 1966;28:1–11.

13. Novak F. *Surg. Gynecol. Tech.* Padova, Italy: Piccin Editore; New York: John Wiley & Sons, Inc; 1978.

14. Boronow RC, Rutledge F. Vesicovaginal fistula, radiation, in gynecologic cancer. *Am J Obstet Gynecol.* 1971;111:85–90.

15. Christ F, Wagner U, Debus G. Early bladder function disorders following Wertheim surgery. Causes and therapeutic consequences. *Geburtshilfe Frauenheilkd.* 1983;43:380–383.

16. Larson DM, Malone JM, Copeland LJ, et al. Ureteral assessment after radical hysterectomy. *Obstet Gynecol.* 1987;69:612–616.

17. Krebs HB, Helmkamp BF, Sevin B-U, Nadji M, Averette HE. Recurrent cancer of the cervix following radical hysterectomy and pelvic node dissection. *Obstet Gynecol.* 1982;59:422–427.

18. Muram D, Curry RH, Drouin P. Cytologic follow-up of patients with invasive cervical carcinoma treated by radiotherapy. *Am J Obstet Gynecol.* 1982;142:350–354.

19. Buchler DA, Kline JC, Peckham BM, Boone MLM, Carr WF. Radiation reactions in cervical cancer therapy. *Am J Obstet Gynecol.* 1971;111:745–750.

20. Kiricuta I, Goldstein AMB. The repair of extensive vesicovaginal fistulas with pedicled omentum: a review of 27 cases. *J Urol.* 1972;108:724–727.

21. Patil U, Waterhouse K, Laungani G. Management of 18 difficult vesicovaginal and vaginal fistulas with modified Ingelman-Sundberg and Martius operations. *J Urol.* 1980;123:653.

22. Becker DW Jr, Massey FM, McCraw JB. Musculocutaneous flaps in reconstructive pelvic surgery. *Obstet Gynecol.* 1979; 54:178–183.

23. Morley GW, Lindenauer SM. Pelvic exenterative therapy for gynecologic malignancy: an analysis of 70 cases. *Cancer.* 1976;38:581–586.

24. Orr JW Jr, Shingleton HM, Hatch KD, et al. Urinary diversion in patients undergoing pelvic exenteration. *Am J Obstet Gynecol.* 1982;42:883–889.

25. Penalver MA, Darwich EB, Averette HE, Donato DM, Sevin B-U, Suarez G. Continent urinary diversion in gynecologic oncology. *Gynecol Oncol.* 1989;34:274–288.

10

Urinary Drainage Devices

W. Glenn Hurt

In 2600 B.C. the Egyptians selected reeds from the Nile to be used as bladder catheters. Catheters were also fashioned from straws, curled-up palm leaves, and dried onion leaves. It is likely that earlier the Sumerians made gold malleable catheters; the Romans made sturdy bronze, flexible lead, and smooth ceramic catheters.[1,2] Despite the long history of bladder catheterization, manufacturers are still in search of the ideal catheter material, which must be evaluated on its strength, flexibility, elongation capacity, surface friction coefficient, memory, biocompatibility, and biodurability.[3]

Ureteral catheters in use now are usually made of polyurethane, silicone, or one of the proprietary products C-Flex (Concept Polymer Technologies, Clearwater, Fla.) or Silitek (Medical Engineering Corporation, Racine, Wis.).[3] Bladder catheters are commonly made of red rubber, latex, or silicone. Catheters are usually coated with polytetrafluoroethylene (Teflon), silicone elastomers, or hydrophilic polymers to protect against mucosal irritation, minimize encrustation and stone formation, and enhance patient comfort.

The design of a catheter depends on its intended purpose. Variables include catheter size, tip configuration, size and shape of balloons, number of channels, length, end connections, and access ports.

URETERAL CATHETERS

In 1875, Gustav Simon, of Heidelberg, Germany, was the first to advocate ureteral catheterization.[2] He performed the procedure by introducing a finger through the urethra to guide a hollow probe up a ureter. About 1900, Joaquin Albarran, a Cuban surgeon working in Paris, France, is thought to have designed and been responsible for the manufacture of the first commercially available ureteral catheter.[3]

In 1967, Zimskind and co-workers[4] revolutionized ureteral catheters by introducing a silicone rubber ureteral catheter that could be introduced cystoscopically. In that same year, Gibbons modified the silicone ureteral catheter by the addition of multiple barbs and a distal flange in an effort to limit its migration.[5] Subsequently, a "J" configuration was added to each end of the silicone catheters; and, in 1978, Finney and Hepperlen and colleagues described the "double-J stent."[5]

Ureteral catheter placement can help normalize renal function, assist in ureteral healing, and prevent ureteral stenosis and kinking. Ureteral catheters also can be of help in identifying the ureters during surgery. Indications for the use of ureteral catheters are listed in Table 10-1.

Table 10-1 Indications for Ureteral Catheters

Ureteral Trauma
Ureteral Surgery
Ureteral Obstruction
Ureteral Fistulas
Urinary Diversion
Ureteral Identification during Surgery

It is imperative to select a ureteral catheter of appropriate length for optimal function and patient comfort. The length can be determined by taking measurements from an intravenous urogram or retrograde pyelogram. If the catheter has coiled ends, the full coil should remain outside both ends of the ureter and should not rest on the trigone.

Patients are often uncomfortable as a result of having an indwelling ureteral catheter. They complain of urinary frequency, nocturia, hematuria, flank pain, suprapubic pain, and dysuria. There appears to be no significant difference in the frequency of these complaints among the commonly used ureteral catheters. Fortunately, these complaints usually disappear within 3 or 4 days after the catheter is removed.

Significant complications may occur with long-term use of indwelling ureteral catheters. They include catheter migration, vesicoureteral reflux, catheter encrustation and stone formation, and ureteral necrosis and fistularization. Catheter migration may occur in either direction. It is more likely to occur with the softer silicone catheter than with the stiffer polyurethane catheter. Full coils on either end of the catheter are less likely to allow migration than is the J configuration. Migration is more often a problem with ureteral catheters that are placed during surgery, because correct placement is facilitated when the catheter is inserted with the aid of fluoroscopy.

Patients with indwelling ureteral catheters should have periodic urine cultures. Asymptomatic bacteriuria does not require treatment. Patients with symptomatic urinary tract or systemic infections should be given appropriate antibiotic therapy.

BLADDER DRAINAGE

Suprapubic Catheters

In 1556, Pierre Franco, of Lausanne, Switzerland, was the first to publish an account of having performed a suprapubic cystotomy.[6] The procedure became more popular after the English anatomist and surgeon, John Hunter, showed that distention of the bladder raises its peritoneal reflection out the pelvis and permits direct, rather than transperitoneal, bladder entry.[2] Gynecologists have used the technique more frequently since 1966, when Hodgkinson and Hodari[7] reported their favorable experience with the use of trocar cystotomy for suprapubic catheter placement as a preferred method of postoperative bladder drainage.

Table 10-2 Advantages of Suprapubic over Transurethral Postoperative Bladder Drainage

Increases patient comfort and convenience.
Requires less nursing care and catheter maintenance.
Assists early ambulation.
Decreases incidence of urinary tract infections.
Does not cause urethritis.
Promotes earlier return of efficient voiding.
Facilitates voiding trials and urinary residual determinations.
Enables patients to participate in catheter care and voiding trials.
Facilitates earlier discharge from hospital.

Advantages of postoperative suprapubic bladder drainage as compared to transurethral bladder drainage are listed in Table 10-2.

Complications of suprapubic bladder drainage include hematuria; wound infection; urinary tract infection; bladder or bowel perforation; and catheter malfunction related to obstruction with blood or debris, displacement, kinking, or fracture. Persons performing needle or trocar cystotomies should prevent bladder and bowel injuries by being aware of Hodgkinson's Ten Commandments for suprapubic bladder catheter insertion (Table 10-3).

Table 10-3 Hodgkinson's Ten Commandments for Instituting Suprapubic Trocar or Needle Bladder Catheter Drainage

1. Always distend bladder to 400 cc.
2. Puncture site should not be more than 3 cm above pubic symphysis.
3. Never insert trocar in vertical direction.
4. Always direct trocar 30° toward bladder.
5. If in doubt, insert needle first for orientation.
6. Watch depth of trocar insertion.
7. Too much pressure on trocar may lead to bladder base damage.
8. Do not let bladder fluid escape before inserting catheter.
9. Be aware of prior abdominal incision as bladder or bowel may be adherent beneath incision.
10. Trocar may be a lethal weapon. Be careful!

Source: Reprinted with permission from *American Journal of Obstetrics and Gynecology* (1969;105:62), Copyright © 1969, CV Mosby Company.

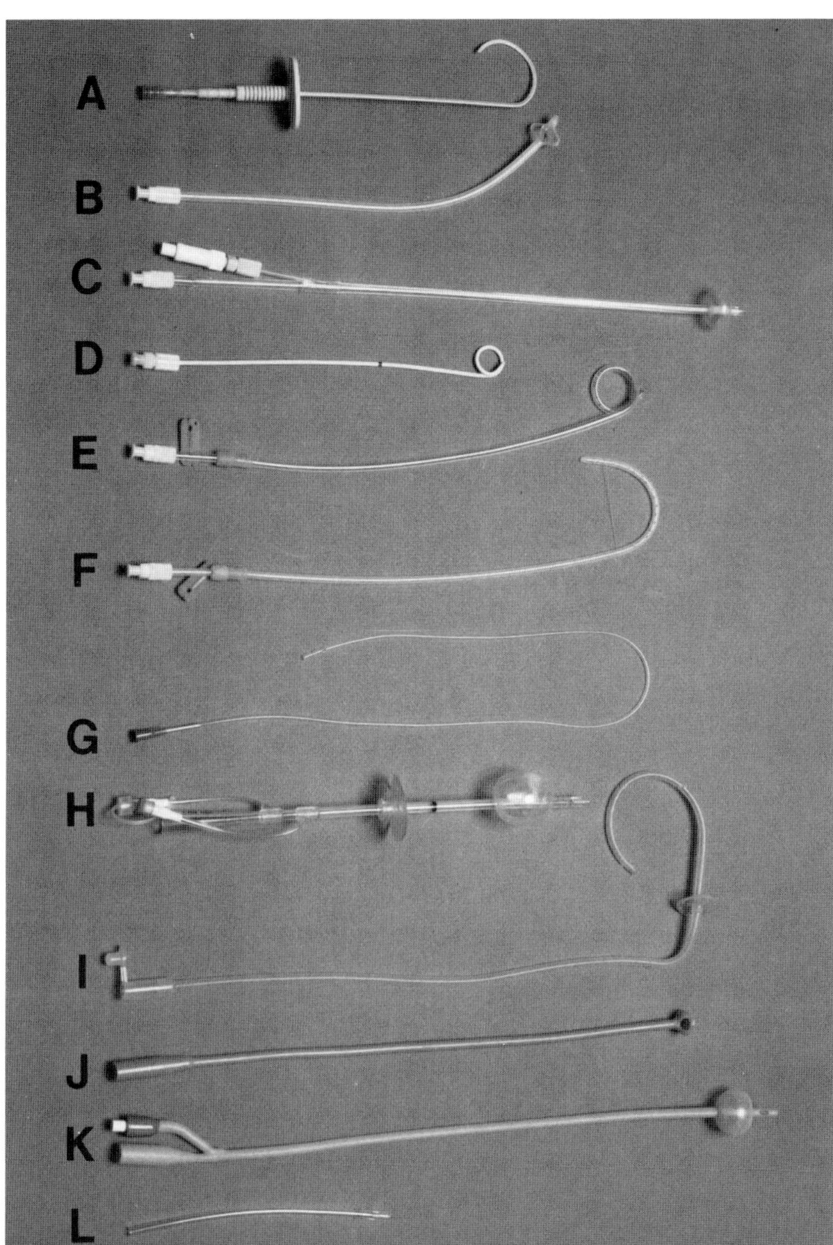

Figure 10-1 Bladder drainage catheters. Suprapubic bladder drainage catheters: **A**, Bonanno, 7F (Becton Dickinson, Rutherford, NJ); **B**, Stamey-Malecot, 12F or 14F; **C**, Rutner balloon, 16F; **D**, Pigtail, 7F; **E**, Sof-flex loop, 14F; **F**, Stamey loop, 12F (B–F Cook Urological Inc, Spencer, Ind); **G**, Cystocath, 8F (Dow Corning Corp, Midland, Mich); **H**, Argyle-Ingram, 12F or 16F (Sherwood Medical Co, St Louis, Mo); **I**, Robertson, 15F (Mentor Corp, Goleta, Calif); **J**, Malecot; **K**, Foley. **L**, Urethral self-catheterization catheter (Mentor Corp, Goleta, Calif or Rusch, Duluth, Ga).

Many prepackaged, commercially available suprapubic bladder drainage devices are available (Figure 10-1). Bard Urological (CR Bard, Covington, Ga.) markets a suprapubic introducer/Foley catheter set complete with stylet and urine collection bag (Figure 10-2). As an alternative, a standard Foley or Malecot catheter may be used for suprapubic bladder drainage either with suprapubic trocar (eg, Ansari or Counsellor) placement or transurethral suprapubic puncture using a fenestrated male urethral sound, uterine packing forceps, or the Robertson catheter introducer (Mentor Corporation, Goleta, Calif.) to draw the catheter into the bladder cavity.

Small lumen suprapubic catheters (<10F to 12F) are satisfactory when the urine is clear. Larger lumen suprapubic catheters (>14F to 16F) are less likely to become obstructed when the bladder contains a significant amount of blood or cellular debris. All catheters should be secured to the skin in a manner that will prevent kinking or displacement.

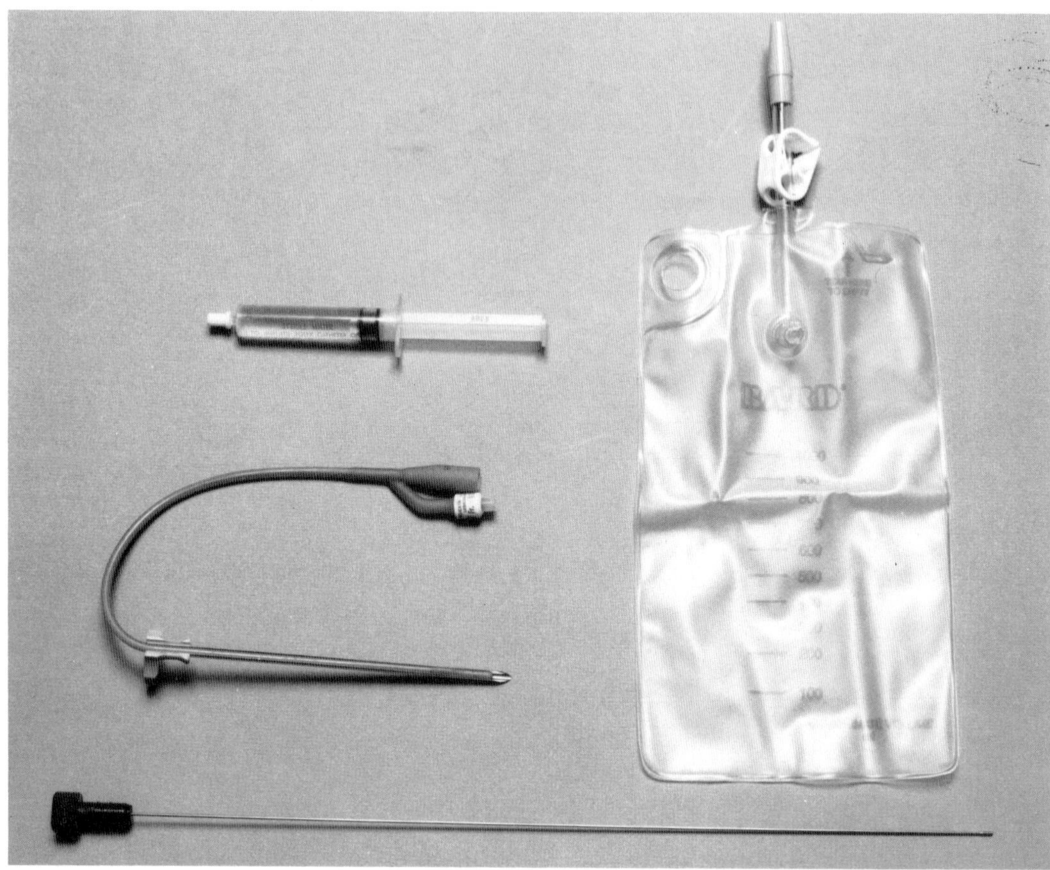

Figure 10-2 Suprapubic introducer/Foley catheter set containing 12F Foley catheter, catheter stylet, syringe for inflation of catheter balloon, and urine collection bag. *Source*: Courtesy of Bard Urological Division, CR Bard Inc, Covington, Ga.

Transurethral Catheters

Goodyear developed the vulcanization process in 1844; about 10 years later, Auguste Nelaton, of Paris, France, introduced the first red rubber catheter. It was made to function as an indwelling catheter by sewing its tubing to the external urethral meatus. Self-retaining urethral catheters did not become practical until Malecot introduced his four-winged catheter in 1892, and Frederic Foley, of St. Paul, Minnesota, introduced his balloon catheter in 1927.[2]

Indwelling urethral catheters in use now are usually made of coated latex or silicone. In women, a 14F or 16F transurethral Foley catheter with a 5 to 10 mL balloon should be adequate for bladder drainage. Larger caliber catheters are likely to damage the urethral mucosa, prevent drainage of the periurethral glands, and interfere with the urethral and periurethral blood supply. Larger balloons increase the urinary residual and cause more urothelial damage. The size of a catheter should not be increased merely to prevent urine from leaking about the catheter.

In 1970, the O'Learys recommended transurethral pediatric feeding tube placement as a method of continuous postoperative bladder drainage.[8] One end of the feeding tube is placed transurethrally into the bladder and the tube is held in place by suturing or taping it to the periurethral skin. The external end of the feeding tube is attached to a urinary collection system. When voiding trials are started, the feeding tube is occluded and the patient is expected to void around the feeding tube. After voiding, the feeding tube can be unclamped to drain the bladder and determine the urinary residual.

In 1972, Lapides and colleagues introduced the concept of clean intermittent self-catheterization.[9] It may be performed by using standard straight catheters or those specifically designed for the purpose (see Figure 10-1). The catheters may be cleaned and reused; they need not be sterilized. Infection is rarely a problem unless there is gross contamination or urothelial damage. Ideally, all patients who are expected to require a significant period of postoperative bladder drainage should be taught self-catheterization. (Resource materials available for this purpose include "Guide to Clean Intermittent Catheterization," Mentor Corporation, Goleta, CA 93117; "Intermittent Self-Catheterization," Eastern Paralyzed Veterans Association, 432 Park Avenue South, New York, NY 10016; "Clean, Intermittent Self-Catheterization for Women," Sacred Heart Medical Center, P.O. Box 45132, Cleveland, OH 44145.)

Complications of transurethral bladder drainage include urinary tract infection, trauma to the urethra and the bladder, and catheter malfunction. In patients treated for gynecologic problems, most hospital-acquired infections involve the urinary tract. Most of these are a result of bladder catheterization. They are responsible for significant postoperative morbidity and are a cause of prolonged hospitalization.

In catheterized patients, the primary sources of contamination are the urethra, the vaginal vestibule, or the catheter drainage and collection system. There is also the possibility of contamination by irrigations, instrumentation, and medical personnel. The incidence of catheter-associated urinary tract infections can be reduced by avoiding unnecessary catheterization, training personnel regarding catheterization and the management of closed drainage systems, and removing indwelling catheters promptly. As long as an indwelling catheter is in place, the patient is likely to have a contaminated urinary tract. Emphasis should not be on antibiotic prophylaxis during the period of catheterization but on catheter removal and subsequent eradication of any urinary tract infection.

Catheter-associated urethral and bladder trauma can be reduced if the catheter size is kept small and the catheter is secured to the patient in a manner that will prevent the catheter from pulling against the neck of the bladder. Catheter maintenance requires careful attention to maintaining a patent, closed drainage system, the contents of which do not become contaminated and do not reflux into the bladder. Periodic urine cultures can be used to determine colonization, but antibiotic treatment is usually not indicated unless the patient becomes symptomatic.

Philosophy of Postoperative Bladder Drainage

It is better to avoid bladder catheter drainage if possible. Any bladder catheter will be uncomfortable, restrict ambulation, and increase the risk of infection. If a limited number of straight, intermittent catheterizations will enable the patient to begin voiding efficiently, that procedure is preferable to inserting an indwelling suprapubic or transurethral catheter. There will always be indications for continuous bladder drainage (Table 10-4), however, and it is up to the physician to determine the method to use.

Under essentially the same circumstances, when there is a need for continuous bladder drainage, there are some physicians who advocate suprapubic bladder drainage and some who advocate transurethral bladder drainage. The choice usually is based on one's experience.

I choose the method of continuous bladder drainage by estimating the anticipated period of drainage. If the patient will require bladder drainage for less than 48 to 72 hours, I am likely to insert a 14F or 16F transurethral Foley catheter. If a longer period of bladder drainage is necessary, I favor insertion of a suprapubic catheter. Patients who have continence surgery and need continuous bladder drainage will most likely have a suprapubic catheter. Such catheters are preferred for use in this particular group of patients because they facilitate voiding trials and urinary residual measurement. Also, they are easily managed by the patient who may have been discharged from the hospital or ambulatory surgery facility with the catheter in place.

Continuous bladder drainage after certain surgical procedures will promote healing and hasten the return of normal bladder function. Although the period of bladder drainage may be a matter of controversy, the objectives should be to promote healing of all incisions and to prevent overdistention of the bladder. A single episode of overdistention of the bladder not only stresses existing suture lines, but also predisposes the patient to urinary tract infection and often delays the return to efficient emptying of the bladder.

Table 10-4 Indications for Continuous Bladder Drainage

Aid in Surgery
Promotion of Healing
- After surgery
- In presence of bladder or urethral injury

Urinary Retention
- Acute
- Chronic

Urinary Diversion
- After surgery
- In presence of
  - intractable incontinence
  - neuropathic bladder dysfunction
  - vulvovaginitis

Urinary Output Monitoring

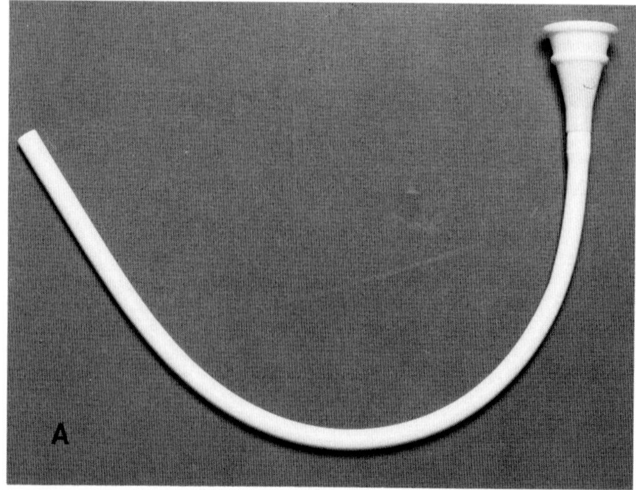

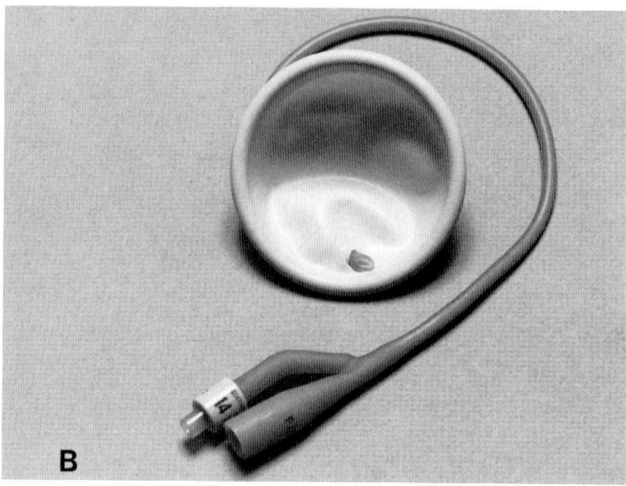

Figure 10-3 **A**, Vaginal urinary drainage device (Urocup, Product No 4300, Urocare Products, Pomona, Calif); **B**, Vaginal urinary drainage device fashioned from contraceptive diaphragm and Foley catheter.

VAGINAL URINARY DRAINAGE

Vaginal urinary drainage is useful in some patients who have genitourinary fistulas. A commercially available drainage device is shown in Figure 10-3A. It is designed to be placed within the vagina and connected to a leg-bag drainage system. A similar vaginal urinary drainage device can be constructed by using a contraceptive diaphragm and urethral catheter (Figure 10-3B).[10]

REFERENCES

1. Ingram JM. Postoperative bladder drainage. In: Buchsbaum HJ, Schmidt JD, eds. *Gynecologic and Obstetric Urology*. 1st ed. Philadelphia: WB Saunders Co; 1978:150.
2. Herman JR. *Urology: A View through the Retrospectroscope*. New York: Harper & Row; 1973:35–40.
3. Mardis HK, Kroeger RM. Ureteral stents: materials. *Urol Clin North Am*. 1988;15:471–479.
4. Zimskind PD, Fetter TR, Wilkerson JL. Clinical use of long-term indwelling silicone rubber ureteral splints injected cystoscopically. *J Urol*. 1967;97:840–844.
5. Saltzman B. Ureteral stents: indications, variations, and complications. *Urol Clin North Am*. 1988;15:481–491.
6. Cumston CG. *Trans Am Urol Assoc*. 1912;6:305–337.
7. Hodgkinson CP, Hodari AA. Trocar suprapubic cystostomy for postoperative bladder drainage in the female. *Am J Obstet Gynecol*. 1966;96:773–781.
8. O'Leary JL, O'Leary JA. The mini-catheter: a reliable indwelling catheter substitute. *Obstet Gynecol*. 1970;36:141–143.
9. Lapides J, Diokno AC, Silber SJ, Lowe BS. Clean intermittent self-catheterization in the treatment of urinary tract disease. *J Urol*. 1972;107:458–461.
10. Banfield PJ, Scott G, Roberts HRM. A modified contraceptive diaphragm for relief of uretero-vaginal fistula. Case report. *Br J Obstet Gynaecol*. 1991;98:101–102.

11

Urinary Diversions

Hugh M. Shingleton and Manuel A. Penalver

Urinary diversion in patients with gynecologic disorders is indicated primarily when excision of the bladder becomes necessary as part of treatment for cancer of the cervix or the vagina. Diversion in women may also be necessary in managing urinary fistulas or relieving ureteral obstruction related to radiation for pelvic tumors. Familiarity with such procedures is essential for gynecologic oncologists and other pelvic surgeons who deal constantly with treatment, treatment effects, and management of complications of genital tract malignancies. In this chapter, we discuss the development of diversionary operations; specific indications and complications for such operations; and techniques of performing the procedures we use.

HISTORICAL PERSPECTIVES

Evolution of Diversion

Developing a suitable substitute for the excised urinary bladder has challenged surgeons for more than a century. The first attempt at diversion was made by Simon,[1] in 1852, in a patient with exstrophy of the bladder; the ureters were implanted into the rectum. After a temporary period of success, the patient died as a consequence of the surgery. This major procedure occurred during the first decade of use of general anesthesia and long before the availability of antibiotics for the inevitable septic consequences. Thus the result is not surprising.

Verhoogen (with de Graeuve),[2] in 1909, was the first to suggest the use of an isolated segment of ileum and ascending colon as a urinary conduit, but the high mortality of major abdominal operations remained a barrier to widespread application. Between 1920 and 1950, the placement of the ureters into the intact sigmoid colon was widely practiced, and Gilchrist and associates,[3] in 1950, reported on the use of ileocolonic segments as bladder substitutes. Ileocolonic conduits, however, failed to ensure continence. Also, reports of hyperchloremic acidosis in up to 70% of patients who had undergone ureterosigmoidostomy,[4] along with reports of ascending infection, rapid deterioration of renal function, and hydronephrosis related to stricturing at the ureteral colonic anastomosis, placed a damper on that operation. The ileal conduit diversion, developed by Bricker in the 1940s and first reported in 1950,[5] offered an attractive alternative (Figures 11-1 and 11-2). Use of isolated segments of colon was advocated by other surgeons. Symmonds and Gibbs[6] pointed out the desirability of using the terminal end of the sigmoid colon during total exenterations to avoid the need for a small bowel anastomosis. This approach resulted in less operating time and less postoperative morbidity, and such segments functioned as well in other respects as did the

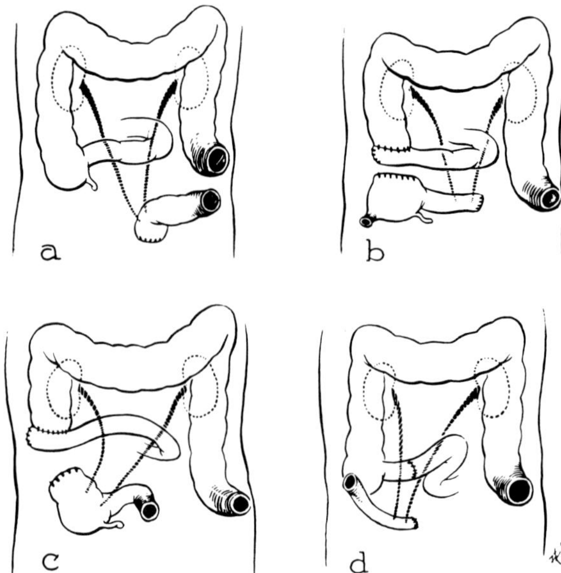

Figure 11-1 Early diversions, as described by Bricker[5]: *a*, Bilateral ureteral anastomosis to an isolated segment of sigmoid colon as practiced in 1940. This procedure places the external stoma of the urinary pouch inconveniently near the colostomy stoma. *b*, Anastomosis of the ureters to the terminal ileum with use of the cecum as a reservoir and drainage of the urine through a cecostomy opening. *c*, Anastomosis of the ureters directly to the cecum and use of the terminal ileum as a tract for drainage of the urine to the outside. Both *b* and *c* have functioned quite satisfactorily, but since one is unable to make these pouches continent it seemed useless to include the cecum and ascending colon in the isolated segment. *d*, Anastomosis of the ureters to an isolated segment of terminal ileum. This appears to be the simplest way to convey the urine from both kidneys to an external stoma. *Source*: Reprinted with permission from *Surgical Clinics of North America* (1950;30:1511), Copyright © 1950, WB Saunders Company.

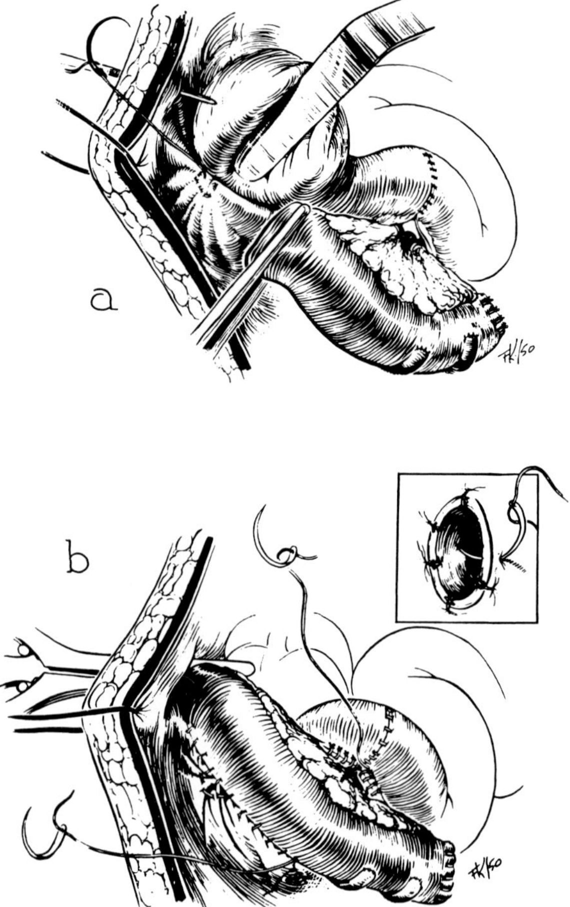

Figure 11-2 Construction of the Bricker pouch as first described. Modifications have occurred, including use of ureteral stents in anastomosis of ureters and irradiated bowel segments, and a raised stoma for ease of appliance use (see Figure 11-7). *Source*: Reprinted with permission from *Surgical Clinics of North America* (1950;30:1511), Copyright © 1950, WB Saunders Company.

ileal conduits. Postoperative conduit leaks and fistulas were associated primarily with the use of irradiated segments of bowel, and these complications emphasized the need for the use of nonirradiated transverse colon segments[7] (Figure 11-3).

Considerations in the choice of an appropriate bowel segment for urinary diversion (Table 11-1) include a history of abdominal or pelvic irradiation, presence of bowel or pelvic adhesive disease, mobility of intestinal segments, ureteral length, plans for partial versus total exenteration, and need for the pelvic sigmoid segment for pelvic closure or vaginal reconstruction.

Evolution of Continent Conduits

In 1978, Kock and associates[8] introduced the continent ileal pouch. They found that an intestinal segment prepared as a reservoir with interruption of the circular muscle fibers accommodates larger urine volumes at lower pressures than a tubular intestinal segment. This principle of detubularization of bowel is central to the issue of continent diversion. The Kock pouch used the principle of intussuscepted nipple valves in an attempt to prevent reflux and to ensure continence. To date, however, the construction of an effective valve that uniformly guarantees lasting urinary continence is far from easy.

The Indiana continent colonic urinary reservoir, created in 1982, was introduced as a simple and relatively reliable pouch to construct. The continence mechanism was achieved by plicating the terminal segment of the ileum and implanting the ureters in a tunneled fashion along the tenia. Daytime continence was achieved in 93% of cases and nocturnal continence in 76%, after a mean follow-up of 14 months.[9]

Thüroff and colleagues,[10] in 1986, described the Mainz pouch, a low-pressure reservoir created from ascending colon, cecum, and two ileal loops. Continence was achieved by accomplishing an isoperistaltic intussusception of the distal segment of the ileum, as

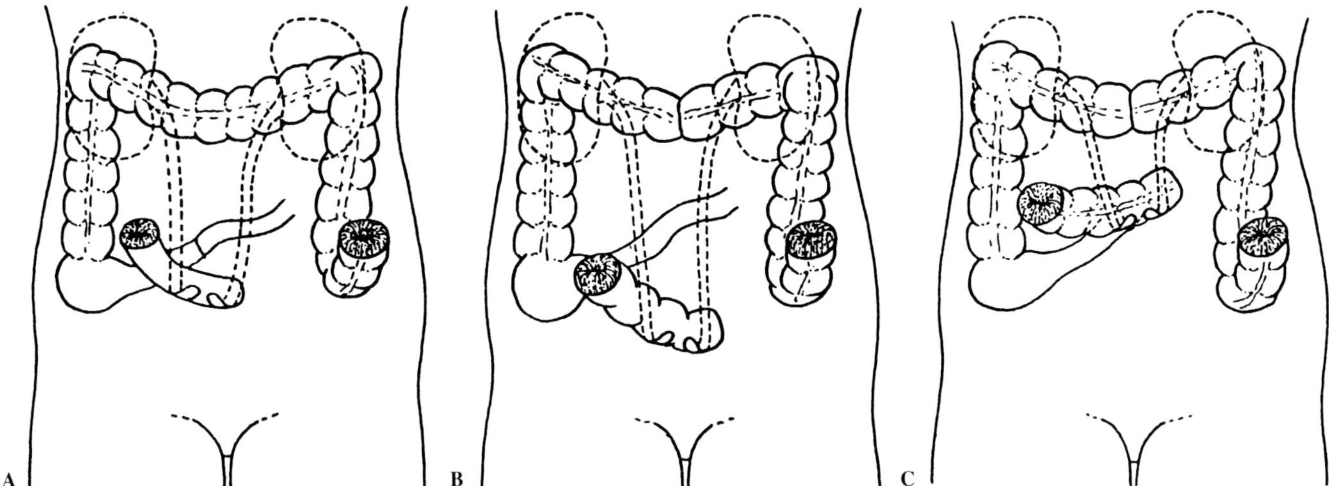

Figure 11-3 The most commonly used methods of supravesical urinary diversion by gynecologic oncologists. (**A**) Ileal conduit, (**B**) sigmoid conduit, and (**C**) transverse colon conduit. *Source*: Reprinted with permission from *Contemporary Ob-Gyn* (1983;22:253–257), Copyright © 1983, Medical Economics Company, Inc.

described by Mansson and co-workers.[11] Ureteral implantation was performed in a nonrefluxing submucosal tunneled technique into the cecum or the ascending colon.

In 1986, Lockhart and Bejany[12] presented the remodeled right colonic segment as an alternative urinary reservoir. The pouch consisted of the terminal ileum, the ascending colon, and the right third of the transverse colon. Continence was achieved by performing a double row plication of the distal segment of the ileum, a modification of the plication technique described by Rowland and associates.[9] Reimplantation of the ureters was done by means of the transcolonic technique of Goodwin and co-workers[13] or the nontunneled modified technique. A later modification that included reinforcing the ileocecal valve with imbricating sutures improved the continence rate.

The Miami pouch was developed by Bejany and Politano,[14] and reported in 1988. The intention of the pouch was to improve the rate of urinary continence, allowing for both increased flexibility in reimplantation of the ureters and an adequate storage system. The alternative to the intussuscepted segment to prevent ureteral reflux was a nontunneled ureterocolonic anastomosis. Continence was achieved by reinforcing the ileocecal segment with three circumferential silk sutures, placed in a purse-string fashion, and tapering the distal segment of the ileum over a 14F catheter.

INDICATIONS AND CHOICE OF PROCEDURE

Indications for urinary diversion in patients with gynecologic disorders vary (Table 11-2). Most urinary diversion procedures are performed in conjunction with operations for recurrent cervical cancer or complications of pelvic radiotherapy. In some cases, women with persistent cancer and acute ureteral obstruction, who otherwise are in good condition, may benefit from per-

Table 11-1 Advantages and Disadvantages of Intestinal Segment Use

Segment	*Advantages*	*Disadvantages*
Ileum	Metabolic complications rare Easy to construct	In radiation field Small bowel* anastomosis required Ureterointestinal anastomosis in pelvis* Stomal stenosis Antireflex anastomosis not possible
Sigmoid colon	Bowel anastomosis avoided Few stomal complications Amenable to antireflex anastomosis	In pelvic radiation field Metabolic complications not uncommon Ureterointestinal anastomosis in pelvis*
Transverse colon	Outside radiation field Metabolic complications rare Ureteral anastomosis not in pelvis* Few stomal complications Amenable to antireflex anastomosis	Large bowel anastomosis required

*During exenterative operations.

Table 11-2 Indications for Urinary Diversion in Patients with Gynecologic Disorders

In Conjunction with Cancer
Pelvic exenteration
Ureteral obstruction*
Complications of Radiotherapy
Bilateral ureteral obstruction
Irreparable vesicovaginal fistula
Severe bladder fibrosis with incontinence
Radiation cystitis (severe)
Urinary Incontinence (Severe)
"Pipestem" urethra
Failed fistula repair*

*Refer to text for full discussion.

cutaneous nephrostomy. In others, particularly after multiple operations for urinary incontinence, supravesical diversion might be considered if severe incontinence persists. This latter approach may also be appropriate in women who have experienced failure with multiple bladder fistula repairs. In most of the gynecologic literature, however, urinary diversion is described as a component of pelvic exenterative operations. The next most common indication relates to bilateral ureteral obstruction, vesicovaginal fistulas, or severe bladder damage as a result of pelvic radiation therapy. Apparently, therefore, most urinary diversions in gynecology are performed in women who have had pelvic irradiation, a major contributor to intraoperative and postoperative morbidity and mortality. In contrast, the urologic and surgical literature primarily addresses urinary diversion in nonirradiated persons, both adults and children.

Several considerations are pertinent to urinary diversion (Table 11-3). If the procedure is indicated in conjunction with cancer, one must determine whether the intent of the surgery is curative or palliative. If the latter, whether the patient is likely to have a sufficient number of months of good quality life remaining to justify a major operation of this type is a factor. The length of the particular operation chosen and the expected morbidity of that surgery must be weighed. The patient's age, medical condition, and ability to comprehend the change in body function and body image are relevant. Her psychologic status in relation to her ability to care for herself in the changed state must be evaluated. In addition to these factors, one must select a particular procedure, plan stomal construction and location, determine the method of ureteral anastomosis, select a proper bowel segment, and consider the use of gastrointestinal stapling instruments as a timesaver during the surgery.

Table 11-3 Considerations Pertinent to Urinary Diversion

Curative versus Palliative Intent
Life expectancy
Prior Radiation Therapy
Length of Required Operation
Expected morbidity
Patient Factors
Age
Medical condition
Ability for self-care
• Comprehension
• Psychologic status
Technical Factors
Selection of procedure
Selection of bowel segment
Stomal construction and location
Method of ureteral anastomosis
Use of stapling instruments

In some situations, temporary measures such as percutaneous nephrostomy are applicable (Table 11-4). Percutaneous nephrostomy may be of special use in persons with cancer and ureteral obstruction who are undergoing (or plan to undergo) pelvic irradiation or chemotherapy as treatment. The tumor shrinkage subsequent to the therapy may allow the urinary tract to return to a more normal condition thereafter. If permanent diversion is needed, however, one might select a urinary conduit. In the absence of a history of pelvic irradiation, ileal conduits retain their popularity for diversion in adults. In conjunction with pelvic exenterations, sigmoid conduits have been advocated by some investigators, so that small bowel anastomosis is not a factor.[15–18] When the colon segment has been subjected to irradiation, however, some investigators report that the early and late complications are similar or identical to those of (irradiated) ileal segments. Users of jejunal conduits[19]

Table 11-4 Modern Methods of Urinary Diversion

Temporary
Percutaneous nephrostomy
Permanent
Incontinent conduits
• Ileal
• Sigmoid colon
• Transverse colon*
Continent conduits
• Kock ileal reservoir
• Gilchrist cecal reservoir
• Indiana cecal reservoir
• Miami ileocolonic reservoir*

*Procedures of choice.

(in an attempt to use less heavily irradiated bowel in persons who have had irradiation to the pelvis) have found that this type of conduit is associated with appreciable (albeit reversible) hypochloremic acidosis with hyponatremia, hypokalemia, and uremia. Although this *jejunal syndrome* is correctable with the administration of salt, it makes the selection of these bowel segments less attractive as a permanent form of diversion.

Transverse colon conduits have gained considerable popularity in use by gynecologic oncologists nationwide.[7,20,21] The advantages of simplicity of performance, use of a nonirradiated bowel segment, and fewer stomal complications have made it the procedure of choice for diversion as part of exenterative operations at The University of Alabama at Birmingham, where 70 procedures have been performed since 1976.

Beginning in February 1988, gynecologic oncologists at the University of Miami have used a continent ileocolonic reservoir as a part of pelvic exenteration operations.[22] The benefits of such a reservoir include continence and improved renal function related to the low pressure system. With this pouch tapered ileum, a reinforced ileocecal valve, and nontunneled ureterocolonic anastomoses are used. Assessment of complications since its creation reveals that it is a technically simple and reliable reservoir when compared to other forms of continent diversion.

COMPLICATIONS AND OTHER CONSIDERATIONS AFTER URINARY DIVERSION

Ileal or Colon Conduits

Patient Adjustment to Stoma

One of the factors in urinary diversion is the patient's adjustment to a urinary ostomy. In our experience, this adjustment has been quite good. Reasons include that a cancer cure may have been made possible by performing the exenterative operation in which the diversion was performed or that the diversion may have resulted in an improvement over the preoperative condition (eg, fistulas or bladder damage).

Sequelae

In any urinary diversion procedure, the complications must also be considered. A number of sequelae are associated with conduit construction or with longstanding urinary diversion with the use of ileal or colon conduits. They are generally classified in six areas:

1. infection
2. leakage of the conduit or the ureteral anastomosis
3. stomal complications
4. small bowel complications
5. formation of stones
6. loss of the renal unit.

Some are associated more with one type of conduit as compared to another.

Infection. Bacterial growth in conduits varies somewhat with the type of diversion. Hill and colleagues[23] reported that at least three fourths of patients with ileal conduits had significant mixed growth of bacteria in the loop urine but slightly less than half of those with colon segments were infected. They consequently attempted to explain the discrepancy between infection rates in colon and ileal loop urines. They believed that, because of the inability to do antireflux anastomoses on segments of ileum and given that most of the patients with ileal conduits have infected urine, eventually the urinary tracts of these patients would fare worse than those of patients with colon conduits (because of the decreased tendency for infection and the possibility of antireflux anastomoses). In gynecologic use, however, antireflux anastomoses typically have not been performed, even on colon segments. Also, Hancock and co-workers,[16] although noting an 18% incidence of infection in a group of patients (about half of whom had ileal conduits and the other half had sigmoid conduits), did not find long-term infections to be different in ileal versus colon conduits.

Acute pyelonephritis is a common problem after conduit construction, occurring in 5% to 20% of patients[17,18,20]; 16 of 115 patients who underwent supravesical urinary diversion at the University of Alabama[20] required one or more readmissions because of pyelonephritis. Preliminary data suggest that risk of pyelonephritis as a late complication may be lower in patients with transverse colon conduits. Also, the use of ureteral stents in the early postoperative period does not seem to increase the incidence of immediate postoperative pyelonephritis.

Urinary Leaks. A serious early postoperative problem relates to urinary leaks. Although a few leaks close spontaneously, that phenomenon is the exception to the rule. Even with spontaneous closure leaking anastomoses often result in the loss of renal units. The incidence of urinary leaks or fistulas varies between 2% and 22%[16,20,24–28] and relates primarily to the percentage of patients in which irradiated bowel segments were used and also to the use or nonuse of ureteral stents in the anastomosis. Second operations for leaks in the early postoperative period after an exenterative procedure are likely to be quite hazardous and are associated with a mortality rate of approximately 33% to 50%.[16,20,29] The use of transverse colon conduits virtually eliminates postoperative urinary leaks when nonirradiated bowel is anastomosed to extrapelvic ureters over indwelling stents.[20]

Stomal Complications. Stomal complications generally are seen in 3.5% to 6% of cases and in most instances relate to retraction, necrosis, or stenosis of the stoma.[17,20,27] Such complications are reported to be less common with the use of large bowel segments, as compared to the use of small bowel,[17,20,21] although Hancock and co-workers[16] reported no significant differences in such a comparison.

Small Bowel Complications. Serious small bowel complications occur in 5% to 15% of patients undergoing ileal conduit diversion.[20,27,30,31] In many of these patients, small bowel fistulas develop, necessitating a second operation for correction. The elimination of the need for small bowel anastomosis by the use of sigmoid or transverse colon segments drastically reduces the chances of small bowel obstruction or fistula and the consequent morbidity and mortality.

Stone Formation. Urinary calculi occur in 2% to 9% of patients with conduits.[20,32,33] Stones are thought to occur because of the metabolic problems of acidosis, increased urinary calcium excretion, chronic urinary stasis, and infection. Some investigators[34] have argued that stapling instruments introduce a foreign body (wire staples) into the conduit, which might increase the incidence of stone formation. This observation has not been proved. Several suggestions have been made to prevent exposed staples at the distal end of the conduit. One is to transect the segment manually. Alternatively, a running suture can be placed in front of the gastrointestinal staple line, so that urine does not contact the staples. The use of a double application of absorbable staples (Polysorb; manufactured by Auto Suture, U.S. Surgical Corporation, Norwalk, Connecticut) for bowel transection may reduce the risk of calculi.[35]

Renal Unit Loss. Conduit diversion is associated with an appreciable chance of the loss of renal function. In the series of Hancock and co-workers[16] with 212 conduits, 17% of patients lost the function of one kidney. This was due in part to strictures developing at the site of the ureter-bowel anastomosis. They reported no significant correlation between the type of conduit used and the subsequent loss of renal function.

Neal,[32] in a study of 111 adults treated for bladder cancer by using ileal conduits, reported a 47% incidence of deterioration of one or both kidneys at long-term follow-up (>5 years). In 16% of these patients biochemical evidence of impaired renal function developed; 4 patients died of renal failure. Bilateral upper tract dilation was noted in 28% of patients. Pitts and Muecke[36] also reported long-term experience with ileal conduits in 172 adults with particular interest in the fate of the kidneys. In their patients, 12 (7%) had damaged renal units, and this percentage increased over time (0 to 5 years, 3%; 6 to 10 years, 11%; 11 to 15 years, 23%; 16 to 20 years, 20%). Six percent of those monitored for 0 to 5 years had renal loss; 19% of those monitored for 11 to 15 years had such findings. The cause of this renal damage was thought to be obstruction of the ureteral-ileal anastomosis (50%), calculi (27%), and progressive deterioration without obstruction (23%). No long-term follow-up data on the fate of kidneys implanted into transverse colon conduits are available, although a study is in progress at the University of Alabama at Birmingham.

Continent Pouches

The Miami Experience

Results from the University of Miami indicate that 19 of 20 evaluable patients with the Miami pouch are continent and wear only an adhesive strip cover for protection. *Continence* is defined as absolute command of the timing of the expulsion of urine from the reservoir. Eleven of 20 patients are able to sleep all night without catheterization. Three patients have had isolated incidents of catheterization difficulty, but none has required stomal revision to date.

Early complications have occurred in 5 patients (36%). The complications necessitated one second operation for a ureterocolonic anastomotic leak, three percutaneous nephrostomy tube placements for ureteral strictures, and one percutaneous drainage of a pelvic abscess. One patient suffered a pulmonary embolism requiring the placement of a prosthetic umbrella device in the vena cava.

The late complication rate is 23%. Complications attributed specifically to the pouch were reflux in two ureters (4.5%), diagnosed by using a pouchogram; stone formation (1 patient); and incontinence at a full pouch. There were two peristomal hernias. In 2 patients stomal stenosis (at the level of the skin) developed; the stenosis in both patients was revised in the office. In addition, rehospitalization was required for 1 patient in whom pyelonephritis developed and 1 patient in whom a small bowel obstruction developed. In none of the patients receiving the Miami pouch have electrolyte abnormalities related to the pouch developed.

Other Experience

Hohenfellner and colleagues[37] have described more than 200 patients treated with the Mainz pouch technique during a 5-year period. The mortality rate associated with the operation was 0.5%. Early complications occurred in 10 patients (5%). They included abdominal wall dehiscence (1 patient), intestinal fistula (1 patient), mechanical ileus (4 patients), need for surgical revision (3 patients), pouch tamponade (1 patient), and nipple necrosis (1 patient). A late complication of stone formation occurred in 12 patients; the patients were treated by using endoscopic therapy (4 patients), nephrectomy (4 patients), and ureteral reimplantation (4 patients).

Rowland and associates[9] reported postoperative pouch leaks in 3 of 29 patients (10.3%). One was treated conservatively, one had percutaneous drainage of an infected urinoma, and one underwent re-exploration with repair of the leak. Four other patients (14%) experienced complications, including the development of small bowel obstruction in 1 patient 1 year after surgery (treated conservatively) and a parastomal hernia (which required surgical repair) in 1 patient.

Somewhat in contrast to the experience with ileocolonic reservoirs summarized earlier is the experience of Skinner and colleagues[38] with the ileal reservoir. In their series, 42 of 250 patients (16.8%) who received Kock pouches experienced early complications, resulting in operative deaths in 2%. One or more late complications required 85 revisions in 77 patients (31%). Urinary leaks occurred in 18 patients (7.2%), 7 of whom required a second operation. Of the 245 patients who survived the operation, 58 (23.7%) complained of leakage of urine after recovery and, indeed, 44 underwent 55 second operations to correct postoperative incontinence. Seven other patients experienced enteral fistulas or pelvic abscess formation after the surgery.

RECOMMENDED APPROACHES

Construction of Transverse Colon Conduits

Preoperative Preparation

Preoperative preparation focuses on several events. Assessment of any patient who is to undergo diversionary surgery should include an intravenous pyelogram. This study is helpful in determining the normality of each renal collecting system and identifying any anomalies such as double ureters or hydronephrosis. Results of the test will provide baseline data to which findings of studies that may be necessary in later months can be compared.

The location of the stoma site needs to be determined. To do this, the physician evaluates the patient's abdomen with the patient in the standing position. A stomal therapist (if available) can assist the physician in this decision and, at the same time, can orient the patient regarding the changes that will occur with surgery.

Bowel preparation is mandatory. Mechanical preparation consists of a clear-liquid diet for 2 or 3 days, followed by the administration of magnesium citrate and cleansing enemas. A quicker method is to use colonic lavage solutions.

Finally, prophylactic antibiotics are recommended. Suggested regimens include oral erythromycin and neomycin sulfate, intravenous metronidazole, or an intravenous cephalosporin.

Technique

In preparation for isolating the segment of transverse colon for use as a conduit, the omentum is dissected away from its attachment to the colon. The mesentery of the transverse colon is transilluminated, allowing visualization of the middle colic artery and, thus, identification of adequate vessel arcades to ensure adequate blood supply for the isolated segment. The colon segment should be approximately 15 to 20 cm in length, but this varies somewhat with the size of the patient and the thickness of the abdominal wall. With the use of a GIA stapling instrument (United States Surgical Corporation, Norwalk, Connecticut), the colon is transected at the previously identified areas (Figure 11-4), following which the mesentery of that segment is transected to allow mobility. Bowel continuity is reestablished using the GIA stapling instrument and TASS (U.S. Surgical Corporation) staples. After this, the mesentery of the reanastomosed colon is reapproximated with a few interrupted absorbable sutures above the conduit.

For the ureteral anastomosis, the ureters on each side are transected at the level of the common iliac vessels. The pelvic ureters are not used because, in all likelihood, they have received high radiation doses (in previously irradiated patients) and thus are subject to poor healing. If possible at the time of transection of the ureter, a segment of overlying and attached peritoneum is taken for use later in covering the anastomosis. The ureters are brought ventrally through the small bowel mesentery for anastomosis to the colon segment. Silastic ureteral stents (outside diameter 0.078 in, inside diameter 0.0125 in) are placed in the ureter to the renal pelvis and secured with an absorbable suture (Figure 11-5). A long Kelly

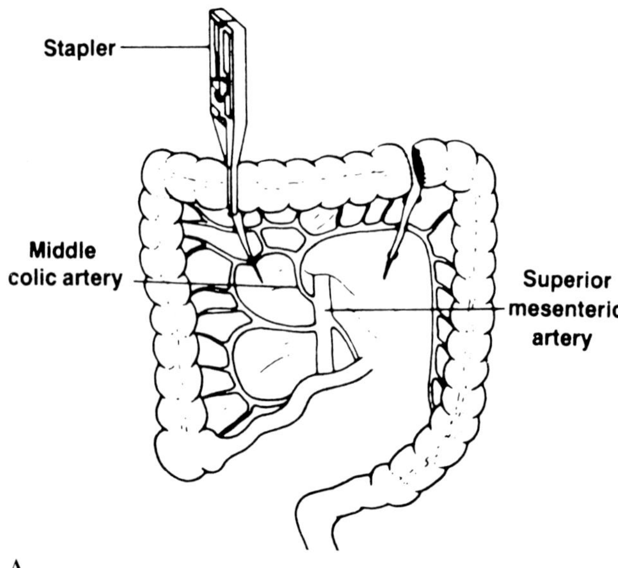

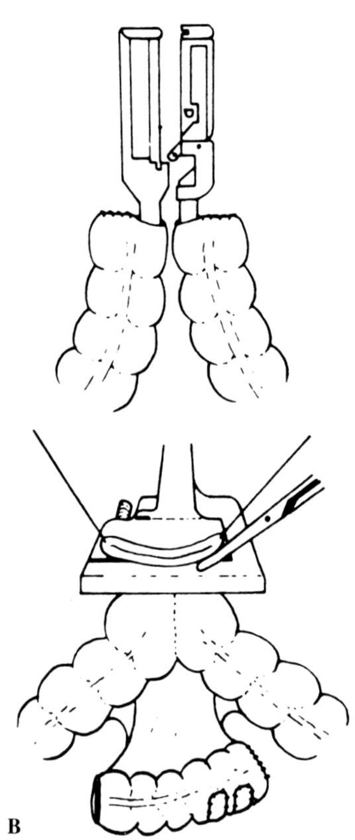

Figure 11-4 **A**, Major blood supply to transverse colon conduit is shown. Middle colic artery (branch of superior mesenteric artery) has been visualized and isolated. **B**, For reanastomosis of transverse colon, isolated conduit segment is placed below anastomosis, just above small bowel mesentery. GIA and TASS (U.S. Surgical) staples allow for a reproducible anastomotic technique. *Source*: Reprinted with permission from *Contemporary Ob-Gyn* (1983;22:253–257), Copyright © 1983, Medical Economics Company, Inc.

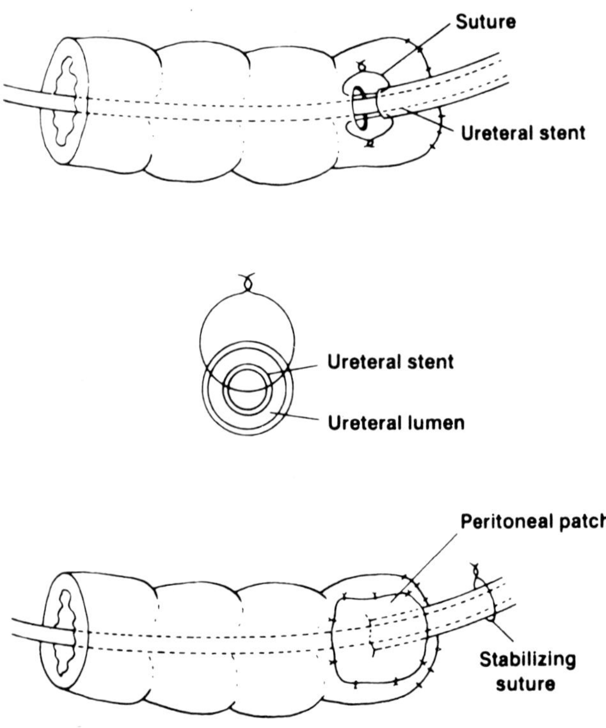

Figure 11-5 For stabilizing effect, ureteral stent has been placed in ureter and pulled through incision in distal end of conduit (*top*). Absorbable suture anchors stent (*center*). After single-layer anastomosis, peritoneal patch is sutured to intestinal segment (*bottom*). *Source*: Reprinted with permission from *Contemporary Ob-Gyn* (1983;22:253–257), Copyright © 1983, Medical Economics Company, Inc.

clamp is passed retrograde through the distal end of the conduit to bring the tip to the point of anastomosis, 3 to 4 cm from the proximal end of the conduit. A cut-down on the tip of this clamp will facilitate creating an adequate opening in the bowel and will allow one to pull the ureteral stent from that opening through the distal end of the conduit. The ureteral anastomosis is then accomplished by using a single layer, full-thickness, ureter-to-bowel anastomosis with 4-0 absorbable sutures. The second ureter is anastomosed in the identical manner, and the peritoneal flap (if available) is used to seal the anastomosis by securing it to the serosal surface of the colon.

The isolated segment with anastomosed ureters and stents protruding from the distal end (Figure 11-6) is now ready for the final portion of the conduit construction (ie, creation of the stoma). Before performing this, the closed end of the conduit is stabilized to the peritoneum of the bowel mesentery with one or two sutures to decrease tension on the ureteral anastomoses and limit mobility of the bowel segment. The conduit is now ready for the final step of stomal formation.

At the preselected stomal site on the abdomen, an Allis clamp is used to grasp the center of the desired stoma. After elevating the skin at this point, a large knife blade is used to make a circular skin incision. A Kelly

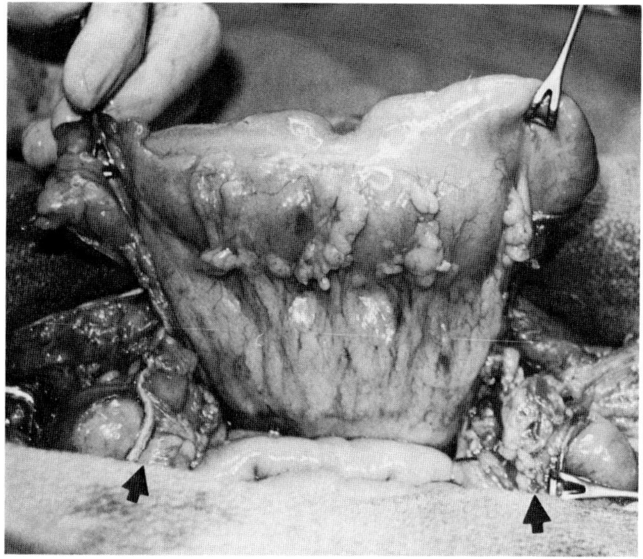

A

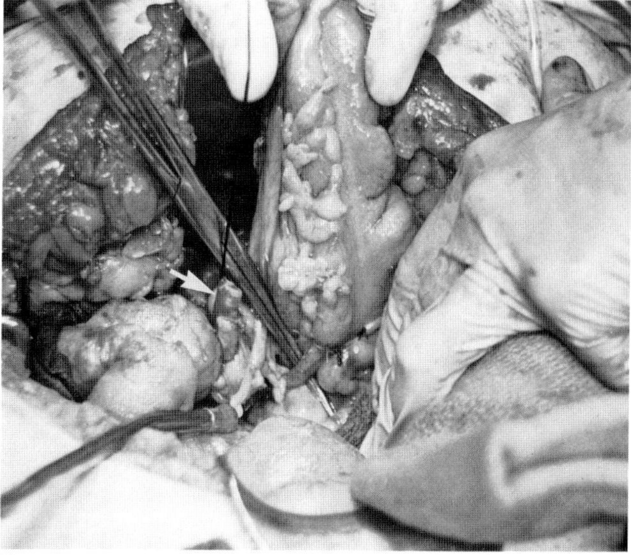

B

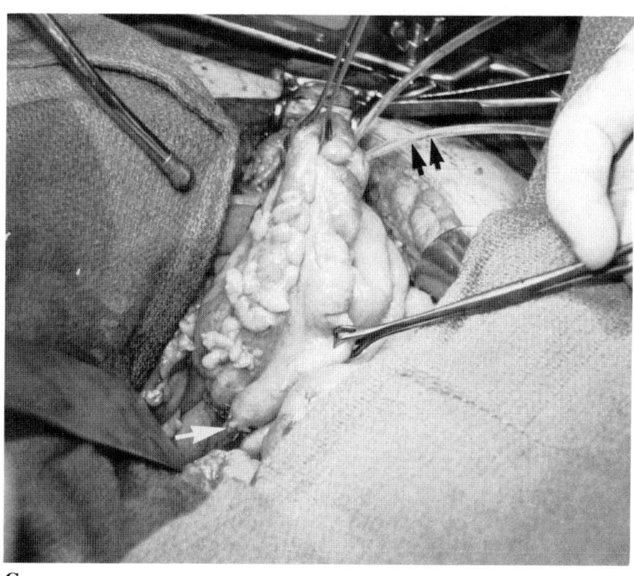

C

Figure 11-6 The transverse colon conduit is technically straightforward and is associated with a low incidence of immediate and delayed postoperative complications. **A**, The conduit segment is isolated using the GIA stapler device. The *arrows* indicate the colon segments to be reanastomosed behind the conduit segment. **B**, One ureter has been anastomosed as described (indicated by the Kelly clamp). The contralateral ureter (*white arrow*), suspended by a silk suture, will be similarly anastomosed to the bowel. **C**, The *white arrow* indicates the complete ureterointestinal anastomosis. The *double black arrows* show the silastic stents exiting through the open end of the conduit. *Source*: Reprinted from *Female Genital Cancer* (p 582) by SB Gusberg, HM Shingleton and G Deppe (editors), with permission of Churchill Livingstone, copyright © 1988.

clamp is passed through the abdominal wall from the peritoneal side to this site. With the use of Mayo scissors, the fascia is incised centrally, equidistant from the stomal margins, to allow the passage of two fingers easily through the abdominal wall. Two Babcock clamps passed into the peritoneal cavity through the stoma are used to grasp the distal end of the conduit (with protruding stents); these are pulled gently through the abdominal wall opening for suturing. A rosebud technique is used (Figure 11-7) with incorporation of both the serosa and the distal edge of the bowel segment such that once the sutures are tied, the stoma protrudes 2 or 3 cm. This is quite important in allowing ease of management of the stomal appliances by the patient. A stoma that can be seen by the patient while lying down allows a better fit of the appliance and, thus, decreases extravasation of urine under the appliance and excoriation of the skin as a

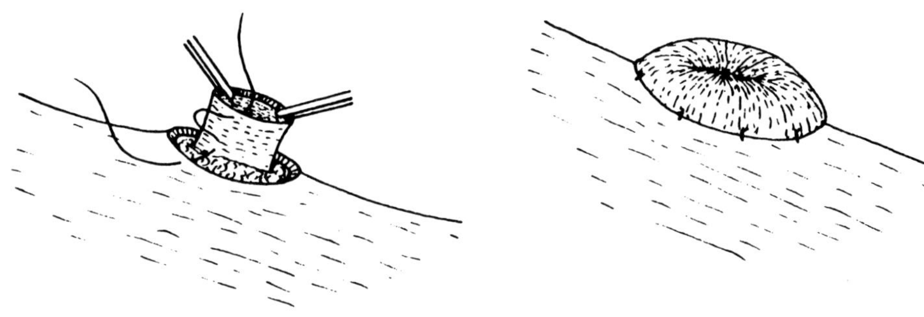

Figure 11-7 Creation of everted stoma requires that bowel protrude above skin surface for approximately 3 to 4 cm. Placement of absorbable sutures as illustrated folds bowel on itself, resulting in rosebud stoma. *Source*: Reprinted with permission from *Contemporary Ob-Gyn* (1983;22:253–257), Copyright © 1983, Medical Economics Company, Inc.

consequence.[39,40] After closure of the abdominal wall at the end of the procedure, the ureteral stents are trimmed such that they protrude a few centimeters into a temporary urinostomy bag. No manipulation is necessary because they are extruded spontaneously by the 10th to 15th postoperative day.

Use of Ureteral Stents

Leaks at the anastomosis of the ureter and the bowel segment have presented problems since the earliest days of bowel segment urinary diversion. Because of this problem, Coffey[41] introduced the technique of constructing submucosal tunnels for ureters in the wall of the intact sigmoid colon. Such tunnels were not practical in ileal segments, and leaks or fistulas at the anastomosed site in irradiated ileum constituted significant problems before the introduction of ureteral stents.

Use of ureteral stents has become almost routine in the gynecologic oncology community.[16,20,42] Hancock and co-workers[16] summed up their advantages as follows:

1. They ensure passage of urine during the immediate postoperative period.
2. They provide an access for irrigation of the renal pelvis or injection of radiopaque dye for urograms.
3. They permit the recording of the output of each kidney separately if required.

One of us (H.M.S.) has routinely used stents for more than two decades in ileal, sigmoid, and transverse colon conduits after a number of unfortunate experiences with unstented anastomoses in ileal conduits.

Advantages of Transverse Colon Conduits

Schmidt and co-workers[21] summarized the advantages of transverse colon conduits as follows:

1. This segment of bowel (ie, transverse colon) is not likely to be affected by pelvic irradiation.
2. High ureteral anastomoses can be achieved, thus also excluding the irradiated pelvic portion of the ureter from the anastomosis.
3. Colon segments are less frequently complicated by stomal stenosis.
4. The effects of absorption of urine across the colon wall on renal function are minimized because of the mass contraction method of emptying the segment and the small residual volumes within the bowel segment.

They also pointed out that one could optionally use an antireflux anastomosis if desired. Transverse colon conduits, however, are not ordinarily performed by gynecologic oncologists because there are no convincing data that they prevent subsequent renal deterioration. An additional benefit of the colon conduit is that the newly constructed conduit lies in the mid to upper abdomen, decreasing the likelihood of the conduit lying in an infected area of the denuded pelvis.

Construction of the Miami Continent Pouch

Preoperative Preparation

All patients undergo mechanical and antibiotic bowel preparation. The stoma site can be located lower on the abdominal wall because avoidance of skin folds is not essential. In general, it should be placed where it will be concealed by the patient's underwear, several centimeters above the pubis.

Technique

The distal ileum is transected 10 cm proximal to the ileocecal valve. The cecum and the segment of ascending colon are mobilized up to the right colic flexure, and the transverse colon is transected just distal to the middle colic artery (Figure 11-8). Continuity of the bowel is restored with an ileotransverse colostomy. If an appen-

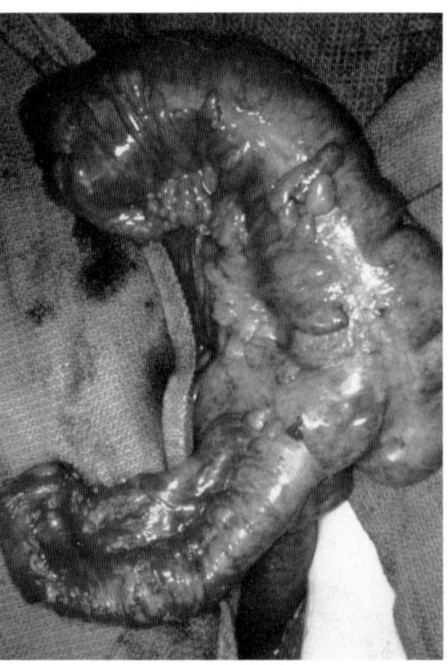

Figure 11-8 Distal segment of ileum is transected 10 cm proximal to ileocecal valve, and cecum and ascending colon are mobilized. Transverse colon is transected just distal to middle colic artery. *Source:* Reprinted with permission from *Gynecologic Oncology* (1989;34:274–288), Copyright © 1989, Academic Press, Inc.

dectomy has not been performed, it should be done during the procedure. The cecum, the ascending colon, and the segment of transverse colon are used to create the reservoir. The colon is opened with cautery along the tenia (Figure 11-9) and folded onto itself to create a U-shaped intestinal plate. The legs of the U are shaped in a side-to-side fashion with absorbable staples (Figure 11-10) to form the posterior wall of the reservoir. This detubularizes the segment of bowel and reduces the potential for high pressure in the colon segment.

The continence mechanism is created by tapering the segment of distal ileum and placing purse-string sutures at the level of the ileocecal valve. The distal ileum is intubated with a 14F red rubber catheter (Figure 11-11). Allis clamps are placed on the antimesenteric border of the ileum and pulled to provide mild traction. A GIA stapling instrument (U.S. Surgical Corporation) is applied to the ileum longitudinally to reduce the lumen down to the underlying 14F catheter in an attempt to increase the pressure of this ileal segment (Figure 11-12A). The excess tissue is excised (Figure 11-12B). Three purse-string sutures (0.5 cm apart) of 2-0 silk are placed in the seromuscular layer of the ileal segment at the level of the ileocecal valve to increase the closure pressure and achieve urinary continence (Figure 11-13). The tapered ileal segment is exteriorized as a stoma to the right lower quadrant of the abdomen for future self-catheterization by the patient.

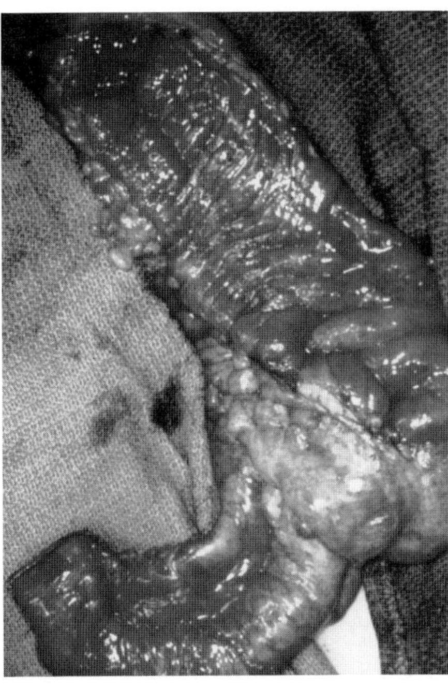

Figure 11-9 Segment of colon is opened along tenia, and colonic mucosa is visualized. *Source*: Reprinted with permission from *Gynecologic Oncology* (1989;34:274–288), Copyright © 1989, Academic Press, Inc.

A hiatus is created in the posterior wall of the colon, through which the ureters are brought into the reservoir. The left ureter is passed through the sigmoid mesocolon before entering the reservoir. A mucosal incision is made

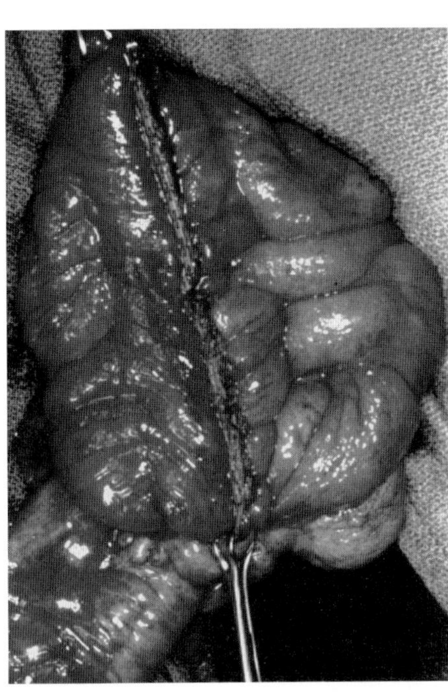

Figure 11-10 Opened colon is folded in U-shaped fashion, and walls are anastomosed with absorbable staples. Posterior wall of reservoir is visualized. *Source*: Reprinted with permission from *Gynecologic Oncology* (1989;34:274–288), Copyright © 1989, Academic Press, Inc.

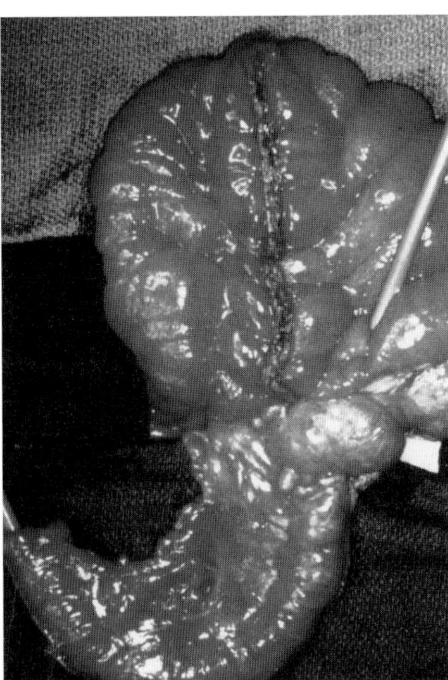

Figure 11-11 Ileum is untubated with 14F red rubber catheter, which can be seen entering reservoir. *Source*: Reprinted with permission from *Gynecologic Oncology* (1989;34:274–288), Copyright © 1989, Academic Press, Inc.

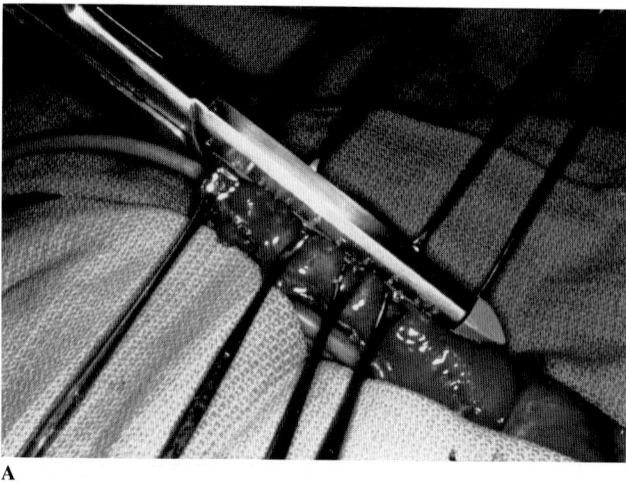

A

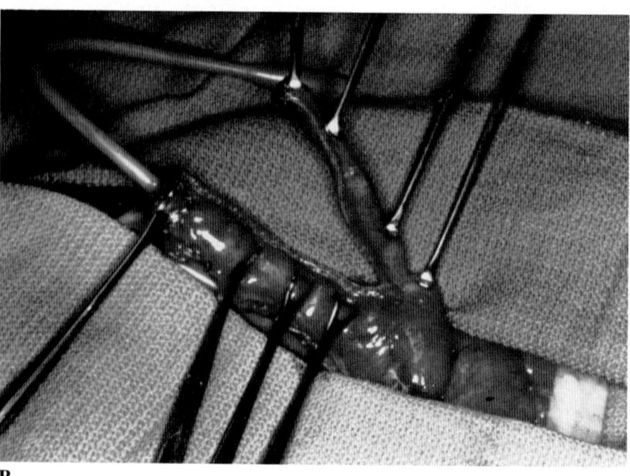

B

Figure 11-12 **A**, GIA stapling instrument (United States Surgical Corp., Norwalk, Conn.) is applied to ileum to reduce the lumen. **B**, Excess tissue of ileum is excised. *Source*: Reprinted with permission from *Gynecologic Oncology* (1989;34:274–288), Copyright © 1989, Academic Press, Inc.

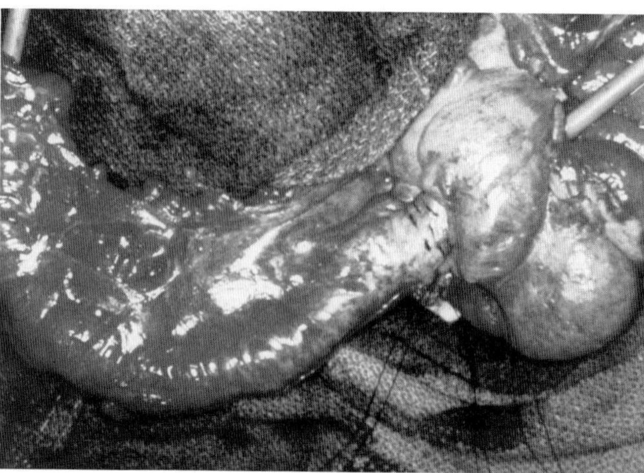

Figure 11-13 Three purse-string sutures of 2-0 silk are placed at level of ileocecal valve. *Source*: Reprinted with permission from *Gynecologic Oncology* (1989;34:274–288), Copyright © 1989, Academic Press, Inc.

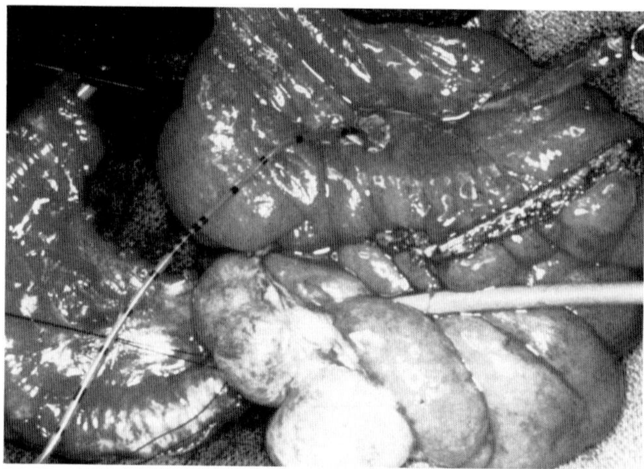

Figure 11-14 Ureterocolonic anastomosis. A 2-cm segment of ureter is brought into reservoir and is demonstrated by clamp. Ureter on right side of picture has been spatulated and anastomosed to submucosal layers of bowel. Ureteral stents are inserted. *Source*: Reprinted with permission from *Gynecologic Oncology* (1989;34:274–288), Copyright © 1989, Academic Press, Inc.

to create a sulcus in which the ureters will be anastomosed. The distal ends of the ureters are spatulated and, with 4-0 polyglycolic acid sutures, anastomosed to the submucosal layers of the colon (Figure 11-14). The muscular wall of the colon and the low-pressure reservoir provide the antireflux mechanism. Extraluminally, the ureteral adventitia is fixed to the bowel serosa. The ureters are stented with single J ureteral diversion stents that are secured distal to the ureterocolonic anastomosis with absorbable sutures. The stents are left in place for 2 weeks and then removed. The nontunneled nonrefluxing ureteral anastomosis has worked well in the colon. Incidence of reflux and obstruction has been similar to that recorded with other forms of intestinal anastomosis. The nontunneled ureterocolonic anastomosis is an advantage over the tunneled implantation, as described by Goodwin and associates,[13] in that it can be performed in any segment of the colon. The success rate at the University of Miami with the ureterocolonic anastomosis has been 90%.

The anterior wall of the reservoir is closed with absorbable staples (Figure 11-15). The reservoir is secured to the abdominal wall; the 14F catheter and single J stents are secured to the skin.

Reinforcing the ileocecal valve is considered essential for maintaining continence. The ileocecal junction normally acts as a valve, thus preventing reflux of colonic contents into the lumen. If a urinary reservoir becomes distended, the ileocecal valve alone may not be sufficient

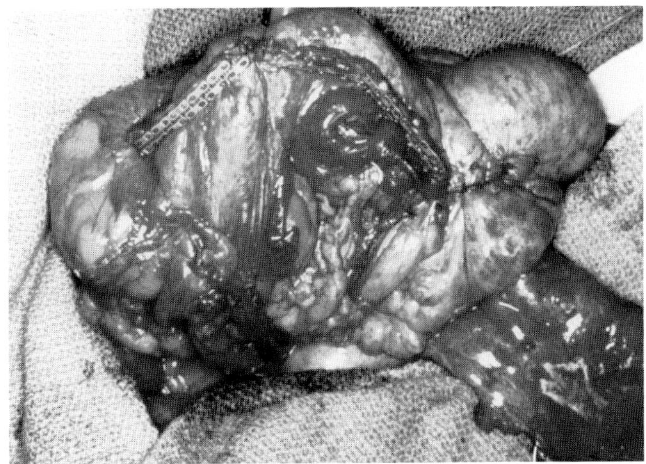

Figure 11-15 Anterior wall of reservoir is closed with absorbable staples. *Source*: Reprinted with permission from *Gynecologic Oncology* (1989;34:274–288), Copyright © 1989, Academic Press, Inc.

to prevent leakage. By tapering the segment of the distal ileum and placing purse-string sutures at the ileocecal valve, the pressure of this segment of bowel exceeds the reservoir pressure at all times, thereby resulting in full continence.

Approximately 2 weeks after surgery, a contrast study of the reservoir and an intravenous urogram (IVU) are performed to evaluate for leakage, reflux, or upper tract obstruction (Figure 11-16). If the radiographs show normal findings, the ureteral stents are removed, and the patient is taught to irrigate and catheterize the pouch. Initially, the patient catheterizes the stoma every 2 to 4 hours and irrigates it 4 times a day. The patient gradually decreases the frequency of catheterization and irrigation if continence and obstruction of the catheter by mucus are not a problem. Patients describe a feeling of fullness or slight cramping in the right lower quadrant of the abdomen, indicating the need to empty the reservoir. The average frequency of catheterization is 5 to 6 catheterizations in 24 hours. The time needed for emptying the reservoir is about 3½ minutes. The amount of urine for each catheterization averages 365 mL (range, 250 to 500 mL). Urodynamic evaluation of the reservoir reveals that the basal pressure fluctuates between 10 and 20 cm of water, whereas in the tapered ileum it varies between 50 and 60 cm of water (Figure 11-17).

CONCLUSION

Urinary diversion in gynecology is performed primarily in conjunction with cancer operations but, at times, is required for women with intractable urinary

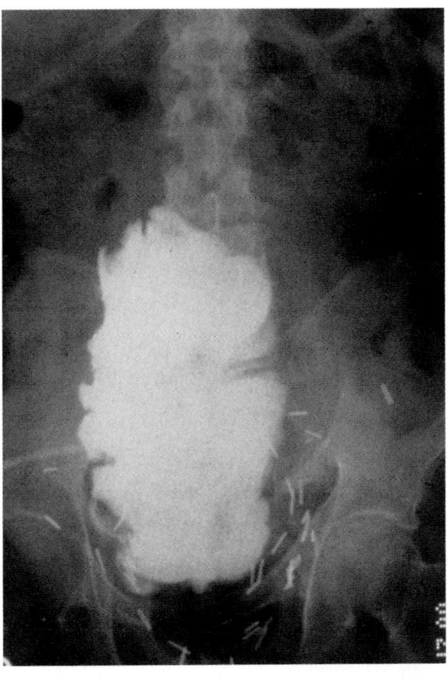

Figure 11-16 Contrast study of reservoir. *Source*: Reprinted with permission from *Gynecologic Oncology* (1989;34:274–288), Copyright © 1989, Academic Press, Inc.

fistulas or other urologic disorders. After 1950, ileal conduits replaced ureterosigmoidostomy as the most widely used form of urinary diversion. Transverse colon conduits have gained popularity among gynecologic oncologists because these nonirradiated bowel segments offer less chance of postoperative urinary leaks and small bowel complications associated with bowel and ureteral

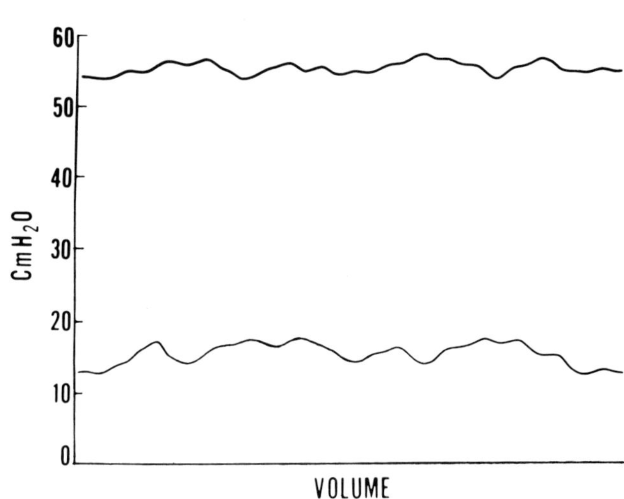

Figure 11-17 Urodynamic evaluation. With filling of reservoir with normal saline, pressure in tapered ileum fluctuated between 50 and 60 cm of water and, in colonic reservoir, between 10 and 20 cm of water. *Source*: Reprinted with permission from *Gynecologic Oncology* (1989;34:274–288), Copyright © 1989, Academic Press, Inc.

anastomoses in radiation-damaged ileum. In 1978, Kock and associates[8] described the use of detubularized segments of ileum and the intussuscepted nipple valves to create a continent pouch that is still advocated by urologists in some centers. Ileocolonic continent pouches, originally suggested in 1908, have received considerable attention in the past 10 to 15 years because of ease of construction, lower revision rates, and higher continence rates as compared with the Kock ileal pouches.

Women who are in need of urinary diversion can be offered at least two major choices: (1) the traditional conduit, which requires external ostomy appliance; or (2) a continent pouch such as the Miami ileocolonic reservoir. Transverse colon conduits offer significant advantages over ileal conduits, especially when performed in women who have had pelvic irradiation. These include fewer urinary tract infections, urinary leaks, and stomal and small bowel complications, as well as less stone formation and subsequent renal loss. In choosing between incontinent and continent conduits, the woman must be made aware that the continent pouches are available in only a few centers in the United States and, in less experienced hands, may add to the length, complexity, and morbidity of exenterative operations. The age and general health of the woman and the likelihood of her long-term survival after diversion weigh heavily in the decision.

REFERENCES

1. Simon J. Ectopia vesica (absence of the anterior walls of the bladder and pubic abdominal partietes): operation for directing the orifices of the ureters into the rectum; temporary success; subsequent death; autopsy. *Lancet.* 1852;2:568.

2. Verhoogen J, de Graeuve A. La cystectomie totale. *Folia Urol.* 1909;3:629.

3. Gilchrist RK, Merricks JW, Hamlin MH, Rieger IT. Construction of a substitute bladder and urethra. *Surg Gynecol Obstet.* 1950;90:752–760.

4. Ferris DO, Hodel HM. Electrolyte pattern of the blood after bilateral ureterosigmoidostomy. *J Am Med Assoc.* 1950;142:634–640.

5. Bricker EM. Bladder substitution after pelvic evisceration. *Surg Clin North Am.* 1950;30:1511–1521.

6. Symmonds RE, Gibbs CP. Urinary diversion by way of sigmoid conduit. *Surg Gynecol Obstet.* 1970;131:687–693.

7. Nelson JH. *Atlas of Radical Pelvic Surgery.* New York: Appleton-Century-Crofts; 1969:181–191.

8. Kock NG, Nilson AE, Norlen L, Sundin T, Trasti H. Urinary diversion via a continent ileum reservoir. Clinical experience. *Scand J Urol Nephrol Suppl.* 1978;49:23–31.

9. Rowland RG, Mitchell ME, Bihrle R, Kahnoski RJ, Piser JE. Indiana continent urinary reservoir. *J Urol.* 1987;137:1136–1139.

10. Thüroff JW, Alken P, Riedmiller N, Engelmann U, Jacobi GH, Hohenfellner R. The Mainz pouch (mixed augmentation ileum and cecum) for bladder augmentation and bladder diversion. *J Urol.* 1986;136:17–26.

11. Mansson W, Colleen S, Sundin T. Continent caecal reservoir in urinary diversion. *Br J Urol.* 1984;56:359–365.

12. Lockhart JL, Bejany DE. The antireflux ureteroileal reimplantation in children and adults. *J Urol.* 1986;135:576–579.

13. Goodwin WE, Harris AP, Kaufman JJ, Beal JM. Open transcolonic ureterointestinal anastomosis: a new approach. *Surg Gynecol Obstet.* 1953;97:295–300.

14. Bejany DE, Politano VA. Stapled and nonstapled tapered distal ileum for construction of a continent colonic urinary reservoir. *J Urol.* 1988;140:491–494.

15. Altwein JE, Hohenfellner R. Use of the colon as a conduit for urinary diversion. *Surg Gynecol Obstet.* 1975;140:33–38.

16. Hancock KC, Copeland LJ, Gershenson DM, Saul PB, Wharton JT, Rutledge FN. Urinary conduits in gynecologic oncology. *Obstet Gynecol.* 1986;67:680–684.

17. Lindenauer SM, Cerny JC, Morley GW. Ureterosigmoid conduit urinary diversion. *Surgery.* 1974;75:705–714.

18. Morales P, Golimbu M. Colonic urinary diversion: 10 years of experience. *J Urol.* 1975;113:302–307.

19. Golimbu M, Morales P. Jejunal conduits: technique and complications. *J Urol.* 1975;113:787–795.

20. Orr JW Jr, Shingleton HM, Hatch KD, et al. Urinary diversion in patients undergoing pelvic exenteration. *Am J Obstet Gynecol.* 1982;142:883–889.

21. Schmidt JD, Buchsbaum HJ, Jacobo ED. Transverse colon conduit for supravesical urinary tract diversion. *Urology.* 1976;8:542–546.

22. Penalver MA, Bejany DE, Averette HE, Donato DM, Sevin B-U, Suarez G. Continent urinary diversion in gynecologic oncology. *Gynecol Oncol.* 1989;34:274–288.

23. Hill MJ, Hudson MJ, Stewart M. The urinary bacterial flora in patients with three types of urinary tract diversion. *J Med Microbiol.* 1983;16:221–226.

24. Schoenberg HW, Mikuta JJ. Technique for preventing urinary fistulas following pelvic exenteration and ureteroileostomy. *J Urol.* 1973;110:294–295.

25. Fallon B, Loening S, Hawtrey CE, Lifshitz SG, Buchsbaum HJ. Urologic compiications of pelvic exenteration for gynecologic malignancy. *J Urol.* 1979;122:158–159.

26. Barber HRK, Brunschwig A. Urinary tract fistulas. *Obstet Gynecol.* 1966;28:754–763.

27. Sullivan JW, Gradstald H, Whitmore WF Jr. Complications of ureteroileal conduit with radical cystectomy: review of 336 cases. *J Urol.* 1980;124:797–801.

28. Wrigley JV, Prem KA, Fraley EE. Pelvic exenteration: complications of urinary diversion. *J Urol.* 1976;116:428–430.

29. Hensle TW, Bredin HC, Dretler SP. Diagnosis and treatment of a urinary leak after ureteroileal conduit for diversion. *J Urol.* 1976;116:29–31.

30. Lichtinger M, Averette H, Girtanner R, Sevin B-U, Penalver M. Small bowel complications after supravesical urinary diversion in pelvic exenteration. *Gynecol Oncol.* 1986;24:137–142.

31. Swan RW, Rutledge FN. Urinary conduit in pelvic cancer patients. *Am J Obstet Gynecol.* 1974;119:6–13.

32. Neal DE. Complications of ileal conduit diversion in adults with cancer followed up for at least five years. *Br Med J.* 1985;290:1695–1697.

33. Podratz KC, Angerman NS, Symmonds RE. Complications of ureteral surgery in the non-radiated patient. In: Delgado G, Smith JP, eds. *Management of Complications in Gynecologic Oncology*. New York: John Wiley; 1982.

34. Bergman SM, Sears HF, Javadpour N. Complication with mechanical stapling device in creation of ileo conduit. *Urology.* 1978;12:71–73.

35. Baker VV, Shingleton HM. Urinary diversion. In: Gusberg SB, Shingleton HM, Deppe G, eds. *Female Genital Cancer*. New York: Churchill Livingstone; 1988:chap 24.

36. Pitts WR, Muecke EC. A 20-year experience with ileal conduits: the fate of the kidneys. *J Urol.* 1979;122:154–157.

37. Hohenfellner R, Müller SC, Riedmiller H, Thüroff JW. Continent urinary diversion: the Mainz pouch technique. In: Knapstein PG, Friedberg V, Sevin B-U, eds. *Reconstructive Surgery in Gynecology*. New York: Thieme Medical Publishers, Inc; 1990.

38. Skinner DG, Lieskovsky G, Boyd SD. Continuing experience with the continent ileal reservoir (Kock pouch) as an alternative to cutaneous urinary diversion: an update after 250 cases. *J Urol.* 1987;137:1140–1145.

39. Jeter KF. The flush versus the protruding urinary stoma. *J Urol.* 1976;116:424–427.

40. Jones MA, Breckman B, Hendry WF. Life with an ileal conduit: results of questionnaire surveys of patients and urological surgeons. *Br J Urol.* 1980;52:21–25.

41. Coffey RC. Transplantation of the ureters into the large intestine in the absence of a functioning urinary bladder. *Surg Gynecol Obstet.* 1921;32:383.

42. Schlesinger RE, Berman WL, Balloon SC, et al. The choice of an intestinal segment for a urinary conduit. *Surg Gynecol Obstet.* 1979;148:45–48.

Index

A

B

C

Note: Page numbers in *italics* indicate material found in figures, tables, and exhibits.

D

E

F

G

P

Q

R

S

V

W